Systematic Approach to
DESCRIBE INSTRUMENTS AND OPERATIVE PROCEDURES IN
Surgery, Orthopedics and Anesthesia

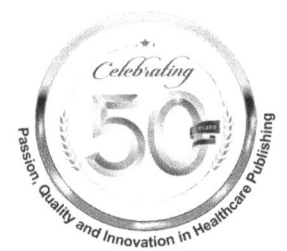

Systematic Approach to

DESCRIBE INSTRUMENTS AND OPERATIVE PROCEDURES IN

Surgery, Orthopedics and Anesthesia

Second Edition

Vinod Pusdekar
MBBS MS (General Surgery) FMAS
Assistant Professor
Department of General Surgery
Government Medical College
Gondia, Maharashtra, India

Forewords

Jagadish B Hedawoo
Varsha Sagdeo

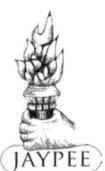

JAYPEE BROTHERS MEDICAL PUBLISHERS
The Health Sciences Publisher
New Delhi | London

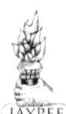 **Jaypee Brothers Medical Publishers (P) Ltd**

Headquarters
Jaypee Brothers Medical Publishers (P) Ltd
4838/24, Ansari Road, Daryaganj
New Delhi 110 002, india
Phone: +91-11-43574357
Fax: +91-11-43574314
Email: jaypee@jaypeebrothers.com

Overseas Office
J.P. Medical Ltd
83 Victoria Street, London
SW1H 0HW (UK)
Phone: +44 20 3170 8910
Fax: +44 (0)20 3008 6180
Email: info@jpmedpub.com

Website: www.jaypeebrothers.com
Website: www.jaypeedigital.com

© 2020, Jaypee Brothers Medical Publishers

The views and opinions expressed in this book are solely those of the original contributor(s)/author(s) and do not necessarily represent those of editor(s) of the book.

All rights reserved. No part of this publication may be reproduced, stored or transmitted in any form or by any means, electronic, mechanical, photocopying, recording or otherwise, without the prior permission in writing of the publishers.

All brand names and product names used in this book are trade names, service marks, trademarks or registered trademarks of their respective owners. the publisher is not associated with any product or vendor mentioned in this book.

Medical knowledge and practice change constantly. This book is designed to provide accurate, authoritative information about the subject matter in question. However, readers are advised to check the most current information available on procedures included and check information from the manufacturer of each product to be administered, to verify the recommended dose, formula, method and duration of administration, adverse effects and contraindications. It is the responsibility of the practitioner to take all appropriate safety precautions. Neither the publisher nor the author(s)/editor(s) assume any liability for any injury and/or damage to persons or property arising from or related to use of material in this book.

This book is sold on the understanding that the publisher is not engaged in providing professional medical services. If such advice or services are required, the services of a competent medical professional should be sought.

Every effort has been made where necessary to contact holders of copyright to obtain permission to reproduce copyright material. If any have been inadvertently overlooked, the publisher will be pleased to make the necessary arrangements at the first opportunity. The **CD/DVD-ROM** (if any) provided in the sealed envelope with this book is complimentary and free of cost. **Not meant for sale.**

Inquiries for bulk sales may be solicited at: jaypee@jaypeebrothers.com

Systematic Approach to Describe Instruments and Operative Procedures in Surgery, Orthopedics and Anesthesia

First Edition: 2013
Second Edition: **2020**
ISBN: 978-93-89776-17-1
Printed at

Dedicated to

My grandfather
Late Shri Jaideorao Pusdekar

List of Reviewers

Asmita Dhurve
Associate Professor
Department of Surgery
Government Medical College
Gondia, Maharashtra, India

Jagadish B Hedawoo
Professor
Department of Surgery
Government Medical College
Nagpur, Maharashtra, India

Manik Gedam
Associate Professor
Indira Gandhi Government Medical College
Nagpur, Maharashtra, India

Nandkishor Jaiswal
Professor and Head
Department of Surgery
Government Medical College
Gondia, Maharashtra, India

Ritesh Bodade
Associate Professor
Department of Surgery
Government Medical College
Gondia, Maharashtra, India

Varsha Sagdeo
Ex-Professor and Head
Department of Surgery
Government Medical College
Nagpur, Maharashtra, India

FOREWORD TO THE SECOND EDITION

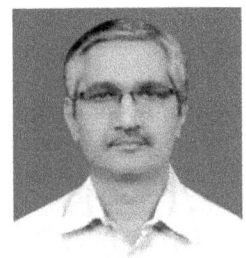

Knowing about the surgical instruments is an integral part of surgical training. Along with the instruments, it is necessary to know about sterilization of instruments. As an undergraduate student, one must know the broad guidelines as well as the methods of sterilization. But for the postgraduate students and practicing surgeons, it is essential to know about the details about sterilization as well as disinfection.

Many of the surgical textbooks do not give the account on instruments, suture materials, as well as the details about the sterilization also. I have gone through this book written by Dr Vinod Pusdekar. This book will make a mark among the books written on this topic of instruments. It has not only covered the instruments of routine use in general surgery, but it also covers the instruments commonly used in the field of orthopedics. He has classified the instruments in a beautiful way, e.g., cutting instruments, holding instruments, instruments for tissue dissection, retractors, etc., as well as the instruments for special surgery such as instruments for thoracic surgery, neurosurgery, plastic surgery, etc. This book describes the instruments in a very simple way in a pointwise manner, with bullets for each statement. So, it becomes easy for a student to remember for the examination.

Along with the instruments the book nicely covers the information about various commonly-used anesthesia methods and drugs used for it. Intravenous fluids are an essential part of surgery as well as anesthesia. The book has good coverage for intravenous fluids, various drugs used for anesthesia as well as different equipment needed for ventilation also.

The important section of this book is dedicated to operative procedures. It nicely covers the topics from preoperative preparation of the patient, commonly done major and minor operations. It has taken due note of simple operations such as circumcision, venesection to today's popular operations such as laparoscopic cholecystectomy to hernia repair also. Besides these procedures, a special mention of bedside procedures like catheterization, putting Ryle's tube, proctoscopy, etc. Considering these as routine bedside procedures, larger textbooks do not have a mention of it; but, it is very necessary for the undergraduate students to know. The writer has a taken a due note of it.

Keeping updated is an essential part of learning in the medical field. Considering this aspect, the author has added a good information about the laparoscopic instruments, its sterilization, including small account on energy sources and robotic surgery also. Approach to trauma patients based on advanced trauma life support (ATLS) guidelines, primary survey, airway, breathing, circulation, disability, exposure (ABCDE) approach, etc., needs special mention. It also gives the guidelines for management of abdominal trauma, thoracic trauma as well as management of burns. Guidelines to treat the acute abdominal conditions such as acute appendicitis, intestinal obstruction, perforation peritonitis and obstructed hernia as well as topics such as acute urinary retention will help the postgraduate students to treat the patients while they are on emergency duty.

I must say this book is a good combination of information on operative surgery, instruments as well as necessary topics in anesthesia. Common instruments in the orthopedic surgery chapter will help the students of orthopedic surgery also. I admire the efforts taken by the author and wish him great success for this second edition.

Jagadish B Hedawoo
MBBS MS (General Surgery) MBA (Hospital Administration) PGDHHM Yoga Therapist
Fellowship by ACRSI Fellowship by IASG
Professor (General Surgery)
Government Medical College, Nagpur
Ex-Professor and Head (General Surgery)
Government Medical College, Akola, Maharashtra
Ex-Medical Superintendent
Government Medical College
Nagpur, Maharashtra, India

FOREWORD TO THE FIRST EDITION

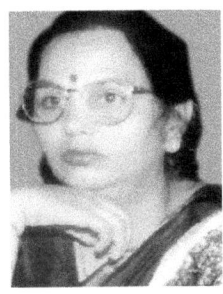

This book is a project that has spanned over a decade. This book is extended to serve as a ready source of necessary information about all surgical instruments which are routinely used in surgical practice in most of the teaching institutes. It also includes practical knowledge about instruments used in surgery, orthopedics and brief description about anesthesia needed for undergraduate level. This book emphasizes on a quick recall of all features of surgical instruments and brief description of surgical procedures. Students will find this book extremely useful for introduction to surgery as it is taught and practiced at major teaching institutes. This book will also help junior residents for their everyday procedures for on-the-spot duty.

The organization of this book is very interesting. It starts with preparation for surgery such as sterilization of the surgical instruments and step-by- step introduces the instruments as they are used in surgery. For easy understanding of the students, topics are divided in sections which are again divided into chapters. Section one provides brief information regarding sterilization, types and parts of surgical instruments. Chapters are divided depending on the use of various instruments, like second chapter deals with sponge holder, its uses, various ways of holding and using it. It proceeds in the same manner likewise in description of instruments, types of instruments, various parts of instruments, its uses and the way it has to be held. Same is true about all instruments. Full section is devoted to tubes, catheters, and drains used in surgical practice. A full section is devoted to anesthesia, which describes all anesthetic equipments, which are routinely used while giving anesthesia. This section also deals with commonly used anesthetic drugs and preanesthetic medications in brief. Similarly, a full section is devoted to orthopedic instruments and implants.

After a brief introduction to preoperative preparation of patient on the operation table and draping, section dealing with surgical procedures are divided into two parts, major and minor operative procedures. It includes almost all major surgeries, which an undergraduate student is expected to know. The description is stepwise, so it is easy to understand and recall. At the same time, alternative laparoscopic procedures are also mentioned wherever done. It also deals with postoperative care of the various surgical procedures. All minor and bedside procedures are well described. It also deals with fluid and electrolyte management.

OUTSTANDING FEATURES OF THIS BOOK

This book is extensively updated for latest equipments and procedures.

The illustrations which has been chosen perfectly and photographs of actual instruments help for quick recall while preparing for examination. Thorough coverage is provided for the equipments used in operation theater.

An undergraduate student can rely on this book as a single source of information on surgical instruments, various bedside procedures, major and minor surgeries, brief necessary information on anesthesia, orthopedic instruments and implants, and fluid and electrolyte management.

Varsha Sagdeo
MBBS MS (General Surgery) DNB (Pediatric Surgery) FICS
Director Medical Education
In-Charge of Breast Care Centre
Cancer Counselor, Shri Radhakrishna Hospital and
Research Institute, Nagpur
Ex-Dean, Government Medical College and
Indira Gandhi Medical College, Nagpur
Maharashtra, India

Preface to the Second Edition

It is observed that students, especially undergraduates, often find it difficult to prepare themselves for practical examination after the theory papers. They need to know instruments in general surgery, anesthesia and orthopedics, basic bedside and operative procedures in general surgery, sterilization procedures, etc., while preparing for table viva in practical examination. This book covers all these aspects in a comprehensive manner.

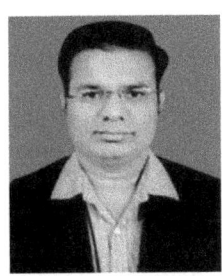

Keeping this in mind, this book is written to help the undergraduate students prior to practical viva examination. This book is also helpful to the postgraduate students of general surgery, orthopedics and anesthesia.

Every attempt has been made in this book to provide a condense information by framing it pointwise.

In general surgery section, relevant points for the identification of the instruments and its uses are mentioned. While discussing the use of instruments, emphasis has been given to mention the particular operation where the instrument is commonly used.

Almost all of the surgical instruments used in general surgery and super specialty surgeries such as neurosurgery, urosurgery and plastic surgery are described in detail along with illustrative photographs.

In orthopedics section, various instruments, their identification along with their uses are discussed. Orthopedic implants used in different fractures are also discussed along with their photographs.

Different sterilization procedures are discussed in details and also mentioned individually along with every instrument.

Anesthesia section includes equipments for general as well as regional anesthesia.

Commonly used drugs in anesthesia and emergency drugs are also described.

Major and minor operative and bedside procedures in general surgery are described in a step-by-step approach and only covers the important procedures commonly asked in examinations.

Preoperative preparation of the patient prior to surgical procedures is described in details.

Different types of surgical suture materials, needles and the basic surgeries where they have been used are discussed thoroughly in the section of the suture materials.

Different types of perurethral catheters, tubes and drains used in general surgery are described.

This book also covers the basic knowledge of different intravenous fluids and intravenous cannulas used in clinical practice.

In view of the recent advances that are taking place in the surgical field, the second edition has included chapters on robotic surgery, instruments used for laparoscopic surgical procedures and a brief description of the energy sources in surgery.

A chapter on approach to diagnose common surgical emergencies presenting at the emergency room and its subsequent management has been added.

I hope that this book will earn its value in its own way in the student's circle.

I apologize for any inadvertent mistakes, which might have been overlooked by me during editing this book.

I am very grateful to the whole team of M/s Jaypee Brothers Medical Publishers (P) Ltd, New Delhi, India, especially Shri Jitendar P Vij (Group Chairman), Mr Ankit Vij (Managing Director), Mr MS Mani (Group President).

I am open to receive comments, any critics and suggestions for the improvement of this book in future from students and teachers. The comments and the suggestions may please be sent to me on my email address: *drvinodpusdekar20@ymail.com.*

Vinod Pusdekar

Preface to the First Edition

It is observed that students, especially undergraduates, often find it difficult to prepare themselves for practical examination after theory papers. They need to know instruments in general surgery, anesthesia and orthopedics, basic operative and bedside procedures in general surgery, sterilization procedures, etc., while preparing for table viva in practical examination. This book covers all these aspects in a comprehensive manner.

Keeping this in mind, this book is written to help the undergraduate students prior to practical viva examination. This book is also helpful to the postgraduate students of general surgery, orthopedics and anesthesia.

Every attempt has been made to provide a condense information by framing it pointwise.

With five years of extensive hard work, I am able to present this book to the students of surgery.

In general surgery section, relevant points for identification of the instrument and their uses are mentioned. While discussing the use of instruments, emphasis has been given to mention the particular operation where the instrument is commonly used.

Almost all of the surgical instruments used in general surgery and super specialty surgeries such as neurosurgery, urosurgery and plastic surgery are described in details along with illustrative diagrams.

In orthopedics section, various instruments, their identification along with their uses are discussed. Orthopedic implants used in different fractures are also discussed along with their illustrative photographs.

Different sterilization procedures are discussed in details and also mentioned individually along with every instrument.

Anesthesia section includes equipments for general as well as regional anesthesia.

Commonly used drugs in anesthesia and emergency drugs are also described.

Major and minor operative and bedside procedures in general surgery are described in a step-by-step approach, and only covers the important procedures commonly asked in examinations.

Preoperative preparation of the patient prior to surgical procedures is described in detail.

Different types of surgical suture materials, needles and the basic surgeries where they have been used are discussed thoroughly in section of suture materials.

Different types of perurethral catheters, tubes and drains used in general surgery are described.

This book also covers the basic knowledge of different intravenous fluids and intravenous cannulas used in clinical practice.

I hope this book will earn its value in its own way in the students circle.

I apologize for any inadvertent mistakes which might have been overlooked by me during editing this book.

I am very grateful to the whole team of M/s Jaypee Brothers Medical Publishers (P) Ltd, New Delhi, India, who helped me and guided me, especially Shri Jitendar P Vij (Group Chairman).

I am open to receive comments, any critics and suggestions for the improvement of this book in future from students and teachers. The comments and the suggestions may please be sent to me on my email address: *drvinodpusdekar20@ymail.com.*

Vinod Pusdekar

Acknowledgments

No one is able to do anything unless our parents make us do that. I express my sincere gratitude to my parents Mrs Shobha and Shri Prabhakarrao Pusdekar, for making me and giving me the courage to write a book.

My sincere thanks and gratitude to the following persons, for their constant help and encouragement during preparation of this book.

My heartfelt thanks to Dr Jagadish B Hedawoo, Professor (General Surgery), Department of Surgery, Government Medical College, Nagpur, who motivated me for the second edition and also gave valuable guidance for it.

I would like to thank my teachers Dr Varsha Sagdeo, Ex-Professor and Head, Department of Surgery, Government Medical College, Nagpur; Dr Makrand Khubalkar, Associate Professor, Government Medical College, Akola; Dr Niketan Jambhulkar, Associate Professor, Government Medical College, Nagpur, and my colleague Dr Nitinkumar Borkar, Associate Professor, AIIMS, Raipur, who motivated me to become a teacher and arouse my interest in academics by motivating me to take lectures of undergraduates and build my confidence in initial days of teaching.

I wish to express my sincere gratitude to the seniors and colleagues of the Department of Surgery at the Government Medical College, Gondia. I would like to thank Dr Nandkishor Jaiswal, Professor and Head of our department along with Dr Ritesh Bodade and Dr Asmita Dhurve, Associate Professors, who supported and encouraged me to complete the second edition. I would also like to thank Dr Nirmal Patle, Consultant General and Laparoscopic Surgeon, Aureus Hospital, Nagpur, and Dr Vijay Kawalkar, Director, Sanjivan Hospital, Yavatmal, for their help. I would like to express my sincere thanks to Dr Taneshwar Gautam, Medical Officer at Swami Vivekanand Medical Mission Hospital, Nagpur, for his help.

I would also like to thank Dr Javed Saudagar, Consulting Orthopedician at Sanjivan Hospital, Yavatmal; Dr Abhjijeet Fuladi, Consulting Orthopedician at Swami Vivekanand Medical Mission Hospital, Nagpur; Dr Sumedh Chaudhary, Associate Professor, and Dr Pravin Agrawal, Associate Professor, Government Medical College, Nagpur, who helped me in writing the orthopedic section, especially by providing instruments and implants for photographs.

My colleagues from the faculty of anesthesia, Dr Satkar Pawar, Consulting Anesthesiologist, Nagpur; Dr Satyendra Warhade, Consulting Anesthesiologist, Nagpur; Dr Pradip Bhojane, Consulting Anesthesiologist at Sanjivan Hospital, Yavatmal; Dr Rishikesh Awale, Assistant Professor, VN Government Medical College, Yavatmal; Dr Gajanan Maske, Assistant Professor, VN Government Medical College, Yavatmal, and Dr Vishal Sawaimul, Consulting

Anesthesiologist, Umred, helped me in writing the anesthesia section. I am grateful to them, for their contribution.

I am indebted to my wife, Dr Yamini Pusdekar, who helped me during preparation of this book right from motivating me to write this book till the final editing of this book, also for the timely communication between me and the M/s Jaypee Brothers Medical Publishers (P) Ltd, New Delhi, India. Words are not enough to express my gratitude to her and my son Parth, who inspired me for writing this book. I will never forget their sacrifice of long hours of family associations over these years while I was busy in preparing this book.

My special thanks to Shri Jitendar P Vij (Group Chairman), Mr Ankit Vij (Managing Director), Mr MS Mani (Group President), Dr Madhu Choudhary (Publishing Head-Education), Ms Pooja Bhandari (Production Head), Ms Sunita Katla (Executive Assistant to Group Chairman and Publishing Manager), Dr Akanksha Singh (Development Editor), Ms Seema Dogra (Cover Visualizer), Mr Rajesh Sharma (Production Coordinator), Mr Kulwant Singh (Typesetter), Mr Vakil Khan (Proofreader), Mr Anil Kumar (Graphic Designer), and the whole team of M/s Jaypee Brothers Medical Publishers (P) Ltd, New Delhi, India.

My sincere thanks to my enthusiastic students, friends, relatives and well wishers, for their constant support, encouragement and help.

Last but not the least, I am deeply indebted to my patients without whom I would not have been able to carry out this work.

Contents

Section 1: Sterilization, Types and Parts of a Surgical Instrument

Chapter 1.	Sterilization of the Instruments	3
Chapter 2.	Various Types of the Instruments in Common Surgical Practice	5
Chapter 3.	Parts of a Typical Surgical Instrument	7

Section 2: Instruments in General Surgery

Chapter 4. Cutting Instruments — 11
- Bard Parker's Handles (Detachable Handle) 11
- Surgical Blades 11
- Scissors 13
- Mayo's Scissor 13
- Metzenbaum Scissor 14
- Mcindoe Scissor 15
- Heath Suture Cutting Scissor 16

Chapter 5. Holding Instruments — 17
- Rampley's Swab (Sponge) Holding Forceps 17

Towel Clips (Towel Holding Forceps) 18
- Doyen's Cross Action Towel Clip 18
- Mayo's (Backhaus) Towel Clip 19

Hemostatic Forceps (Artery Forceps) 19
- Spencer Wells Hemostatic Forceps 19
- Halsted Mosquito Hemostatic Forceps 22
- Kocher's Hemostatic Forceps 22
- Lister's Sinus Forceps 23
- Allie's Tissue Forceps 24
- Babcock's Tissue Forceps 26
- Lane Tissue Forceps 27
- Cord Holding Forceps (Collingwood–Stewart Cord Holding or Hernia Forceps) 28
- Tongue Holding Forceps (Thompson's) 29
- Duval Lung Forceps 29
- Cheatle Forceps 30

Chapter 6.	**Instruments for Tissue Dissection**	**31**
	❖ Dissecting Forceps 31	
	❖ Vascular Forceps 33	
	❖ Right Angle Forceps (Lahey Forceps) or Mixter Forceps 33	
Chapter 7.	**Stone Holding Forceps**	**35**
	❖ Desjardin's Choledocholithotomy Forceps 35	
	❖ Pyelolithotomy Forceps 36	
	❖ Suprapubic Cystolithotomy Forceps 36	
Chapter 8.	**Needle Holders**	**38**
Chapter 9.	**Modern Techniques of Suturing**	**40**
	❖ Skin Stapler 40	
	❖ Skin Glues for Wound Closure 40	
Chapter 10.	**Retractors**	**41**
	❖ Langenbeck's Right Angled Retractor 41	
	❖ Czerny Retractor 42	
	❖ Morris Retractor 43	
	❖ Deaver's Curved Abdominal Retractor 44	
	❖ Doyen's Retractor 45	
	❖ Malleable Retractor 45	
	❖ Allison Lung Retractor 45	
	❖ Volkmann's Cat's Paw Retractor 46	
	❖ Skin Retractor 47	
	❖ Single Hook Retractor 47	
	❖ Kidney Hilum Retractor 47	
	❖ Self-retaining Retractors 48	
	❖ Self-retaining Retractor (Balfour's Type) with Provision of Third Blade for Attachment 48	
	❖ Self-retaining Retractor with Two Blades (No Provision for 3rd Blade Attachment) 49	
	❖ Mollison's Self-retaining Mastoid Retractor 50	
	❖ Joll's Thyroid Retractor 51	
	Retractors of the Oral Cavity (Mouth Gags) *51*	
	❖ Doyen's Mouth Gag 51	
	❖ Jennings Mouth Gag 52	
Chapter 11.	**Clamps**	**53**
	Gastrointestinal Clamps *53*	
	❖ Doyen's Gastrointestinal Occlusion (Non-crushing) Clamp 53	
	❖ Moynihan's Gastric Occlusion (Non-crushing) Clamp 54	
	❖ Kocher's Gastric Occlusion Clamp 55	
	❖ Payr's Crushing Clamp 55	
	❖ Intestinal Crushing Clamps 56	

Contents **xxi**

Vascular Clamps 56
- Bulldog Vascular Clamp 56
- Satinsky Vascular Clamp 56
- Mayo's Pedicle Clamp 57

Chapter 12. Miscellaneous Instruments in General Surgery   59
- Kelly's Rectal Speculum (Proctoscope) or Anal Speculum 59
- Brodie's Olive Pointed Fistula Director with Frenulum Slit 60
- Malleable Olive Pointed Probe 61
- Trocar and Cannula 63
- Suprapubic Trocar and Cannula 63
- Hydrocele, Trocar and Cannula 64
- Yankauer Suction Cannula 64
- Multihole Suction Cannula 65
- Kidney Tray 66
- Volkmann's Spoon or Scoop 67

Chapter 13. Instruments in Specialized Surgery   68

Instruments Used in Thoracotomy 68
- Doyen Rib Raspatory 68
- Schumacher Rib Shear 69

Instruments Used in Tracheostomy 69
- Tracheal Dilators 69

Instruments Used in Neurosurgery (Craniotomy) 70
- Hudson's Brace/Burr/Perforator 70
- Bone Cutter and Bone Nibbler 70
- Horsley's Dura Mater Separator and Skull Elevator 70
- Dura Separator 71

Instruments Used in Plastic Surgery 72
- Humby's Knife with Guarded Blade (Skin Grafting Knife) 72

Urology Instruments 73
- Metallic Urethral Bougie Lister's Metallic Bougie 73

Section 3: Catheters, Tubes and Drains

Chapter 14. Catheters   77
- Metallic Urethral Catheter for Male 77
- Simple or Plain Rubber Catheter 78
- Foley's Self-retaining Balloon Catheter 79
- Silicone Self-retaining Catheter 81
- Malecot's Catheter 82

Chapter 15. Trocar and Cannula   83
- Suprapubic Trocar Cannula (Supracath) 83
- Intercostal Trocar Cannula 83

Chapter 16.	Tubes	85
	❖ Nasogastric Tube (Ryle's Tube) 85	
	❖ Flatus Tube 86	
	❖ Tracheostomy Tubes 87	
	❖ Suction Tubings 88	
Chapter 17.	Drains	90
	❖ Corrugated Rubber Drain/Sheet 90	
	❖ Suction Drain 91	
	❖ Abdominal Drain 92	
	❖ Urosac Bag 93	

Section 4: Intravenous Cannulas, Intravenous and Blood Sets, Intravenous Fluids

Chapter 18.	Intravenous Cannulas and Sets	97
	❖ Intravenous Cannula (Intracath/Vasofix) 97	
	❖ Scalp Vein Set 98	
	❖ Intravenous Infusion Set 99	
	❖ Blood Transfusion Set 100	
	❖ Three-Way Cannula 101	
Chapter 19.	Intravenous Fluid Bottles (Crystalloid Bottles)	102
	❖ 5% Dextrose Injection 102	
	❖ Ringer Lactate Injection 102	
	❖ Sodium Chloride Solution 103	
	❖ Dextrose Normal Saline 104	
	❖ Sterile Water Vial 105	
Chapter 20.	Syringes and Needles	107
	❖ Syringes 107	
	❖ Hypodermic Needle 108	

Section 5: Orthopedics Instruments and Implants

Chapter 21.	Orthopedics Instruments	111
	❖ Farabeuf's Raspatory or Periosteum Elevator 111	
	❖ Lane's Bone Levers 112	
	❖ Osteotome 113	
	❖ Chisel 114	
	❖ Bone Gouge 114	
	❖ Bone Awl or Bradawl 115	
	❖ Mallet 116	
	❖ Punch 116	

- Bone Holding Forceps   117
- Bone Cutting Forceps or Bone Shears   117
- Bone Nibbler or Bone Nibbling Forceps   118
- Volkmann's Spoon or Scoop   119
- Gigli's Wire Saw   119
- Guidewire   120
- Hand Drill   120
- 'T' Handle or Chuck Handle for Inserting Guidewire   121
- Drill Bit Guide   121
- Tap   122
- K-Wire Bender and Cutter Heavy Duty Plier Nose Plier   123

Chapter 22. Orthopedics Implants   **124**
- Plates   124
- Screws   125
- Prosthesis for Hip Hemiarthroplasty   125
- Austin Moore's Prosthesis   126
- Thompson's Prosthesis   127
- Bipolar Prosthesis   128
- Intramedullary Nails (IM Nails)   128
- Rush Nail   129
- K-Wire   131
- Kuntscher's Intramedullary Nail (K-Nail)   132
- S-P Nail   133
- Stainless Steel Wire   134

Bohler's Pin (Steinmann) with Rotating Stirrup   *134*
- Steinmann Pin   134
- Bohler's Stirrup   135

Chapter 23. Bandages, Crepe Bandages and Plaster of Paris Bandages   **136**
- Cotton Bandages   136
- Cotton Crepe Bandage (Elastocrepe)   136
- Plaster of Paris Bandage   137

Section 6: Suture Materials Used in Surgical Practice

Chapter 24. Classification and Description of Suture Materials   **141**
- Classification or Types   141

Chapter 25. Needles   **145**

Chapter 26. Different Types of Suture Materials   **147**
Absorbable Suture Materials   *147*
- Natural Absorbable Suture Material   147
- Synthetic Absorbable Suture Material   149
- Polyglactin 910 Sutures   149

Nonabsorbable Sutures **151**
- Nonabsorbable Natural Sutures   151
- Nonabsorbable Synthetic Sutures   153

Section 7: Anesthesia Equipments

Chapter 27. **Airways**   **159**
- Guedel's or Oropharyngeal Airway   159
- Nasopharyngeal Airway   160
- Laryngeal Mask Airway   160

Chapter 28. **Equipments for Tracheal Intubation**   **162**
- Laryngoscopes   162
- Endotracheal Tubes   163
- Connector   165
- Stylet   166
- Magill's Forceps   166
- Suction Catheter   167

Chapter 29. **Equipments for Ventilation**   **169**
- Ambu Bag (Ambulatory Manual Breathing Unit)   169
- Oxygen Reservoir   170
- Non-rebreathing Valve   170
- Angle (Universal) Connector   171
- Reservoir Bag   171
- Corrugated Antistatic Rubber Tube   173
- Face Masks   173
- Oxygen Mask and Tubing   175
- 'T' Piece   175

Chapter 30. **Equipments for Regional Anesthesia**   **177**
- Spinal Needle   177
- Epidural Catheter   179

Chapter 31. **Commonly Used Drugs in Anesthesia**   **181**
- Bupivacaine Hydrochloride in Dextrose Injection   181
- Bupivacaine Hydrochloride Injection   182
- Lignocaine Hydrochloride and Dextrose Injection   182
- Lignocaine Hydrochloride   183
- Lignocaine with Adrenaline   184
- Lignocaine Hydrochloride Injection   185
- Lignocaine Spray   185
- Lignocaine Hydrochloride Gel   187
- Adrenaline Tartrate Injection   187
- Atropine Sulfate Injection   189
- Glycopyrrolate (Pyrolate) Injection   189

- Ondansetron 190
- Hydrocortisone Sodium Succinate Injection 191
- Dexamethasone Sodium Phosphate Injection (Dexona) 192
- Furosemide (Lasix) 193
- Midazolam (Mezolam) 193
- Diazepam (Calmpose) 194
- Injection of Etofylline and Theophylline (Deriphyllin) 195
- Thiopentone Sodium (Thiosol Sodium) 195
- Ketamine Hydrochloride Injection (Aneket) 196
- Propofol Injection (Neorof) 196

Muscle Relaxants 198
- Succinylcholine (Sucol) 198
- Atracurium/Pancuronium/Vecuronium/Rocuronium 199
- Atracurium Besylate 199
- Neostigmine Methylsulfate 199

Inhalational Anesthetic Agents 200
- Halothane/Sevoflurane/Isoflurane/Desflurane 200
- Halothane 200
- Isoflurane 201
- Sevoflurane and Desflurane 201

Section 8: Surgical (Operative) Procedures

Chapter 32. Preoperative Preparation of the Patient Prior to Surgical Procedures 205
- Preparation of the Operative and Surrounding Area 205

Chapter 33. Preparation of the Patient on the Operation Table Prior to the Procedures 207

Chapter 34. Major Operative Procedures 209
- Appendicectomy 209
- Open Appendicectomy 209
- Laparoscopic Appendicectomy 214
- Treatment of Appendicular Mass 216
- Treatment of Appendicular Abscess 217
- Cholecystectomy 217
- Open Cholecystectomy 218
- Laparoscopic Cholecystectomy 220
- Circumcision 222
- Operations for Repair of Inguinal Hernia 224
- Herniotomy 225
- Operations for Repair of Adult Inguinal Hernia 226
- Primary Tissue Repairs (Inguinal Herniorrhaphy) 227
- Anterior Tension Free Mesh Repair (Hernioplasty) 233

- Preperitoneal Repairs 234
- Kuntz Operation (Inguinal Orchidectomy) 236
- Herniorrhaphy versus Hernioplasty 236
- Laparoscopic Hernioplasty 237
- Techniques 239

Surgeries for Hydrocele — 240
- Repair of Adult (Acquired) Hydrocele 240
- Lord's Plication of the Sac 241
- Jaboulay's Eversion of the Sac 242
- Subtotal Excision of the Sac 244
- Vasectomy 245
- Suprapubic Cystolithotomy 246
- Modified Radical Mastectomy: MRM (Patey's Mastectomy) 248
- Other Types of Mastectomy 251
- Surgeries for Thyroid Gland 252

Chapter 35. Minor Operative Procedures — 259
- Incision and Drainage of an Abscess 259
- Insertion of an Intercostal Drain 262
- Tracheostomy 263
- Venesection 265
- Excision of the Cyst (Sebaceous or Dermoid Cyst) 267
- Excision of the Lipoma 268
- Lymph Node Biopsy 269

Section 9: Bedside Procedures

Chapter 36. Bedside Procedures — 273
- Periurethral Catheterization 273
- Ryles Tube (Nasogastric) Insertion 275
- Proctoscopy/Anoscopy 276
- Intravenous Cannula Insertion 277

Section 10: Advanced Techniques in General Surgery

Chapter 37. Laparoscopy Surgery and Instruments — 281
- Imaging System 281
- Gas for Pneumoperitoneum 284
- Insufflator 285
- Instrument Trolley 286
- Suction Irrigation Machine 286
- Operative Hand Instruments 286
- Insufflation Cannulas 287
- Trocars 287

- Reducing Sleeve 289
- Operative Hand Instruments 289
- Graspers 290
- Instruments for Sharp Dissection 292
- Different Handles of Hand Instrument 292
- Insulated Outer Tube 293
- Needle Holders 293
- Hook and Spatula 294
- Harmonic Scalpel 294
- Clip Applicator 294
- Suction and Irrigation Hand Apparatus 295
- Port Closure Instrument 295
- Sterilization of Instruments 296

Chapter 38. Robotic Surgery 298

Section 11: Energy Sources in Surgery

Chapter 39. Energy Sources in Surgery 303

Section 12: Approach to Surgical Patients in Emergency Room

Chapter 40. Approach to Trauma Patients in Emergency Room 307
- Approach to Patient Sustaining Head Injury 308
- Approach to Patients Sustaining Chest Injury 310
- Approach to Patient Sustaining Abdominal Injuries 312
- Approach to Patient Sustaining Burns 314

Chapter 41. Approach to Patient of Acute Abdominal Conditions in Emergency Room 316
- Approach to Patient with Acute Appendicitis 316
- Approach to Patient with Intestinal Obstruction 319
- Approach to Patient with Sigmoid Volvulus 320
- Approach to the Patient with Perforation Peritonitis 321
- Approach to Patient with Strangulated or Obstructed Hernia 323

Chapter 42. Approach to Patients of Genitourinary Emergencies in Emergency Room 325
- Approach to the Patient of Torsion of the Testes 325
- Approach to the Patient with Urinary Retention 326
- Approach to the Patient with Paraphimosis 327

Index 329

Section 1

Sterilization, Types and Parts of a Surgical Instrument

Section Outline

1. Sterilization of the Instruments
2. Various Types of Instruments in Common Surgical Practice
3. Parts of a Typical Surgical Instrument

CHAPTER 1

Sterilization of the Instruments

Sterilization is the process of destroying life of all microorganisms causing infection (bacteria, viruses, fungi including bacterial spores).

Disinfection means killing all the microorganisms (infectious agents, except spores) outside the body, by exposing them directly to the chemical or physical agents.

Commonly employed methods for sterilization are **steam sterilization (autoclaving), boiling, chemical and gas sterilization.**

Steam sterilization: Steam sterilization is one of the most common forms of sterilization in general practice. All reusable metal instruments are sterilized by autoclaving at a temperature of 121° C, at 15 pounds per square inch (Ib/sq) pressure for 30-40 minutes and rubber articles like gloves, catheters, rubber drains for 15 minutes, after the desired temperature and pressure is achieved. If sharp instruments have to be autoclaved, their sharp ends must be well padded and covered with cotton pads to preserve their sharpness, as they lose their sharpness by repeated autoclaving. It is cheap alternative and effective too. Before sterilization, all the instruments, tubing, and cords should be wrapped doubly in a cloth to prevent contact with the hot metallic container which is then placed in the autoclave.

Boiling: Metal instruments can be sterilized by boiling them for half an hour (30 minutes) which kills all the bacteria and its spores. Boiling of the instrument should be continued for half an hour after water achieves a temperature of 100° C. But boiling is not suitable for sharp instruments as they lose their sharpness by repeated boiling. It also leads to crust formation over the instruments.

Chemical sterilization (High level disinfection): Sharp instruments like scissors, osteotomes, needles, etc. are sterilized by keeping them dipped in chemicals like lysol or cidex (2% glutarldehyde solution) for a minimum of 4-24 hours (10 hours) for their proper sterilization. Fiberoptic instruments like light cords, laparoscope, cystoscope, arthroscope are sterilized by immersing them in cidex. Other chemical agents used are peracetic acid and 6% stabilized hydrogen peroxide. Formaldehyde also can be used. But its use for sterilizing instruments and other items is not recommended nowadays.

Direct flaming: In case of urgency, when an instrument has fallen down from the operation table and is urgently required for the ongoing surgical procedure, it can be sterilized by direct flaming. The instrument is kept in a bowl and rectified spirit is poured over it and then it is flamed. Direct flaming achieves a temperature of 1400°C to make the instrument sterile.

Gas sterilization: Gas used for gas sterilization is ethylene oxide. It is suitable for all disposable instruments, insulated hand instruments and tubings. Gas sterilization with ethylene oxide causes no damage to instruments, and it is non-corrosive to optics, but it is costly. Fiberoptic instruments like laparoscope, cystoscope, arthroscope can be sterilized by keeping them in a formalin vaporizer chamber for at least 1 hour, in which formalin tablets are kept, which releases the formaldehyde gas. Chamber should be completely closed and airtight.

Note: Students can easily remember the first 4 methods of sterilization by remembering mnemonic ABCD (A: Autoclaving, B: Boiling, C: Chemical sterilization, D: Direct flaming).

CHAPTER 2
Various Types of Instruments in Common Surgical Practice

Instruments in surgical practice, which may be of general surgery, orthopedics, ENT, ophthalmology or obstetrics and gynecology, can be broadly divided into following categories:
- Cutting instruments like scissors, surgical blades, etc.
- Holding instruments like swab holding forceps, tissue holding forceps, needle holder, etc.
- Retractors like Deaver's retractor, right angled retractor, Morris retractor, etc.
- Dissecting instruments like dissecting forceps, Lahey's forceps, etc.
- Clamps are used to clamp the blood vessels like Bulldog vascular clamp or to occlude the hollow organs of gastrointestinal tract like Doyen's gastrointestinal clamp, Payr's crushing clamp, etc.

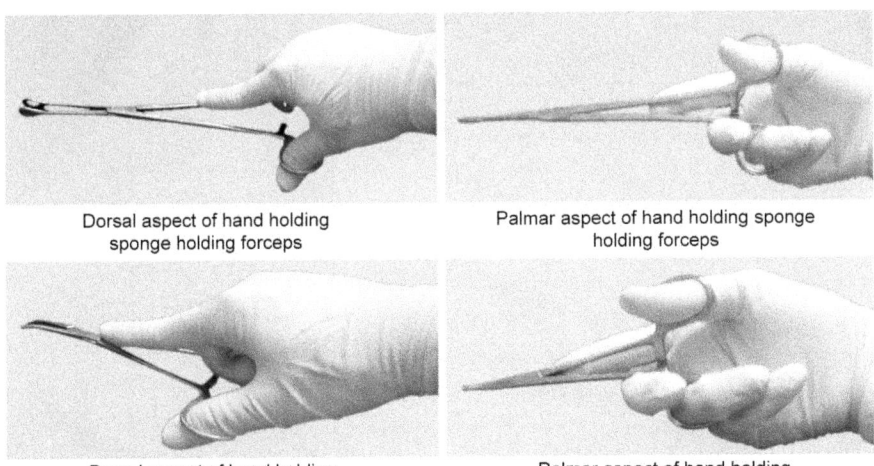

Dorsal aspect of hand holding sponge holding forceps

Palmar aspect of hand holding sponge holding forceps

Dorsal aspect of hand holding hemostatic forceps

Palmar aspect of hand holding hemostatic forceps

Fig. 1: Right hand holding a typical surgical instrument.

How to hold a surgical instrument having finger bows, while using it or working with it?

Insert thumb in one of the finger bows and ring finger into the another one, middle finger rests on the catch, while the index finger has to be kept over the length of the shaft, tip of which directed towards the tip of the blades, while working with most of the instruments commonly used in surgical practice (Fig. 1).

CHAPTER 3

Parts of a Typical Surgical Instrument

A typical long surgical instrument has the following parts (Fig. 1):

Finger bows: Two finger bows (rings) for holding the instrument properly (Commonly the thumb and the ring finger has to be put in the finger bows, while working with most of the surgical instruments).

Shaft: A pair of shaft or handle of the instrument, provides necessary length to the instrument (from catch to the joint).

Catch: A catch or ratchet when locked, the blades are closed and remain closed till the catch is released, making the instrument self-holding for the tissue held between its blades. Catch is meant for tight holding of the tissue held in between its blades without slipping. The instrument can be locked at its 1st, 2nd, 3rd or 4th catch, depending on the purpose of holding the tissue. In some instruments, it may not be present like scissors, sinus forceps, etc. where free movements of the blades are required.

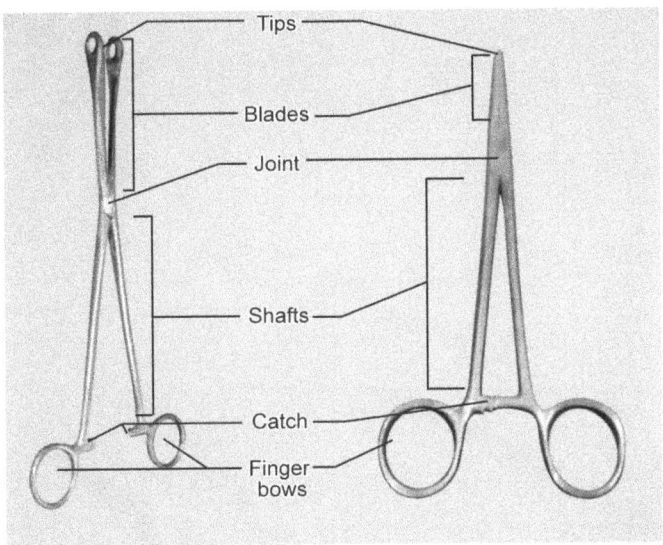

Fig. 1: Parts of a typical long surgical instrument.

Joint or shank: The two parts of the shaft and blades are kept attached by a joint. This joint may be either a box type or pivot type. In box joint, there is a slot in one shaft and the other shaft is passed through this slot (like in hemostatic forceps). In pivot joint, the two shafts are attached with each other at one point by a screw (like in scissors).

Blades: A pair of blades constitutes the terminal part of the instrument (from the joint to the tip of the instrument). The blades are of different varieties and designed as per the use of the instrument.

Tip of the instrument: Terminal part of the blades, which may be sharp or blunt, depending on the purpose of the instrument for which it is commonly used.

Section 2

Instruments in General Surgery

Section Outline

4. Cutting Instruments
5. Holding Instruments
6. Instruments for Tissue Dissection
7. Stone Holding Forceps
8. Needle Holders
9. Modern Techniques of Suturing
10. Retractors
11. Clamps
12. Miscellaneous Instruments in General Surgery
13. Instruments in Specialized Surgery

CHAPTER 4

Cutting Instruments

BARD PARKER'S HANDLES (DETACHABLE HANDLE)
- Flat stainless steel instrument
- One end is narrower with a slot for attaching the scalpel blade
- The handle (shaft) is grooved or having serrations on whole of its length for better gripping of the handle, while using it without slipping
- Number of the handle is written on its shaft which may be of 3, 4 and 5 in number, and blades can be interchanged with standard handles, which fits in their slots, according to the size of the blades
- Sterilization by autoclaving (Fig. 1).

SURGICAL BLADES
- Blades are detachable and disposable
- They have straight back and cutting edge
- The shape of the cutting edge decides its function
- Large selection of blades of different sizes and shapes are available from no.10 to 24
- Blades no. 10, 11, 12 and 15 fits in the Bard Parker's handle number 3 and 5
- Blades no. 18, 19, 20, 21, 22, 23 and 24 fits in the Bard Parker's handle number 4
- Supplied in presterilized pack (Fig. 2).

How to Hold the Bard Parker's Handle after Attaching Surgical Blade to it?

It depends on the procedure for which the handle is used:
- **Dinner knife position:** Making an incision to avoid tailing at the end of the incision
- **Writing position:** Better control over the surgical blade is exercised in this position
- **Grasping position:** Used in amputations. Cutting edge is towards the operating surgeon.

Section 2: Instruments in General Surgery

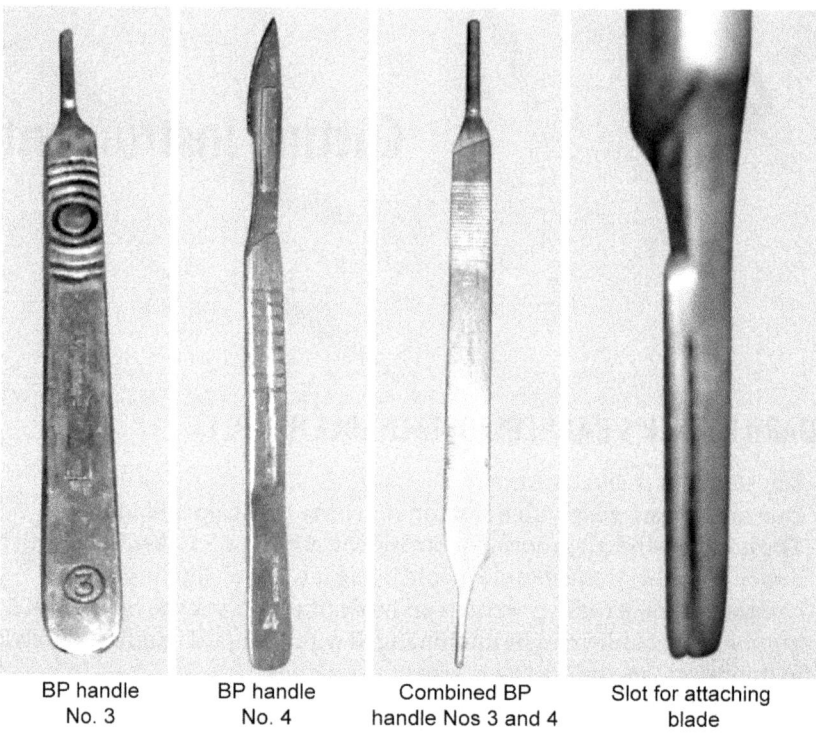

Fig. 1: Different sizes of BP handles.

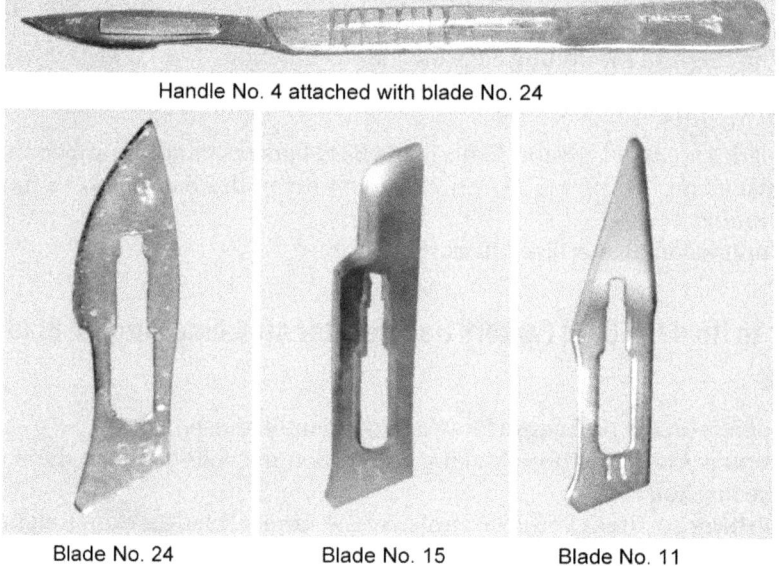

Fig. 2: Different sizes and number of surgical blades.

Uses of Bard Parker's Handles and Surgical Blades

- ❖ To make the skin incision to start any operative procedure surgical blades nos. 20, 21, 22, 23 and 24 have wide shaft, and are used to make larger incisions for laparotomy, mastectomy, etc. They are also used for sharp dissection to raise the skin flaps during modified radical mastectomy, incisional hernia repair, radical neck dissection, etc.
- ❖ Surgical blade no. 15 has narrow shaft and is used to make smaller skin incisions as well as dissection for excision of sebaceous cyst, lipoma, lymph node, during venesection to cut the vein, etc.
- ❖ Surgical blade No. 11 has oblique edge with sharp pointed tip, so known as 'stab knife'. It is commonly used to incise the skin, subcutaneous tissue, deep fascia to open the abscess cavity in a single stroke, during incision and drainage of an abscess. It can also be used to incise the skin, subcutaneous tissue and the muscles while inserting drains like abdominal and intercostal drains.

SCISSORS

- ❖ It has pair of blades, shaft, pivot type of joint and finger bows
- ❖ Length of the scissors is variable as per the purpose of its use
- ❖ Blades of the scissor may be straight or curved. It has a chisel edge with a bevel
- ❖ Bevel varies according to the function and structure which has to be cut
- ❖ Tips of the blades may be blunt or sharp and pointed
- ❖ It has pivot type of joint for free and smooth movements while cutting the tissue
- ❖ Sterilized by keeping them dipped in concentrated lysol for 1 hour to 24 hours in dilute lysol
- ❖ Sterilization by boiling and autoclaving damages the sharpness of the instrument.

MAYO'S SCISSOR

- ❖ It is a long and stout scissor and has various sizes
- ❖ It may be straight or curved with flat blades
- ❖ Tips of the blades may be blunt or sharp, pointed, according to its use (Fig. 3).

Uses

- ❖ Mainly used for cutting the thread or sutures after ligation or suturing
- ❖ To cut the tough structures during dissection like linea alba, external oblique aponeurosis, anterior and posterior rectus sheath, etc.
- ❖ During appendicectomy, curved Mayo's scissor is used to split the internal oblique and transversus abdominis muscle, to reach the peritoneum
- ❖ Rarely used for dissection of tissue.

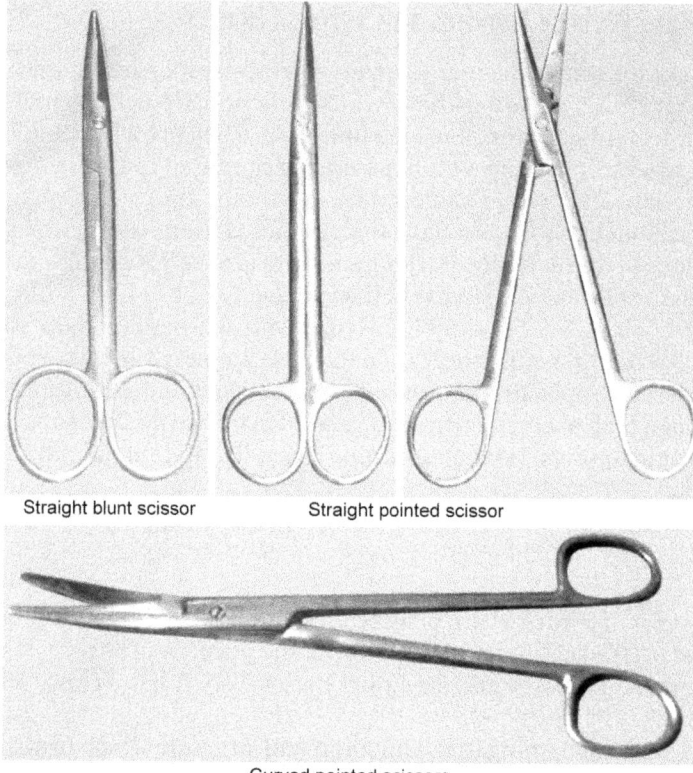

Fig. 3: Mayo's scissors.

METZENBAUM SCISSOR

- It is much lighter than Mayo's scissor
- It is long fine scissor, with long shafts (handles) and short blades
- Blades of the scissor may be straight or curved, delicate and mostly fine tipped (Fig. 4).

Uses of Metzenbaum and Mcindoe's Scissors

- For fine tissue dissection and cutting delicate structures during various surgeries
- To create a plane between tissue while dissecting out a cyst, lipoma, lymph node, etc.
- To open the peritoneum during laparotomy
- To dissect the hernial sac from rest of the cord structures
- To raise the fine skin flaps in thyroidectomy, incisional hernia, modified radical mastectomy, radical neck dissection, etc.

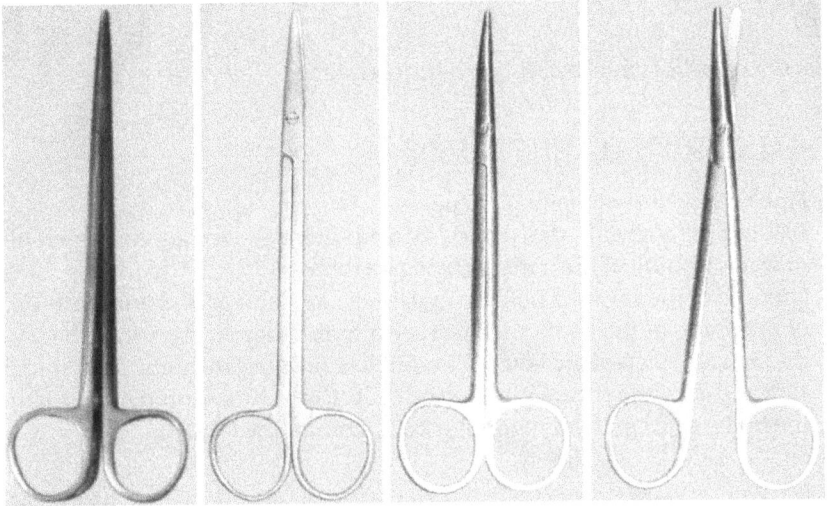

Fig. 4: Metzenbaum dissecting scissors.

- Used during nephrectomy and splenectomy to cut the pedicles after ligating them
- During cholecystectomy, to divide the cystic duct and artery after their ligation
- To cut the intestine, during resection and anastomosis.

MCINDOE SCISSOR

- Same as Metzenbaum scissor, except that blades are smaller than Metzenbaum scissor
- Blades are small as compared to the shaft, which are long (Fig. 5)

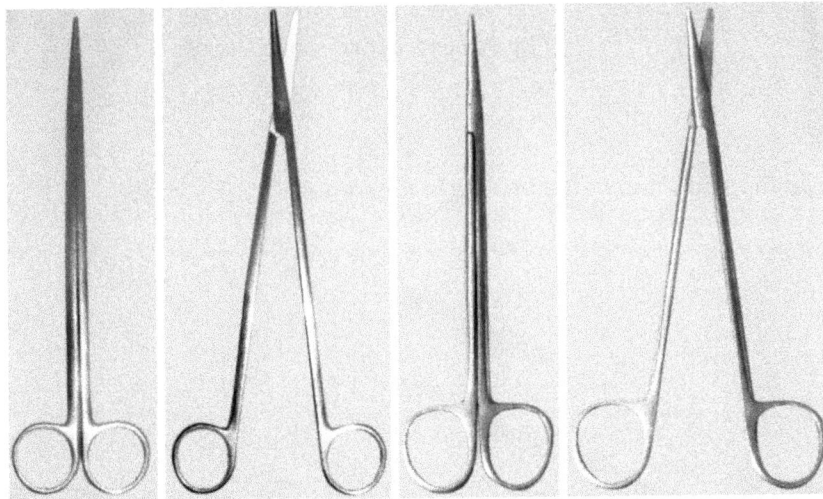

Fig. 5: McIndoe scissors.

Uses

Described earlier same as Metzenbaum scissor.

■ HEATH SUTURE CUTTING SCISSOR

- ❖ Fine scissor curved on angle type
- ❖ Blades are too small, sharp and at the tip there are serrations, which help in firm gripping of the suture during its removal
- ❖ One end of the suture is held up by a dissecting forceps and only part of one of the blade of the scissor is inserted into the loop of the suture between the skin and loop of the stitch. The stitch is cut close to its entrance into the skin and then the suture is pulled outside. Cut suture should not remain in the body, as it can lead to foreign body granuloma (Fig. 6).

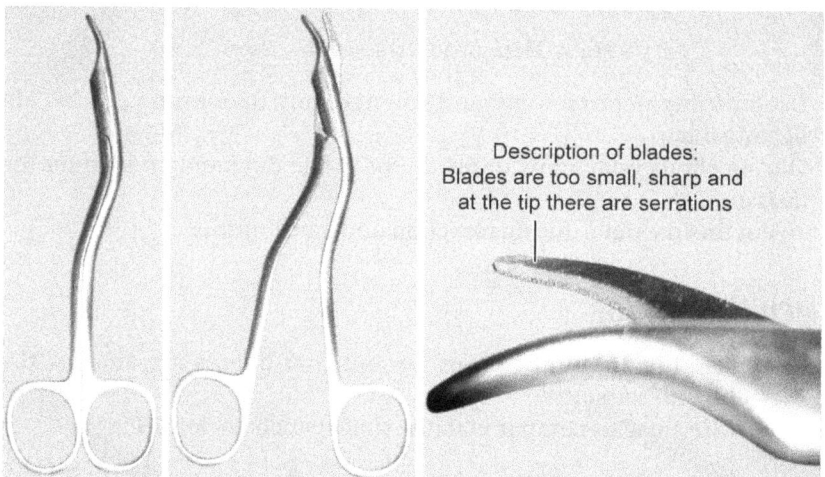

Fig. 6: Heath suture cutting scissor.

Uses

To cut the skin sutures after healing of the wound.

CHAPTER 5

Holding Instruments

- Mostly called as 'forceps'
- It may be tissue holding forceps, swab holding forceps, stone holding forceps, etc.
- Name of the instrument is mostly given as per the purpose for which the instrument is used.

RAMPLEY'S SWAB (SPONGE) HOLDING FORCEPS

- Long instrument (9 and 1/2 inches in length) provided with finger bows, pair of long shafts with catch, a box type of joint and pair of blades
- It may be straight or curved
- Tips of the blades are oval, fenestrated and having transverse serrations on its inner aspect, to hold the swab firmly without slipping while using the instrument and fenestrations in it allows bulging of the swab
- The instrument is made longer by providing it with long shafts and blades to enable the scrubbed surgeon to clean the operative area with antiseptic solution without touching the rest of the unsterile field of the patient's body (non-touch technique)
- Sterilization by autoclaving (Fig. 1).

Uses

Mainly Used as

For preoperative cleansing (scrubbing) of the skin of the operative and nearby surrounding area with swab soaked in antiseptic solution before all operations, to make the area sterile and free of microorganisms before starting any procedure.

Section 2: Instruments in General Surgery

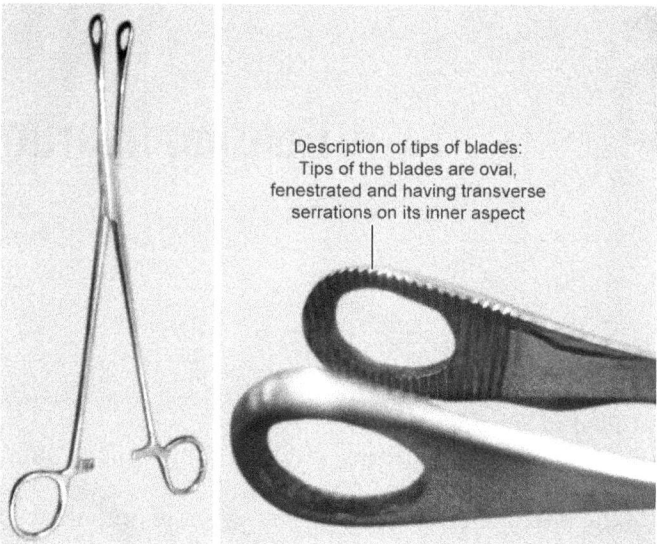

Fig. 1: Rampley's swab holding forceps.

Additional Uses

- To hold the fundus and Hartmann's pouch of the gallbladder to give gentle traction, while dissecting gallbladder from the gallbladder fossa during open cholecystectomy
- As a tongue holding forceps during oral surgeries
- As a pile holding forceps during hemorrhoidectomy
- As an ovum holding forceps
- To hold the cervix of uterus during pervaginal examination
- For removing the laminated membrane and daughter cysts, during hydatid cyst removal from solid organs like liver, lungs, spleen, etc.

TOWEL CLIPS (TOWEL HOLDING FORCEPS)

DOYEN'S CROSS ACTION TOWEL CLIP

- Pincer like instrument
- On pressing the shaft, the blades opens and on releasing it the blades closes and the tips of the two blades meet or cross each other to hold the towel or sheets (drapes) firmly
- Blades are curved and sharply pointed for firmly holding the whole thickness of the drape, without interfering and protruding in the operative field to lie underneath the towel and out of surgeon's sight
- Sterilization by autoclaving (Fig. 2).

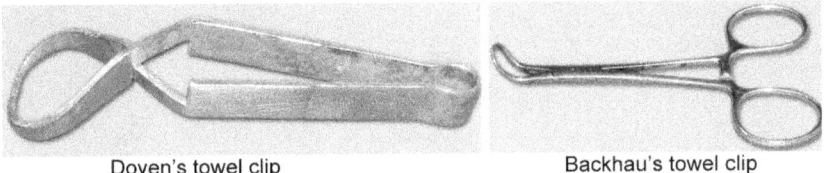

Doyen's towel clip   Backhau's towel clip

Fig. 2: Different types of towel clips.

■ MAYO'S (BACKHAUS) TOWEL CLIP

Blades and tips are same as Doyen's towel clip, but it does not have pincer like action and having the shafts, finger bows and catch similar to that of hemostatic forceps.

Uses

Mainly Used as

For fixing the draping sheets or towels (Draping means placing sterile sheets surrounding the operative field, to isolate the operative area from the adjacent unsterile area. It prevents contamination of the sterile operative area during surgery from the surrounding unsterile area).

Additional Uses

- ❖ For fixing the diathermy cables, suction tubes, camera cables, etc.
- ❖ For holding the fractured ribs, while elevating a depressed flail segment of chest in 'flail chest injury'.
- ❖ As a tongue holding forceps in oral surgery
- ❖ To give external traction in fracture of the small long bones.

HEMOSTATIC FORCEPS (ARTERY FORCEPS)

■ SPENCER WELLS HEMOSTATIC FORCEPS

- ❖ It has finger bows, catch, pair of shafts (handles) and pair of blades
- ❖ It may be straight or curved
- ❖ Blades are usually half the length of the shaft
- ❖ Whole length of the inner sides of the blades are provided with transverse serrations
- ❖ Tips of the blades are conical
- ❖ When catch is locked, blades are opposed and tightly closed
- ❖ As no gap remains between the blades after locking the instrument and due to presence of transverse serrations on both the blades on whole of their length, it firmly holds and crushes the tissue held in between its blades and prevents slipping of tissue
- ❖ Sterilization by autoclaving (Fig. 3).

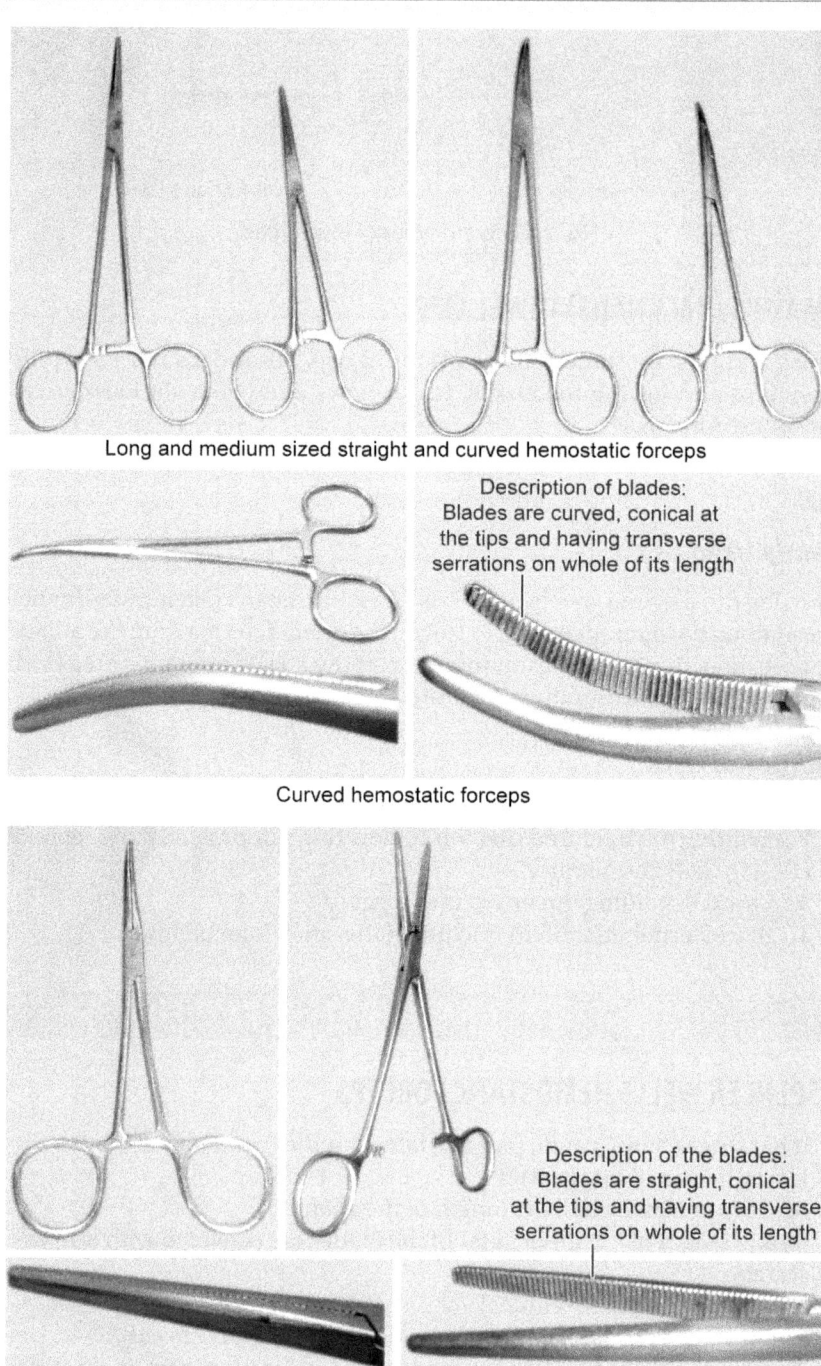

Fig. 3: Spencer Wells type curved and straight hemostatic forceps.

How to Differentiate the Hemostatic Forceps from the Needle Holder?

❖ Hemostatic forceps is a lighter instrument than needle holder. Its blades are longer as compared to the needle holder and having transverse serrations in whole length of its blades
❖ Needle holder is relatively heavier instrument. Its blades are smaller as compared to the shaft and there are criss-cross serrations on the whole of the inner aspect of the blades, along with groove in the center of each blade.

Uses

Mainly Used as

❖ To hold (catch) the bleeding vessels (capillaries, veins, arteries) to stop bleeding from them, while cutting through different layers of tissues, during all operations by catching and crushing or ligating the bleeding vessel, i.e. called as 'hemostatic forceps'
❖ Smaller vessels if left crushed for a couple of minutes, is sufficient to arrest the bleeding. While larger vessel may require ligation, before releasing the vessel.

Additional Uses

❖ During appendicectomy, it is used to split the internal oblique and transversus abdominis muscle to reach the peritoneum. Also used to crush the base of the appendix before cutting it
❖ While doing intestinal resection and anastomosis, mesenteric vessels of the adjacent diseased intestine are held in between the hemostatic forceps before resecting the segment of diseased intestine, to prevent bleeding from the cut mesenteric vessels
❖ For blunt dissection and to create plane between the subcutaneous tissue and the cyst wall or capsule of lipoma, lymph node, while excision of the cyst, lipoma, biopsy of lymph node, etc.
❖ To hold the cut margins of the rectus sheath, linea alba, external oblique aponeurosis, peritoneum, etc. during closure of the laparotomy incisions
❖ As a pedicle clamp, while ligating pedicle of spleen or kidney during splenectomy or nephrectomy respectively
❖ To dissect vein from the subcutaneous tissue, while doing venesection
❖ To hold the end of the ligature while suturing
❖ To tie a knot after suturing, and also to hold the one end of the suture, while removing it
❖ As a dressing forceps
❖ To hold and pass the perurethral catheter by non-touch technique.

■ HALSTED MOSQUITO HEMOSTATIC FORCEPS

- ❖ Similar to Spencer Well's type of hemostatic forceps with exception that it is very light, small, delicate and having fine pointed tips
- ❖ May be straight or curved
- ❖ Sterilization by autoclaving (Fig. 4).

Uses

Mainly Used as

To hold the small, fine bleeding vessels, while cutting through different layers of the tissue during all operations, to stop bleeding from the cut vessels.

Additional Uses

- ❖ During appendicectomy, mesoappendix is poked with curved mosquito forceps at an avascular site and ligature passed through it and ligated before division of the mesoappendix to secure appendicular artery, to prevent bleeding from the appendicular artery
- ❖ During circumcision, to separate adhesions between the glans penis and the inner surface of the prepuce, and also to hold the edges of the prepuce, to give traction while splitting and cutting it
- ❖ For hair lip and soft palate surgery
- ❖ Routinely used, in all the pediatric surgeries by the pediatric surgeon.

■ KOCHER'S HEMOSTATIC FORCEPS

Similar to Spencer Well's type of hemostatic forceps, *except:*
- ❖ May be medium or large sized
- ❖ Blades are slightly longer than Spencer Well's type of hemostatic forceps
- ❖ At the tip of its blades, there is a tooth in one blade and a groove in the other blade, which fits in each other to lock the blades (tips) completely when the catch is closed, giving firm hold of the tissue held in it
- ❖ Sterilization by autoclaving (Fig. 5).

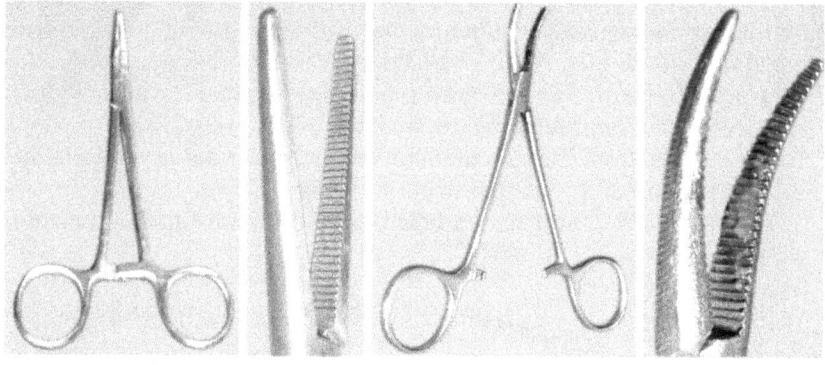

Straight mosquito forceps   Curved mosquito forceps

Fig. 4: Halsted mosquito forceps.

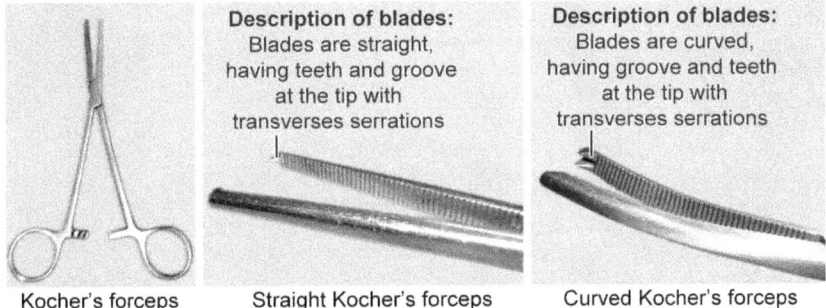

Fig. 5: Kocher's hemostatic forceps.

Mainly Used as

During hemi, subtotal or near total thyroidectomy, it is applied around the margins of the lobe of the thyroid gland to be excised, before excision of that lobe to prevent bleeding from the remnant tissue of the thyroid gland.

Additional Uses

- ❖ Suitable for holding the bleeding vessels in the tough structures like palm, sole and scalp, where the vessels tends to retract in the deep fascia after cutting the overlying skin and subcutaneous tissue. The teeth and the groove at the tip of blades, help to hold the retracting bleeding vessels securely
- ❖ To hold meniscus during meniscectomy
- ❖ To hold the perforating vessels during modified radical mastectomy
- ❖ In obstetric practice, it is used for artificial rupture of the membranes.

■ LISTER'S SINUS FORCEPS

- ❖ It does not hold anything, but is discussed in this section, as students confuse it with Spencer Well's type of straight hemostatic forceps
- ❖ It is a long slender instrument with pair of blades having transverse serrations only at the tip of both the blades and their tips are blunt, olive tipped, non-traumatic. No catch
- ❖ Transverse serrations at the tip are for breaking the loculi and to introduce the corrugated rubber drain or roller pack in the abscess cavity
- ❖ Sterilization by autoclaving (Fig. 6).

How to Differentiate it from the Spencer Well's Type of Hemostatic Forceps?

- ❖ Transverse serrations are present only at the tip and not on the whole of the blades, as that of the hemostatic forceps

Section 2: Instruments in General Surgery

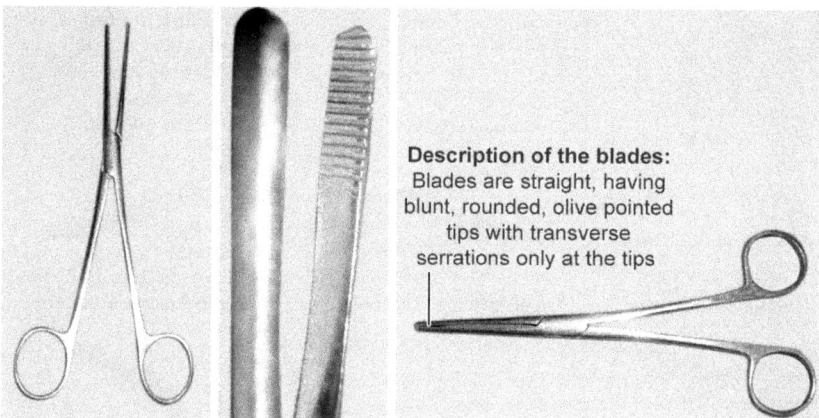

Description of the blades:
Blades are straight, having blunt, rounded, olive pointed tips with transverse serrations only at the tips

Fig. 6: Lister's sinus forceps.

- Tips are olive, rounded and blunt, so non-traumatic to the tissue, when it is poked blindly through the tissue
- Not provided with a catch, so if accidently any important vital structures are grasped in between the blades and their tips, it will not get crushed as that in hemostatic forceps.

Uses

Mainly Used as

For incision and drainage of a deep seated abscess by Hilton's method, to reach and explore the tract of the abscess cavity situated at the neck, axilla, groin and at the other sites where important vital structures are present.

Additional Uses

- To introduce the corrugated rubber drain (CRD), while making blind tract to drain the dead space after any operation like hydrocele, excision of lipoma, cyst, for making counter incision in case of breast abscess, where most prominent part is not most dependent
- For exploring a sinus tract.

ALLIE'S TISSUE FORCEPS

- It is a light instrument having finger bows, catch, box type of joint, pair of shafts and blades
- Blades are long, straight and there is a gap in between whole of their length, to accommodate the tissue grasped at the tips without crushing them in between the two blades
- Tips of the blades are slightly curved or angulated and provided with alternate fine, sharp teeth and grooves, which interlock within each other,

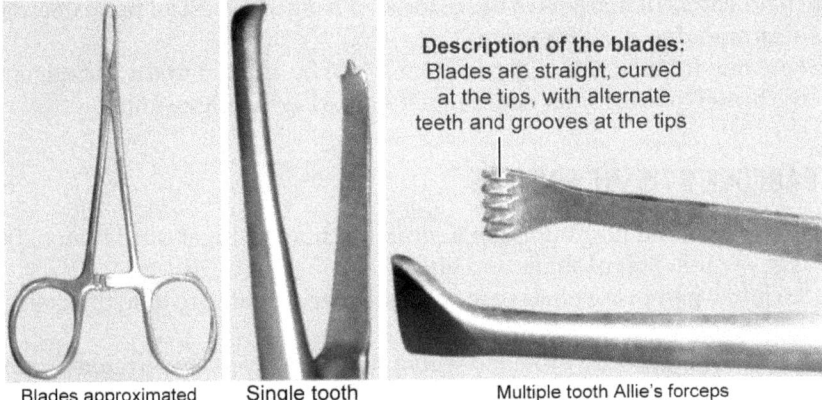

Description of the blades:
Blades are straight, curved at the tips, with alternate teeth and grooves at the tips

Blades approximated   Single tooth   Multiple tooth Allie's forceps

Fig. 7: Allie's tissue forceps.

when the catch is closed for better grip of the tissue held in it. Teeth and alternate grooves may be 1, 2, 3 or 4 in number
- When the catch is closed, teeth at the tip of one blade fits or gets locked in the groove of the tip of the other blade and vice-versa
- It minimally crushes the tissue hold in between the tips. The remaining portion of the blades allows the tissue to bulge through the gap between the blades
- Skin flaps should be held from inner side of it along with the subcutaneous tissue rather than directly holding the skin from outside, to prevent teeth marks on the skin surface
- Sterilization by autoclaving (Fig. 7).

Uses

- To hold the skin and subcutaneous tissue flaps for retraction, while dissecting the capsule or wall of a cyst during excision of lipoma, cyst, lymph node, etc.
- To hold the tough tissue like fascia or aponeurosis, in order to approximate them while suturing
- To hold the tough galea aponeurotica of the scalp, while raising skin flaps during craniotomy
- During thyroidectomy, radical neck dissection, modified radical mastectomy, to hold the margins of skin while raising the skin flaps
- In the repair of incisional, epigastric or umbilical hernia, to hold the margins of fascial gap (defect) through which the hernial sac is herniating, while dissecting the sac from the surrounding tissue. Also used to hold the skin margins while raising the skin flaps
- During laparatomy via midline incision, to retract the skin margins while incising the linea alba to reach the peritoneum. Also while closing the midline incision, linea alba held up by the Allie's tissue forceps while suturing it

- To hold the cut margins of the bladder, during transvesical prostatectomy or suprapubic cystolithotomy
- Fine one toothed Allie's tissue forceps can be applied to the cut edges of the bowel to bring their edges together, during their anastomosis.

BABCOCK'S TISSUE FORCEPS

- It is a light and nontraumatic instrument having finger bows, catch, box type of joint, pair of shafts and blades
- Terminal part of the blades are curved and fenestrated to hold the delicate structures
- Tip of the blades are provided with a ridge (transversely serrated) on one blade and groove on the other, so when the catch is closed, the ridge of one blade fits in the groove of the other blade, for better apposition and firm grip of the tissue held in it, without slipping of the tissue
- Fenestration in the blades makes the instrument light and also allows the held tissue to bulge in between them, even after locking the catch, without crushing the tissue
- Sterilization by autoclaving (Fig. 8).

Uses

Mainly Used as

- To hold the tubular and delicate structures in the body
- During appendicectomy, two Babcock's forceps are used, one to hold the base of the appendix and the other is applied to its apex
- To hold the other tubular structures like ureter during pyelolithotomy or ureterolithotomy, fallopian tubes during tubal ligation, spermatic cord during hernia surgery, etc.

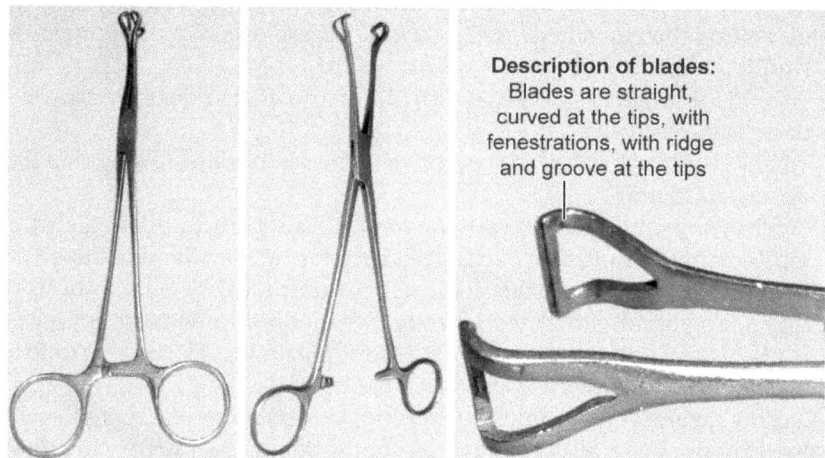

Description of blades: Blades are straight, curved at the tips, with fenestrations, with ridge and groove at the tips

Fig. 8: Babcock's forceps.

Additional Uses

- During small and large bowel resection and anastomosis, to hold the cut margins of the ends of the intestine, to bring them together during their anastomosis
- During gastrectomy, gastrojejunostomy, to hold the cut margins of the stomach and jejunum during their anastomosis
- During feeding gastrostomy or jejunostomy, to hold the stomach or jejunum while applying the purse string suture to fix the feeding tube to the serosa
- To hold the cut margins of the bladder, during transvesical prostatectomy or suprapubic cystolithotomy.

▌LANE TISSUE FORCEPS

- It is short, thick, bulkier and heavy instrument
- It has finger bows, catch, box type of joint, pair of shafts and blades
- Blades are small as compared to the shafts, and curved and fenestrated, which permits the bulky tissue to accommodate within it and allows them to bulge without crushing, when the instrument is locked
- At the tip, there is a sharp interlocking teeth, which fits in each other when the instrument (catch) is closed and provides firm grip of the tissue held in between them without slipping, while giving gentle traction to the tissue held in it for dissection
- Sterilization by autoclaving (Fig. 9).

Uses

Mainly Used as

- To hold the bulky and slippery tissue
- To hold the subcutaneous tissue and fat in obese patients during surgeries
- During mastectomy, it is used to hold the breast tissue while dissecting it off from the pectoral fascia or chest wall

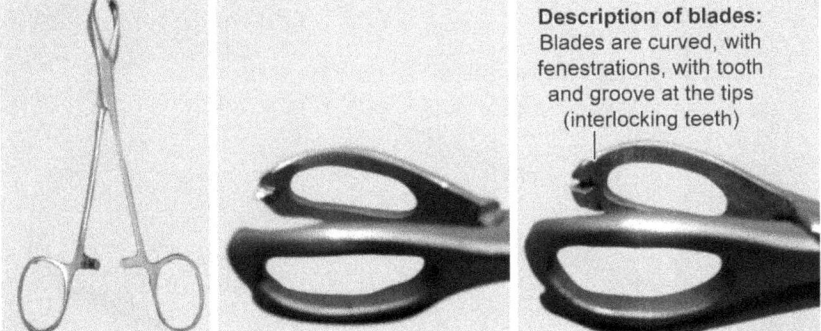

Description of blades: Blades are curved, with fenestrations, with tooth and groove at the tips (interlocking teeth)

Fig. 9: Lane tissue forceps.

❖ During submandibular or parotid gland excision, to hold the gland during dissection from the surrounding tissue.

Additional Uses

To fix the draping sheets and to fix the suction tubes and diathermy cables.

■ CORD HOLDING FORCEPS (COLLINGWOOD-STEWART CORD HOLDING OR HERNIA FORCEPS)

- ❖ It is also called as 'hernia ring'
- ❖ It has finger bows, catch, pair of shaft along with two semicircular blades, which makes a circular opening in the blades, when the catch is closed
- ❖ Sterilization by autoclaving (Fig. 10).

Uses

During hernia repair, to isolate the spermatic cord from the operative area during dissection of the sac, and also to retract the cord away from the site of the repair (from the posterior wall of the inguinal canal).

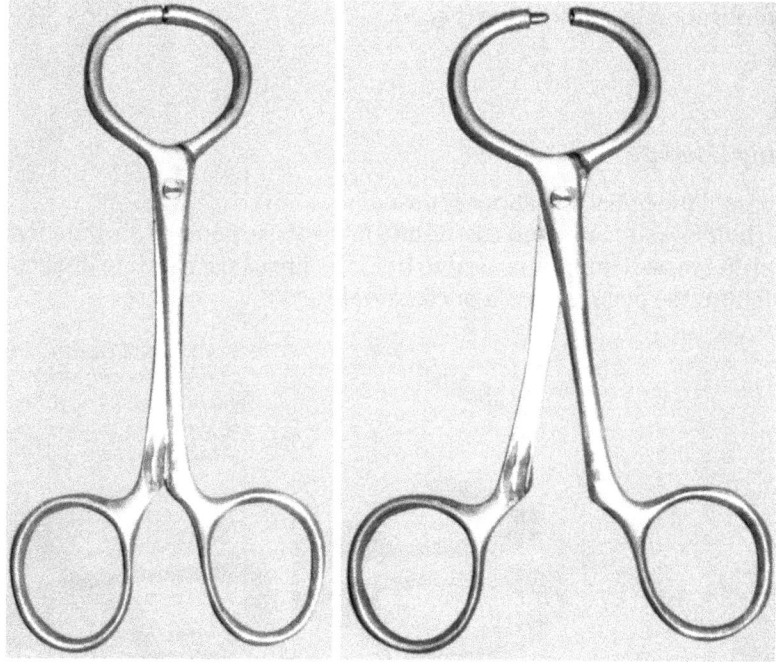

Fig. 10: Cord holding forceps.

TONGUE HOLDING FORCEPS (THOMPSON'S)

- It has finger bows, catch, pair of blades and shaft and box type of joint
- The tip of the blades are triangular, fenestrated and having transverse serrations
- It is not commonly used nowadays, due its crushing effect and fear of pressure necrosis of the portion of the tongue held in it
- It is substituted by towel clips, tongue stitch or by holding tongue between two gauze pieces by assistants hand (Fig. 11).

Uses

To hold the tongue during operations of the oral cavity and tongue.

DUVAL LUNG FORCEPS

- It is a delicate instrument having finger bows, catch, pair of shafts and blades
- The tip of the blades has broad, triangular, fenestrated jaws with ridge and groove at the tips
- Available in various sizes
- Nontraumatic to the tissue held in it, as the grip is spread over a wide area, and only the distal edges of the triangular blades meet when the catch is locked (Fig. 12).

Uses

To hold the lung tissue, while performing operations on the lung like pneumonectomies, excision of lung hydatid, etc.

May be Used

- To hold the cut edges of the intestines, during resection and anastomosis
- To hold the bladder wall, during suprapubic cystolithotomy.

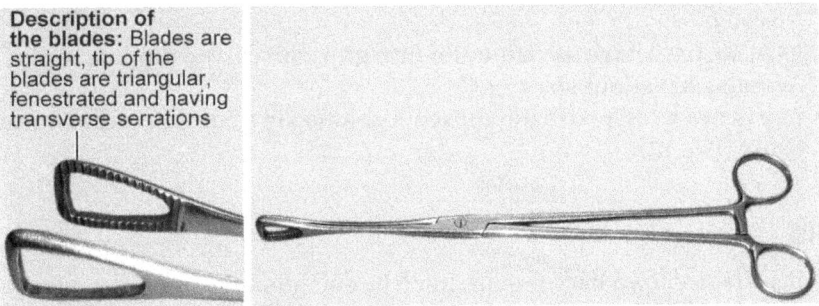

Description of the blades: Blades are straight, tip of the blades are triangular, fenestrated and having transverse serrations

Fig. 11: Tongue holding forceps.

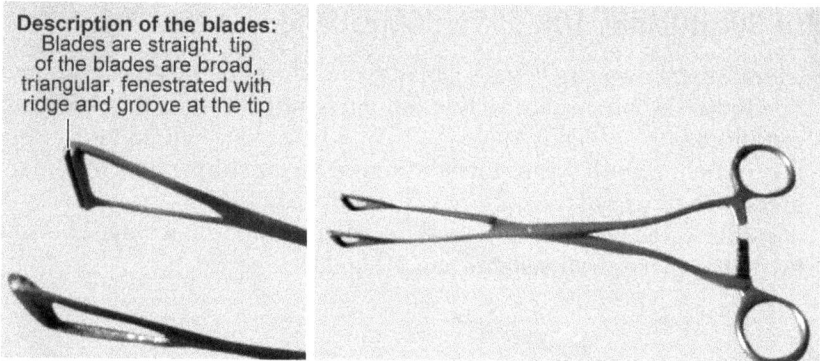

Fig. 12: Duval lung forceps.

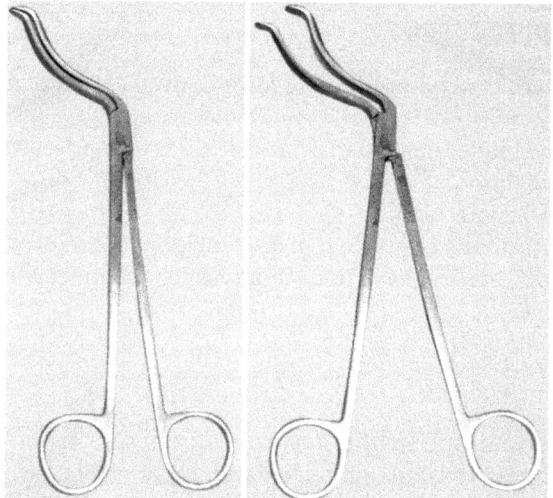

Fig. 13: Cheatle forceps.

CHEATLE FORCEPS

- It is a large instrument, with finger bows, joint, pair of shaft and blades. No catch
- Its blade have large serrations for firm grip with curved dipping blades
- Available in various sizes
- As it is always dipped in the antiseptic solution in a bottle, it is always ready to use (Fig. 13).

Uses

To pick the sterilized instruments, linen by operation theater assistant who is not scrubbed during the surgery to avoid their handling to make them unsterile.

CHAPTER 6

Instruments for Tissue Dissection

■ DISSECTING FORCEPS

Two armed instrument with spring like action.

Plain (Non-Toothed) Dissecting Forceps

- ❖ May be medium or long sized plain dissecting forceps or fine tipped, short plain dissecting forceps
- ❖ It is delicate and inflicts minimal tissue damage, so used while handling delicate structures
- ❖ Two limbs of the shaft are attached to each other at one end, and designed such that it provides a spring like action, and keeps the blades apart when the instrument is not in use
- ❖ Pressing the shafts brings the tips of the blades together and grips the tissue between them without traumatizing (as it does not have the tooth and socket at their tips like toothed forceps)
- ❖ There are transverse serrations at the tip of the blades, which gives firm grip and helps in lifting the tissue while dissection and also picking up the needle through the tissue while suturing them
- ❖ Some have guard between the blades, which prevents over approximation of the blades
- ❖ Grooves or ridges on the outer surface of the shaft provides firm grip of the instrument, without slipping of the fingers holding them (Fig. 1).

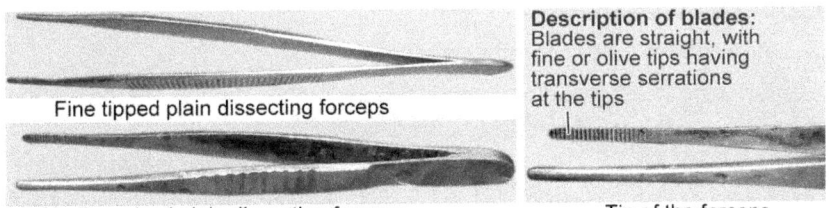

Fine tipped plain dissecting forceps

Description of blades: Blades are straight, with fine or olive tips having transverse serrations at the tips

Medium sized plain dissecting forceps

Tip of the forceps

Fig. 1: Plain dissecting forceps.

Uses

- To hold the delicate and friable structures during dissection in any surgery, as it inflicts minimal tissue damage to the tissue that is held in it
- Used during almost all surgeries to hold the structures like peritoneum, intra-abdominal viscera, vessels, nerves, and muscles during dissection and suturing
- Fine tipped forceps are used during nerve repair, vascular anastomosis and cardiac surgeries
- During hernia surgeries, to hold and dissect the sac from the rest of the cord structures
- During resection and anastomosis of the intestine, to hold the cut margins of the intestine during their anastomosis
- During appendicectomy, to bring the cecum out of the wound to deliver the appendix
- While burying the base of the appendix. After appendicectomy, stump has to be held with the plain forceps and pushed in the cecal wall as the purse string suture is tied.

Toothed Dissecting Forceps

- Configuration is same as the plain forceps, except that there is a tooth at the tip of one blade and groove at the tip of other blade, so when the blades are approximated toothed tip fits into the groove of other tip
- Because of the presence of tooth and groove at the tips, tissue held in it is better gripped, and there are less chances of slipping of the tissue. But it is traumatic to the tissue (Fig. 2).

Uses

- Applied to the bulky, slippery, heavy and tough tissue in the body during dissection
- For holding and retracting the skin flaps during venesection, excision of the lipoma, cyst, lymph node, etc.

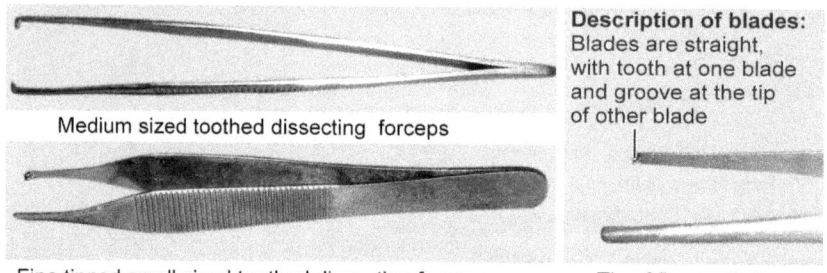

Medium sized toothed dissecting forceps

Description of blades: Blades are straight, with tooth at one blade and groove at the tip of other blade

Fine tipped small sized toothed dissecting forceps

Tip of fine tooth forceps

Fig. 2: Tooth dissecting forceps.

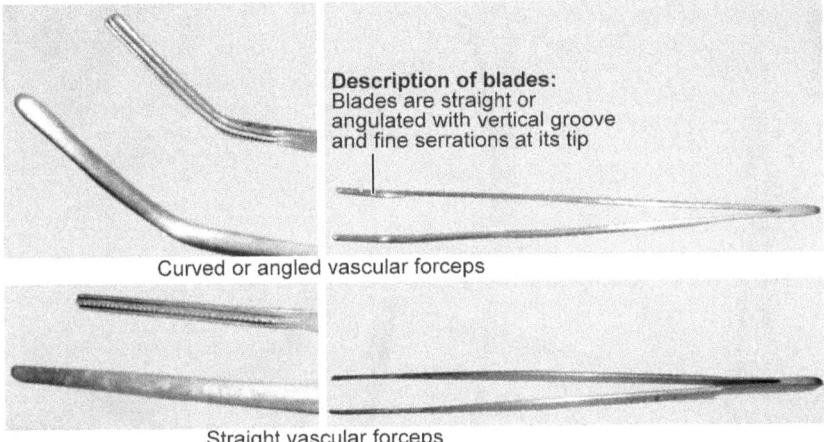

Fig. 3: Vascular forceps.

- Used during almost all operations, to hold the tough structures like skin, fascia, and aponeurosis
- To hold the cut margins of the skin, during suturing of the incision or the wound
- To hold the linea alba, during closure of midline laparotomy incision.

VASCULAR FORCEPS

- These are designed like plain dissecting forceps, but they are very fine and delicate
- They are having vertical groove with fine serrations at the tip like vascular clamps, which holds the vessel without inflicting even slight trauma to the vessel wall (Fig. 3).

Uses

- To hold the vessels (arteries or veins) during vascular anastomosis and their repair
- To hold the delicate structures like pancreas during pancreaticojejunostomy.

RIGHT ANGLE FORCEPS (LAHEY FORCEPS) OR MIXTER FORCEPS

- It is a long instrument available in different sizes
- It is having finger bows, a catch, a pair of shaft and blades
- Terminal parts of the blades are bent at right angle to the rest of the blade
- Transverse serrations are present in both the blades in whole of their length
- Sterilization by autoclaving (Fig. 4).

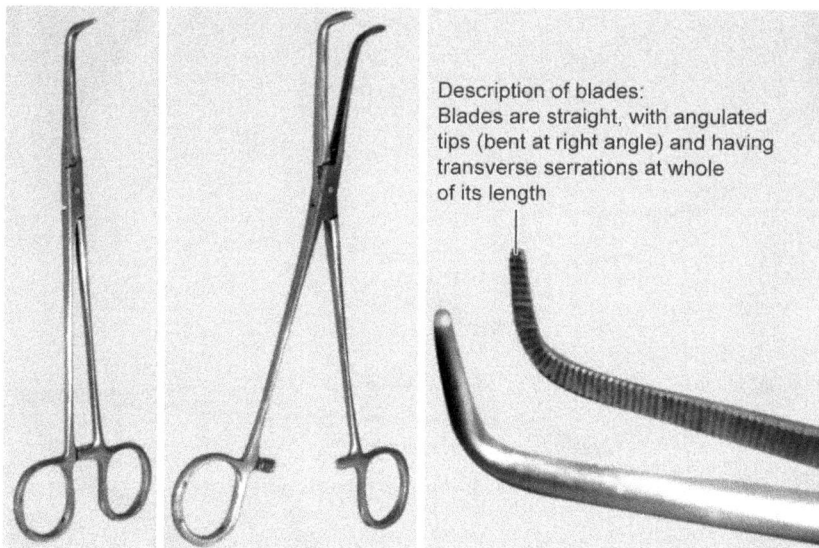

Fig. 4: Lahey forceps or Mixter forceps.

Uses

- To dissect the pedicles of solid organs like spleen, kidney, etc. from the adjacent tissue and then for passing ligatures around the dissected vessels, for ligating the pedicles
- During nephrectomy, to ligate the renal artery and vein separately in the renal pedicle, isolating and passing ligature around them, and tying them before cutting them
- During splenectomy, to isolate the splenic artery and vein in its pedicle, passing ligature around them, and tying them before cutting them
- During thyroid surgery, to dissect the middle thyroid vein, superior thyroid and inferior thyroid pedicles, passing ligature around them and then tying them before division of the pedicles
- During cholecystectomy, to dissect the cystic duct and artery, passing ligature around them and then tying them before their division
- Also used as a hemostatic forceps to hold the bleeding vessel in the depth.

CHAPTER 7

Stone Holding Forceps

DESJARDIN'S CHOLEDOCHOLITHOTOMY FORCEPS

- It is a long, slender, delicate instrument designed to avoid trauma to the common bile duct while stone removal
- It has finger bows, screw type of joint, pair of shafts and blades
- Shafts are curved with no catch, so that stone should not get crushed during its removal
- Blades are also gently curved for working in depth in minimum space, with flat and fenestrated tips to hold the stone properly without crushing
- No serrations in the blade and at the tips
- Sterilization by autoclaving (Fig. 1).

Uses

Mainly Used as

During choledocholithotomy, it is inserted into the common bile duct and the stones in the duct removed, by holding them in the fenestrated tips.

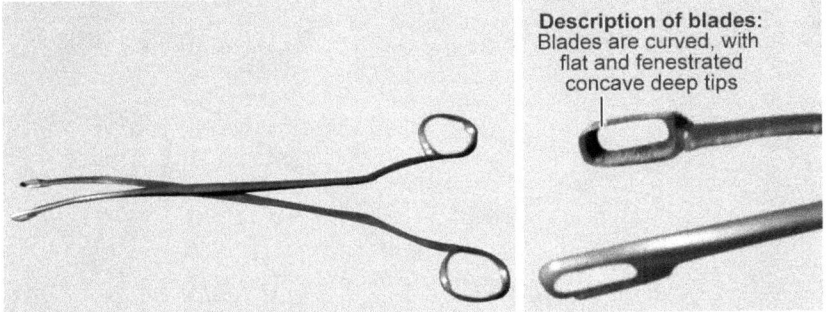

Description of blades: Blades are curved, with flat and fenestrated concave deep tips

Fig. 1: Desjardin's choledocholithotomy forceps.

Can be Used as

During removal of the stones from the kidney (nephrolithotomy), pelvis (pyelolithotomy) or also from the ureter (ureterolithotomy).

■ PYELOLITHOTOMY FORCEPS

- ❖ It is a long instrument with finger bows, pair of shaft and blades. No catch in the shaft
- ❖ Blades are curved or angulated and having various shapes as per the angulations with oval, fenestrated tips, with transverse serrations on the inner side of the tip of the blades
- ❖ Sterilization by autoclaving (Fig. 2).

Uses

To hold the stone during its removal from the kidney during nephrolithotomy, from the renal pelvis during pyelolithotomy and from the ureter during ureterolithotomy.

■ SUPRAPUBIC CYSTOLITHOTOMY FORCEPS

- ❖ It has pair of blades and shafts, screw type of joint but, having a single finger bow
- ❖ Shaft (handle) is peculiar. One finger bow (ring) for the thumb is like bows of other instruments, whereas the other shaft has incomplete ring and is hook like to accommodate the remaining four fingers. This type of handle provides adequate grip without crushing pressure of the fingers on the stone held in the forceps
- ❖ Blades are spoon shaped, concave and their inner surface are provided with fine spicules or blunt serrations, which helps in firm gripping of the stone, without crushing it

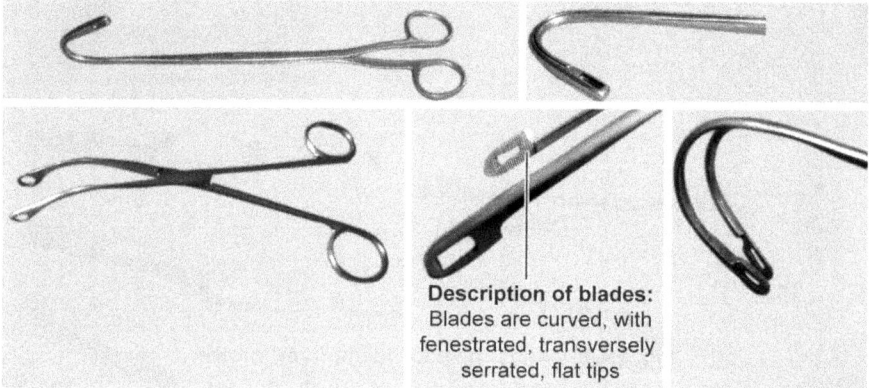

Description of blades: Blades are curved, with fenestrated, transversely serrated, flat tips

Fig. 2: Pyelolithotomy forceps with different angulations.

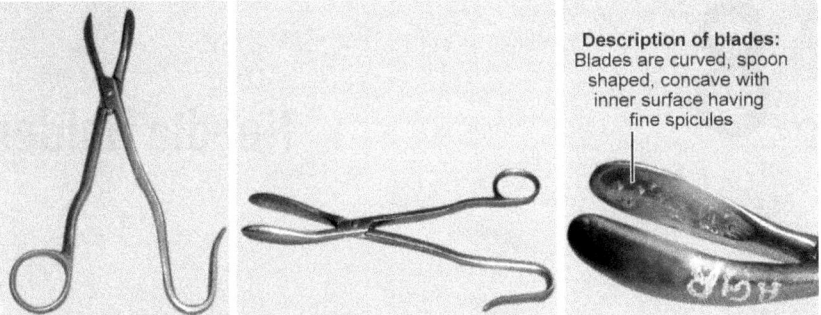

Fig. 3: Suprapubic cystolithotomy forceps.

- No catch, to prevent accidental locking of the instrument during the stone removal. It may crush the stone and incomplete removal of it and its fragments if break accidently, which may act as a nidus for future stone formation. Also distance between the blades is adjustable even for large stone, as with catch it is always fixed.
- Sterilization by autoclaving (Fig. 3).

Uses

To remove the bladder stone (vesical calculus) during suprapubic cystolithotomy.

CHAPTER 8

Needle Holders

INTRODUCTION

* It has finger bows, catch, box type of joint, and pair of shafts and blades
* Needle holder is a relatively heavier instrument than most of the instruments, used in surgery
* It may be long, medium or short, depending on the operative areas where it has to be used
* Blades are always straight, but shaft may be straight or curved, in long needle holders not to obstruct the vision of the surgeon, while suturing tissue in the depth
* Blades are too short as compared to the shaft (long shaft), and heavy for better grip and control over the needle gripped between them
* There are criss-cross serrations on the inner aspect of the blades, which allows firm grip of the needle and prevent it from rotation or slipping, while suturing
* Most of the them have a central groove in the center of the blades, to minimize crushing effect on the needle and also prevent straightening out of the curved needle
* Needle should be held by the needle holder, at the junction of anterior 2/3rd and posterior 1/3rd of the needle (at its neck)
* Sterilization by autoclaving (Fig. 1).

Uses

* To hold the different types of needles while suturing and ligation
* Short and straight needle holders are used for superficial and skin suturing
* Long and curved needle holders are used for suturing in depth, i.e. inside the abdominal cavity or in the pelvis

Chapter 8: Needle Holders

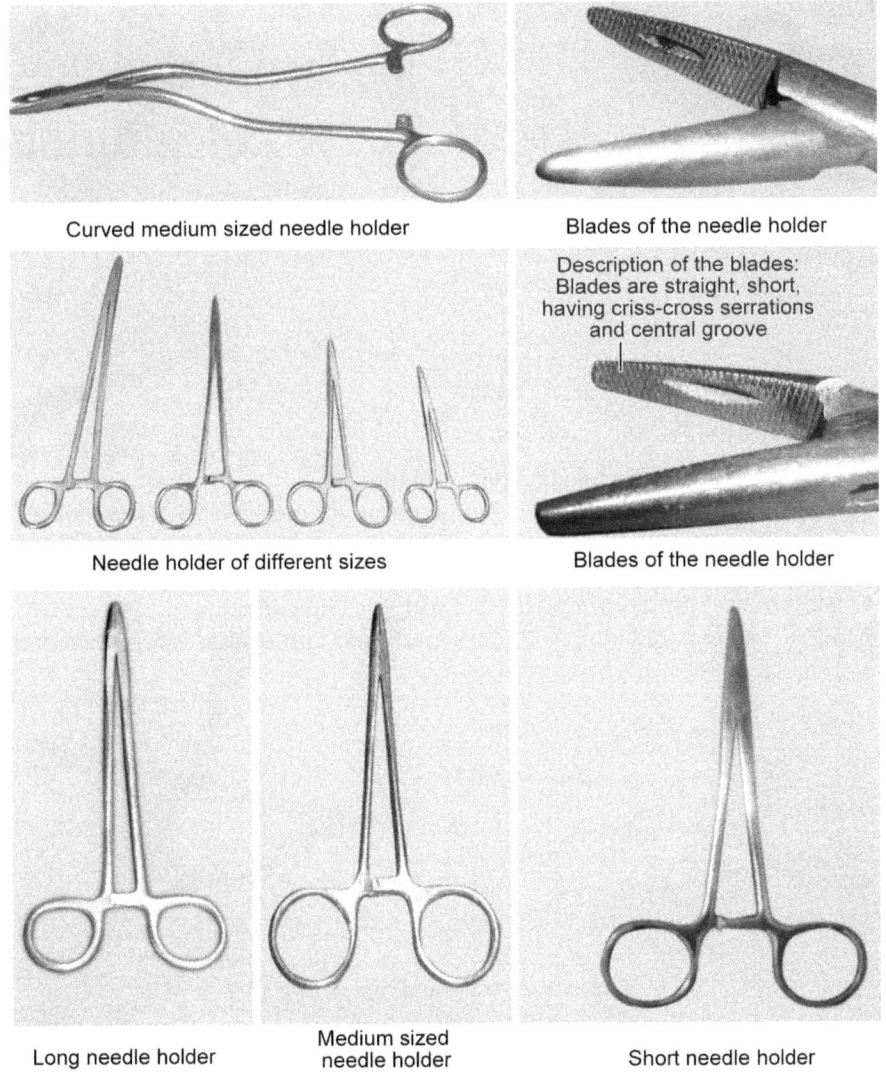

Fig. 1: Needle holders.

- Medium sized needle holder used in suturing peritoneum, linea alba, repairing posterior wall of the inguinal canal, etc.
- Short sized fine tipped needle holder used in pediatric surgeries.

CHAPTER 9

Modern Techniques of Suturing

SKIN STAPLER

- ❖ It works on the principle of a paper stapler
- ❖ The two cut edges of the incision are brought together with the toothed tissue forceps and the metal clip is applied at the closely approximated edges, by pressing the handles of the stapler
- ❖ Most of the staplers are preloaded with the clip cartridge
- ❖ Clips are removed after 7–10 days after their application by clip removal (Fig. 1).

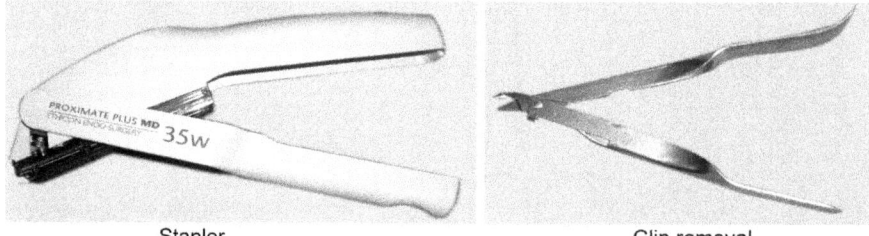

StaplerClip removal

Fig. 1: Skin stapler and clip removal.

SKIN GLUES FOR WOUND CLOSURE

- ❖ Skin glue is special medical glue used to close superficial clean wounds
- ❖ Skin glues are safe and effective new method to close selected wounds
- ❖ They are cost effective and also help to prevent infection
- ❖ Not all wounds are suitable to be closed by glue
- ❖ Ideal wounds for using glue for skin closure are wound less than 4 cm, not contaminated or infected and have skin edges that are not under tension
- ❖ Wounds should be closed within 12 hours
- ❖ Good for children with short clean wounds
- ❖ Glues are painless to apply and good better cosmetic results with less scar than stitches
- ❖ Skin glues are cyanoacrylates.

CHAPTER 10

Retractors

INTRODUCTION

Designed and used mainly to get adequate exposure of the operative area, adjacent organs and tissues by retracting the edges of the incision, adjacent tissue and organs without undue increase the length of the incision. If bleeding present, it will be better seen and controlled under direct vision. It also prevents unnecessary tissue handling and their inadvertent damage.

LANGENBECK'S RIGHT ANGLED RETRACTOR

- It has a handle to hold the instrument, long shaft to provide necessary length to the instrument and flat solid blade for retraction. It has different sizes
- It may be single or double bladed. Blade is curved at right angle to the shaft
- Tip of the blade is also curved at right angle to the rest of the blade for better retraction of the tissue without slippage of the tissue which has been retracted
- In double bladed retractor, there is another flat solid blade at the other end of shaft
- The handle is serrated or grooved for better grip of the retractor while retracting. It is fenestrated to reduce the weight of the retractor, so that the assistant holding the retractor will not get exhausted
- Sterilization by autoclaving (Fig. 1).

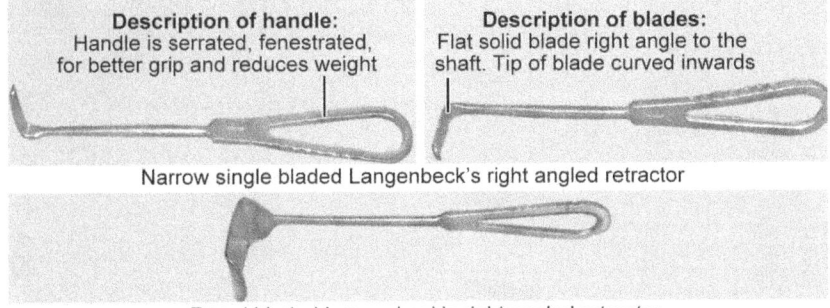

Fig. 1: Langenbeck's right angled retractors.

Uses

- To retract the edges of the incision during dissection
- For retracting the skin, subcutaneous tissue and fat, muscles for better visualization of the operative area in surgeries like excision of lipoma, cyst, lymph node biopsy, etc.
- During thyroid surgery, they are applied to the strap muscles from each side in the midline, to expose the thyroid gland
- During modified radical mastectomy, to retract the pectoralis major muscle for complete excision of all levels of the axillary lymph nodes
- During appendicectomy, to retract the internal oblique and transversus abdominis muscle to reach the peritoneum
- During inguinal hernia repair, to retract the different layers in the operative area, while repairing the posterior wall of the inguinal canal
- During suprapubic cystolithotomy, to retract the recti from the midline to reach the bladder wall.

CZERNY RETRACTOR

- It is somewhat same as double bladed Langenbeck's retractor, except one blade is having double hook
- At one end, there is flat, solid blade at right angle to the shaft like
- Langenbeck's retractor, while at the other end, there is a biflanged hook (double hook blade) facing in exactly opposite direction that of the other blade
- Shaft is fenestrated, to reduce the weight of the instrument to make it light weight
- Sterilization by autoclaving (Fig. 2).

Uses

Uses of the Biflanged Blade:

- To retract the ends of the incision, while approximating (suturing) the incision layer by layer in midline laparotomy. The tissue to be sutured will

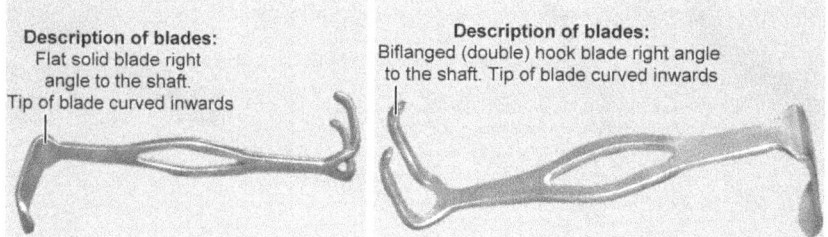

Fig. 2: Czerny retractors.

be seen in between the biflanged blade, and so the ends of the cut edges can be sutured under direct vision.

Uses of the Flat Blade

Same as Langenbeck's retractor.

MORRIS RETRACTOR

- ❖ Designed like L. It is a large and strong retractor, having various sizes
- ❖ Designed same as Langenbeck's retractor, but the blade is wider and slightly concave than the Langenbeck's retractor providing more space for work
- ❖ The tip of the blade (lip) is more curved inward for retracting the tissue firmly and prevents it from slipping, while retracting the tissue
- ❖ The handle is serrated or grooved for better grip of the retractor while retracting. It is fenestrated to reduce the weight of the retractor, so that the assistant holding the retractor will not get exhausted early
- ❖ Sterilization by autoclaving (Fig. 3).

Uses

Mainly Used as

- ❖ During laparotomy, to retract the cut edges of the strong anterior abdominal wall for better visualization of the operative area, exposing the peritoneal cavity and intra-abdominal viscera
- ❖ To retract the intra-abdominal viscus like the coils of the intestine, kidney, etc.

Additional Uses

- ❖ For tissue retraction in different operations
- ❖ While making and closing different abdominal incisions.

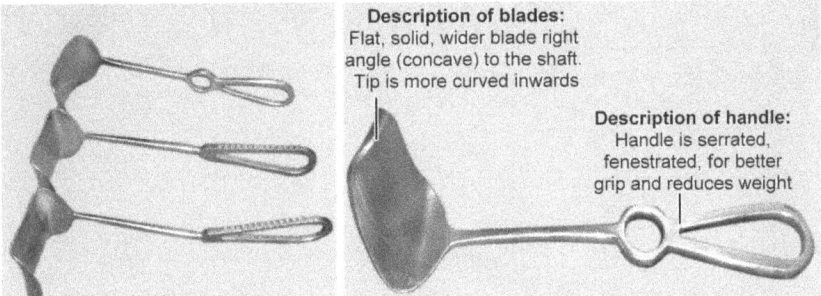

Fig. 3: Morris retractors.

DEAVER'S CURVED ABDOMINAL RETRACTOR

- It is a large curved retractor shaped like 'S' with flat curved blade at one end in the concavity of which the structure to be retracted gets accommodated
- It has long handle ending like a hook for firm grip
- Available in various different sizes depending upon the width of the blades
- Organs to be retracted must be protected by a sponge to prevent iatrogenic injury to the retracted organ by the edges and tip of the blade
- Sterilization by autoclaving (Fig. 4).

Mainly Used as

- Commonly used retractor in all abdominal surgeries
- For retraction of the solid intra-abdominal organs like liver, spleen, kidney, etc.
- For retraction of solid organs like liver during cholecystectomy, truncal vagotomy, gastrectomy, etc.

Additional Uses

- To retract the stomach during Whipple's procedure
- To retract the small intestine during resection anastomosis, right or left hemicolectomy, abdominoperineal resection, etc.
- To retract the urinary bladder in male and uterus in female in abdominoperineal resection
- To retract the cut edges of the anterior abdominal wall during laparotomy.

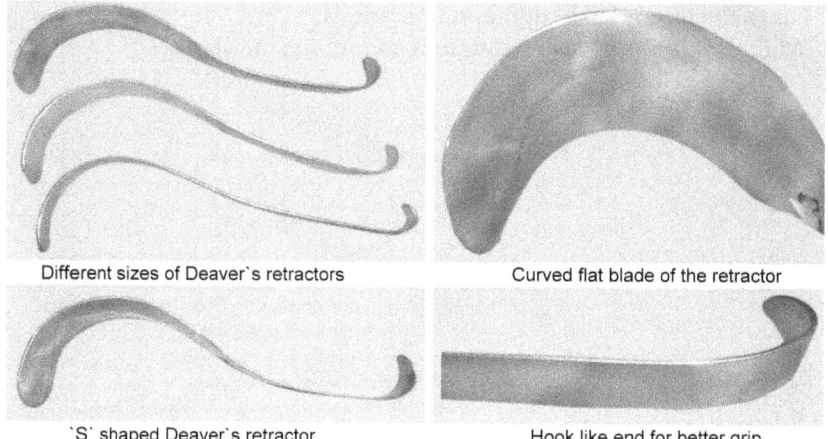

Fig. 4: Deaver's retractors.

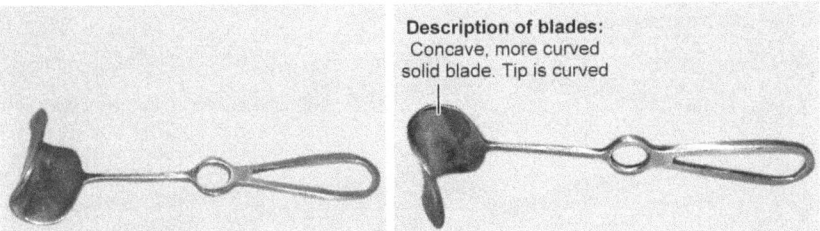

Fig. 5: Doyen's retractors.

DOYEN'S RETRACTOR

- ❖ Similar to the Deaver's retractor, with slight modification in its blade and blade is made like that of Morris retractor, but is more curved inwards
- ❖ Sterilization by autoclaving (Fig. 5).

Uses

In pelvic surgery like abdominoperineal or anterior resection to retract the bladder, uterus, etc.

MALLEABLE RETRACTOR

It is made of malleable metal, which can be bend to take various different shapes (Fig. 6).

Uses

To retract any intra-abdominal viscus during laparotomy, as it can be bent to take various shapes as per requirement of the surgeon to retract the organs.

ALLISON LUNG RETRACTOR

- ❖ It has special blade made up of wires in the form of a net which prevents damage to the retracted lung

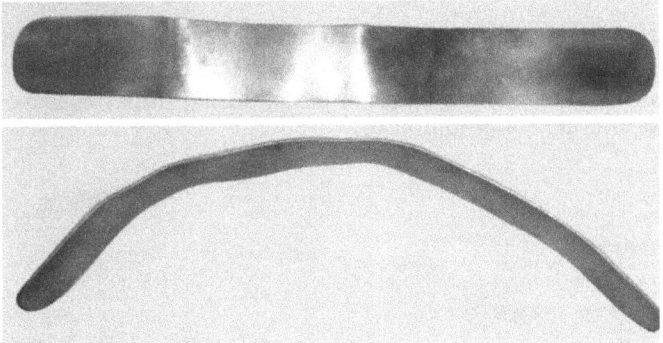

Fig. 6: Malleable retractor.

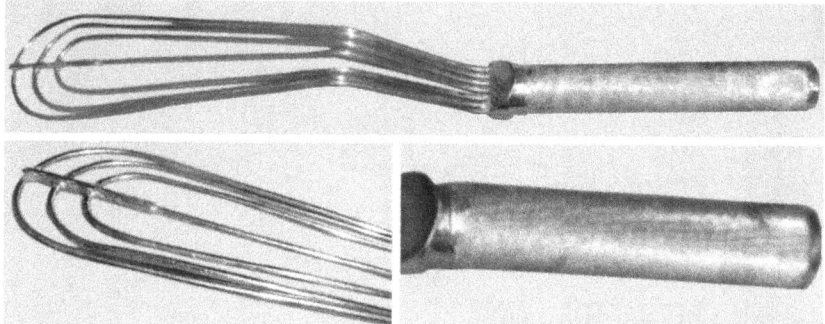

Blade made up of metal wires in a form of net — Long, curved cylindrical handle

Fig. 7: Allison lung retractor.

- It has long curved cylindrical handle, for firm gripping of the retractor without slipping it
- Blade is attached to the handle at an angle, not to obstruct the vision of surgeon
- Sterilization by autoclaving (Fig. 7).

Uses

To retract the lung, during lung surgeries and also in esophageal resection for carcinoma esophagus.

VOLKMANN'S CAT'S PAW RETRACTOR

- It has a handle, and two ends
- One blade is in the form of multiple hooks with pointed sharp edges, while the other end may have serrated handle or may be like
- Langenbeck's right angled retractor
- Pointed hook like edges are helpful for firm retraction
- Sterilization by autoclaving (Fig. 8).

Uses

- To retract the tough structures like fascia of palm, sole and scalp during surgery
- For retraction of the skin edges or fascia during surgeries like excision of the cyst, lipoma, lymph node, etc.

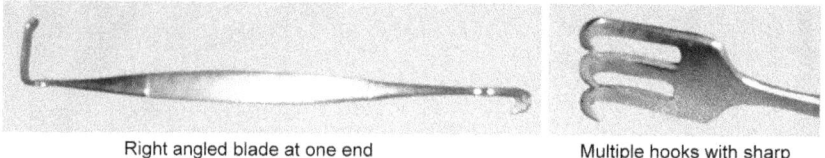

Right angled blade at one end — Multiple hooks with sharp edges like cat's paw

Fig. 8: Volkmann's cat's paw retractor.

Chapter 10: Retractors **47**

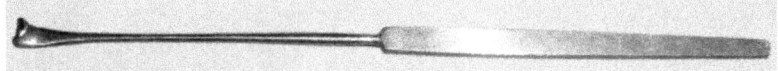

Fig. 9: Curved blade skin retractor.

SKIN RETRACTOR

- It has handle, shaft and blade
- Blade is curved inwards for firm retraction without slipping of the tissue retracted
- Sterilization by autoclaving (Fig. 9).

Uses

To retract the skin, subcutaneous tissue while operating on the skin surface like excision of the sebaceous cyst, lipoma, lymph node, etc.

SINGLE HOOK RETRACTOR

- It is a delicate instrument having long blade and handle
- The tip of the blade is like a hook, which may be sharp or blunt
- Sterilization by autoclaving (Fig. 10).

Uses

- For operations at the skin surface, to retract the skin flaps or edges during operations in the subcutaneous plane like excision of lipoma, cyst, venesection, etc.
- To retract the isthmus of the thyroid gland and strap muscles of the neck during tracheostomy
- To retract or lift the nerve, to avoid injury to it while dissecting the adjacent structures
- To retract edges of the skin flaps while raising skin flaps during radical mastectomy.

KIDNEY HILUM RETRACTOR

- It is having handle and blade
- Handle is cylindrical with serrations for better grip

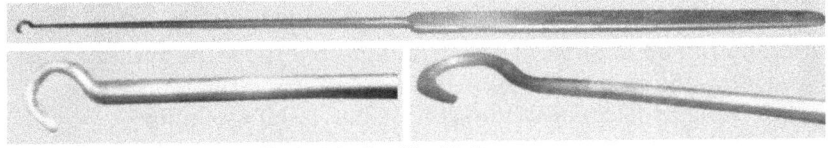

Hook at the tip of the blade

Fig. 10: Single hook retractor.

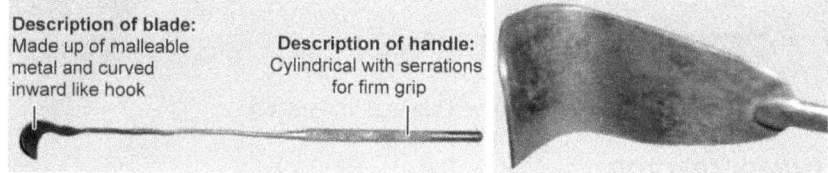

Description of blade: Made up of malleable metal and curved inward like hook

Description of handle: Cylindrical with serrations for firm grip

Fig. 11: Kidney hilum retractor.

- Blade is long, having flat, curved hook like tip
- The blade is made up of malleable metal, to mould it to increase or decrease the angle of curved tip, according to the shape of the hilum of the kidney to be retracted (Fig. 11).

Uses

To retract the hilum of the kidney during pyelolithotomy, while removing difficult impacted staghorn calculus from the calyces.

SELF-RETAINING RETRACTORS

These retractors usually have two blades for retraction (some may have three) and a locking arrangement, to make the retractor self-retaining. Assistant's hands remain free, so it can be applied for long time, without relaxation at crucial movements and also when the assistant get exhausted.

SELF-RETAINING RETRACTOR (BALFOUR'S TYPE) WITH PROVISION OF THIRD BLADE FOR ATTACHMENT

- There is horizontal bar or frame on which one of the two blades of the retractors slides, while the other blade is fixed to one end of the bar
- Sliding retractor blade can be fixed to the horizontal bar by means of a screw, by tightening the screw after desired retraction of the tissue is achieved
- Another screw in between the blades, keeps the third blade in position
- Advantage of this retractor is that, when it is used assistant's hands remain free
- Sterilization by autoclaving (Fig. 12).

How to Use

- While applying the retractor, the two blades are kept close to each other in the midline, and then the screw is tightened to retract the cut edges of the anterior abdominal wall from midline, to expose the peritoneal cavity and intra-abdominal viscera
- Tightening and fixation of the screw makes it self-retaining
- Third blade is used to retract the costal margin or mostly used towards the pelvis, during pelvic operations like abdominoperineal or anterior resection, to retract the bladder and uterus.

Chapter 10: Retractors **49**

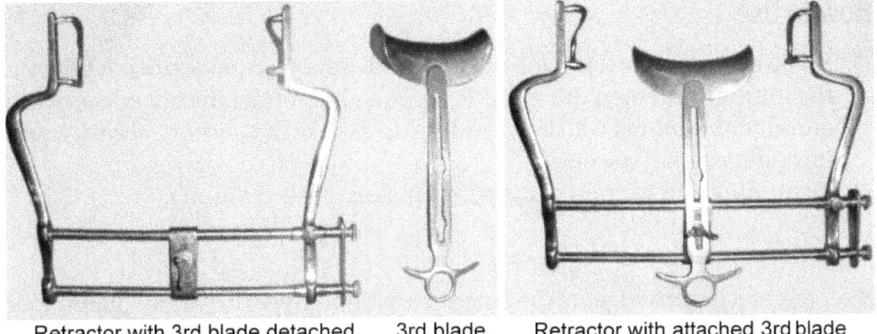

Retractor with 3rd blade detached   3rd blade   Retractor with attached 3rd blade

Fig. 12: Balfour's self-retaining retractor.

Uses

- To retract the cut edges of the anterior abdominal wall in major abdominal surgeries like gastrectomy, liver resections, etc. to keep the assistants hand free from holding the retractors
- Third blade used in the pelvic operations like abdominoperineal or anterior resection for carcinoma rectum, to retract the bladder and uterus.

■ SELF-RETAINING RETRACTOR WITH TWO BLADES
(No Provision for 3rd Blade Attachment)

- There is horizontal bar, on which one of the two blades of the retractors slide, while one of the blade is fixed to one side of the bar
- Sliding retractor blade can be fixed to the horizontal bar by means of screw, by tightening the screw, after desired retraction of the tissue is achieved
- Advantage of this retractor is that, when it is used assistants hands remain free
- Sterilization by autoclaving (Fig. 13).

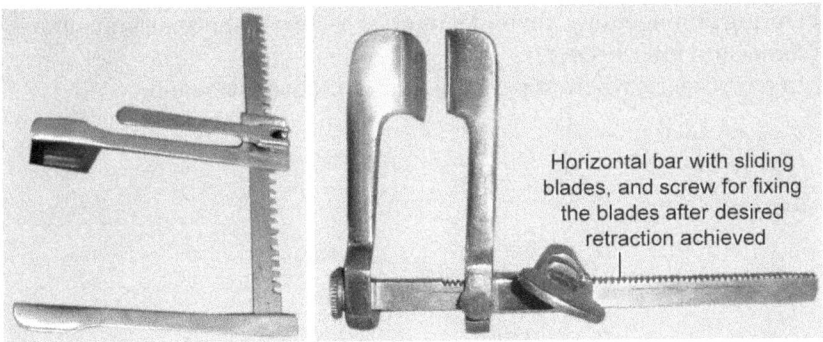

Horizontal bar with sliding blades, and screw for fixing the blades after desired retraction achieved

Fig. 13: Self-retaining retractor.

How to Use

- While applying the retractor, the two blades are kept close to each other in the midline and then the screw is tightened to retract the cut edges of the anterior abdominal wall from midline to expose the peritoneal cavity and intra-abdominal viscera
- Tightening and fixation of the screw makes it self-retaining.

Uses

- To retract the cut edges of the anterior abdominal wall in various abdominal operations like gastrectomy, liver resections, etc. to keep assistants hand free from holding the retractors
- To retract the ribs forcibly during thoracotomy for operations for lung hydatid, pneumonectomies, etc.

■ MOLLISON'S SELF-RETAINING MASTOID RETRACTOR

- It has pair of blades and shafts, rachet lock mechanism in the shaft for locking the blades and finger bows
- Blades has many hooks (4 or 5) with curved tips, which gives firm retraction of the tough tissue like skin, muscles, fascia, etc.
- Two flanges can be adjusted by means of screw mechanism
- Self-retaining when the rachet is closed
- Sterilization by autoclaving (Fig. 14).

Uses

Mainly Used in

Mastoid surgery to retract the scalp.

Additional Uses

- To retract the scalp during craniotomy. Retraction of the scalp allows retraction and compression of the blood vessels at the cut edges achieving hemostasis
- During laminectomy, thyroid surgeries to retract the skin, subcutaneous tissue and muscles, etc.
- In any surgery, where superficial skin retraction is needed.

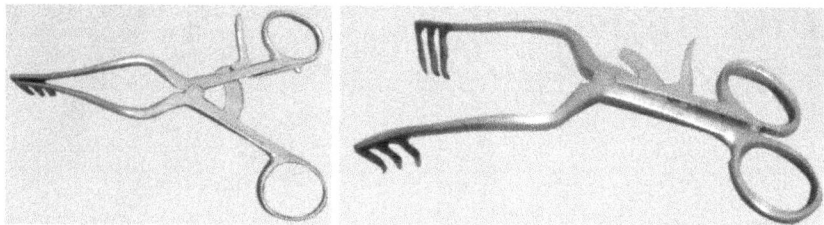

Fig. 14: Mollison's self-retaining retractor.

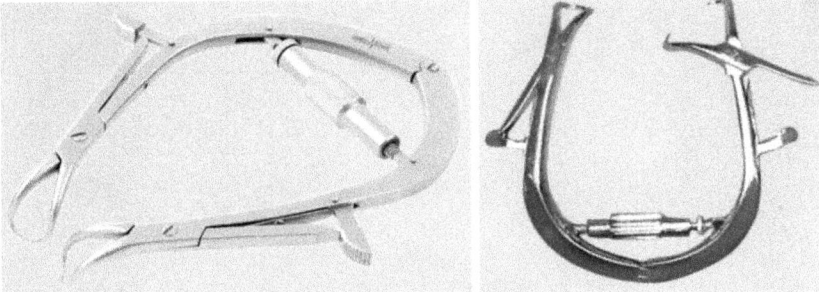

Fig. 15: Joll's thyroid retractor.

JOLL'S THYROID RETRACTOR

- There are 2 towel clips like forceps at the either end of the retractor for retraction
- Two flanges can be adjusted by means of screw mechanism
- Self-retaining
- Sterilization by autoclaving (Fig. 15).

Uses

To hold and retract the upper and lower skin flaps during thyroid surgeries.

RETRACTORS OF THE ORAL CAVITY (MOUTH GAGS)

DOYEN'S MOUTH GAG

- The blades are semicircular in shape and curved or bent in their terminal parts at their tips
- It becomes self-retaining, when the rachet (catch) is closed
- It has pair of semicircular blades, shafts (handles), rachet lock mechanism in the shaft for locking the blades and finger bows
- When the finger bows are kept apart the tips of the blades are closed, and when the finger bows are approximated the blades are separated and the instrument is opened up
- Tips of the blades rest on the teeth
- Sterilization by autoclaving (Fig. 16).

Uses

- To keep the mouth open, during intraoral operations like glossectomy, cleft palate operation, excising of intraoral ranula, biopsy of an intraoral suspicious lesion, etc.
- Also used during nasopharyngeal surgeries, to keep the mouth open for surgeries.

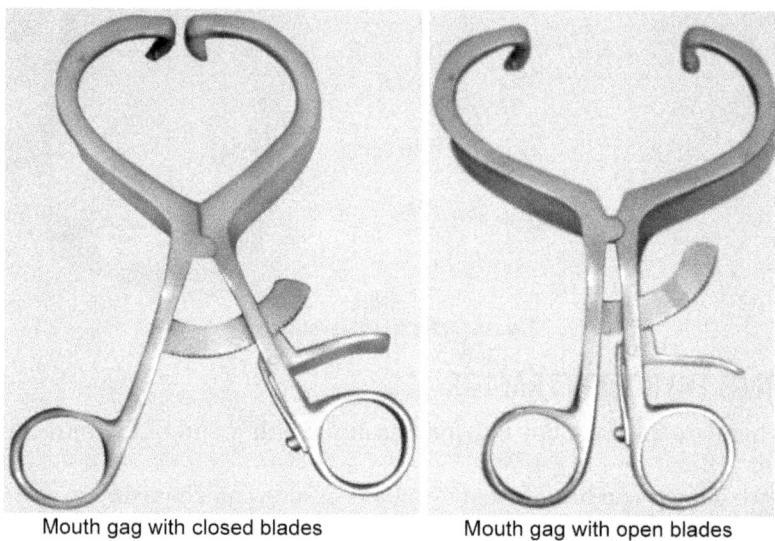

Mouth gag with closed blades Mouth gag with open blades

Fig. 16: Doyen's mouth gag.

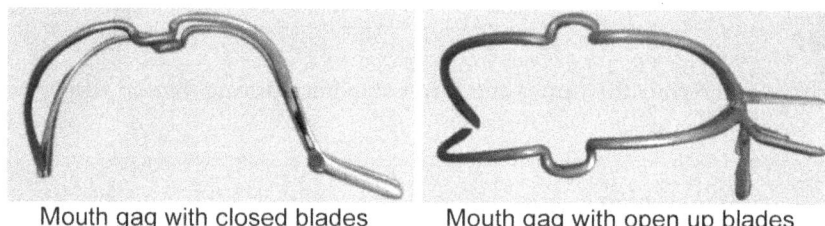

Mouth gag with closed blades Mouth gag with open up blades

Fig. 17: Jennings mouth gag.

JENNINGS MOUTH GAG

- It is self retaining, when the rachet is closed
- It is having pair of blades and handles, rachet lock mechanism in the shaft for opening the blades
- The tip of the blades are attached at the tips, and the remaining portion of the blades come close and goes apart as per the approximation of the handles. When the handles are approximated the blades are separated
- Sterilization by autoclaving (Fig. 17).

Uses

- To keep the mouth open, during intraoral operations like glossectomy, cleft palate operation, excising intraoral ranula, biopsy of an intraoral suspicious lesion, etc.
- Also used during nasopharyngeal surgeries to keep the mouth open, for surgeries.

One more other type of mouth gag is Davis mouth gag.

CHAPTER 11

Clamps

GASTROINTESTINAL CLAMPS

■ DOYEN'S GASTROINTESTINAL OCCLUSION (NON-CRUSHING) CLAMP

- ❖ It has finger bows, catch, and pair of shaft with pair of long blades
- ❖ Its blades are flat, light weight, thin and springy, which may be straight or curved
- ❖ Blades have vertical serrations in whole of their length and they are superficial in depth, to hold the intestine without slipping. As they are superficial, they are occluding, but crushing effect is minimal. Tips are blunt and rounded
- ❖ Blades may be long or short with slight concavity, which meet at the tips, with slight gap between the blades even though all the catches (slots) are closed, which allows slight bulging of the intestine and occlude the intestine nicely without crushing it
- ❖ Its shafts are relatively short, as compared to the blades
- ❖ Sterilization by autoclaving (Fig. 1).

Uses

- ❖ To clamp the intestine, to prevent spillage of intestinal contents and contamination of the peritoneal cavity, during intestinal resection and anastomosis
- ❖ Its hold and steadies the cut ends of the viscera during anastomosis
- ❖ It prevents bleeding from the cut ends of the resected intestine, making the anastomosis easier.

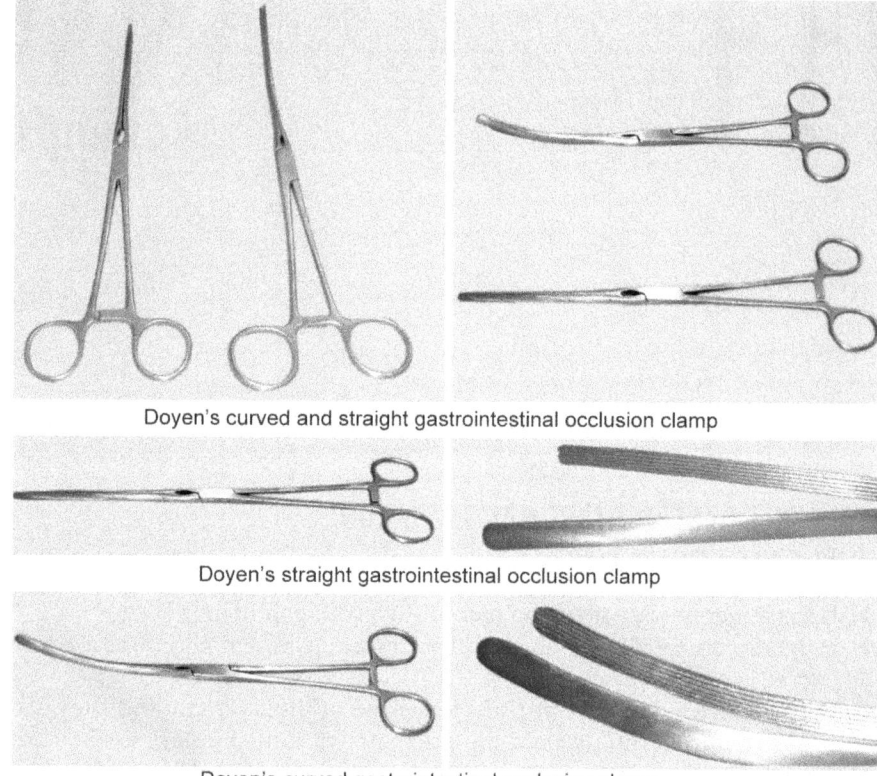

Doyen's curved and straight gastrointestinal occlusion clamp

Doyen's straight gastrointestinal occlusion clamp

Doyen's curved gastrointestinal occlusion clamp

Fig. 1: Doyen's gastrointestinal occlusion clamp.

MOYNIHAN'S GASTRIC OCCLUSION (NON-CRUSHING) CLAMP

- Same as intestinal clamp but having transverse or oblique serrations in its blades
- Its blades are long and may be straight or curved, and having a linear fenestration in the center of each blade, along whole of its length
- Fenestration make the instrument lighter, increases elasticity, and allows the part of intestine to bulge, thus minimizing the crushing effect on the occluded stomach
- Sterilization by autoclaving (Fig. 2).

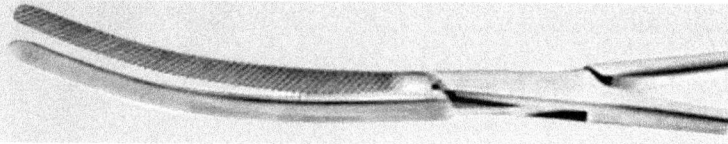

Fig. 2: Moynihan's gastrointestinal occlusion clamp.

Uses

To clamp the stomach during gastric resections like partial gastrectomy, to prevent spillage of gastric contents into the peritoneal cavity. It also prevents bleeding from the cut ends of the resected stomach and makes the anastomosis easier.

■ KOCHER'S GASTRIC OCCLUSION CLAMP

Same as Doyen's gastrointestinal clamp.

■ PAYR'S CRUSHING CLAMP

- ❖ It is a heavy instrument
- ❖ Handle is stout and there is double lever arrangement, so with minimum force maximum crushing effect is obtained. First lever opposes the blade firmly, and the second lever near the handle multiplies the exerted pressure and crushes the viscus
- ❖ Mucosa crushed and curls up after applying it, so these clamps are applied to the part of the diseased stomach, which has to be resected and removed from the body. The portion of the stomach which has to be saved and has to be kept in the body should be clamped by gastric occlusion clamp, which occludes the stomach without crushing it
- ❖ Its blades may be long (in gastric clamp) or short (in duodenal and small intestinal clamp)
- ❖ Its blades are heavy and have vertical serrations (serrations parallel to the length of the blades), on whole of its length and are deep for crushing the tissue held in it
- ❖ Its one tip is having a blunt tooth, while the other having a groove, which interlocks, to lock the blades fully, when the levers are closed
- ❖ Sterilization by autoclaving (Fig. 3).

Uses of Payr's Gastric Crushing Clamp

Applied during gastric resections (partial gastrectomies) done for gastric carcinoma, carcinoma of lower third of the esophagus, chronic gastric ulcer, large perforated peptic ulcer, gastric injuries, etc.

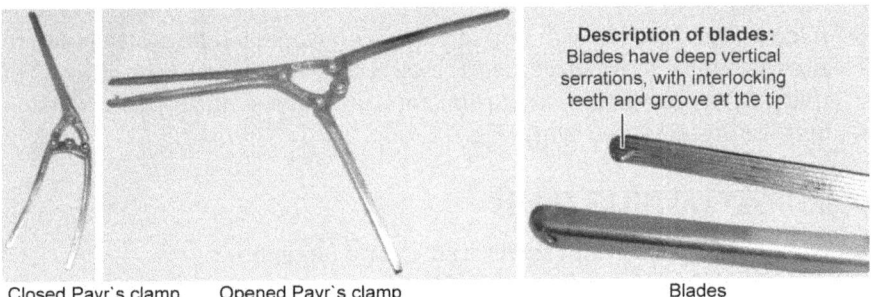

Closed Payr's clamp   Opened Payr's clamp   Blades

Fig. 3: Payr's gastric crushing clamp.

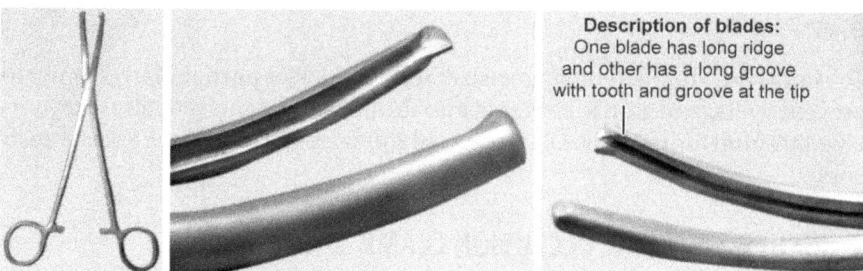

Fig. 4: Intestinal crushing clamp.

INTESTINAL CRUSHING CLAMPS

- It has finger bows, catch with pair of shafts and blades
- It is a stout and heavy instrument
- The blades mostly have oblique or transverse serrations, while some may have long ridge on whole of the length of inner aspect of one of the blade which fits into the groove of other blade along with single teeth and socket at the tips, like Kocher's forceps, when the catch is closed
- The blades gets approximated even before the catch is locked, and after locking the catch, no gap remains between the blades like gastrointestinal occlusion clamps
- It crushes and damages the tissue clamped in between its blades, and also occludes its blood supply
- Sterilization by autoclaving (Fig. 4).

Uses

Applied as a crushing clamp in intestinal resection to the portion of the intestine, which has to be resected.

VASCULAR CLAMPS

BULLDOG VASCULAR CLAMP

- It is a clamp, having spring like action. Its blades get opened, after pressing the shaft
- It has vertical groove with fine serrations on whole length of its blades, to prevent injury to the occluded vessel, which may lead to thrombosis of that part of the vessel, if its portion gets traumatized during the occlusion
- Sterilization by autoclaving (Fig. 5).

SATINSKY VASCULAR CLAMP

- It has pair of blades and shafts, a catch and finger bows
- The blades has vertical groove with fine serrations, to avoid injury to the occluded vessel

Chapter 11: Clamps

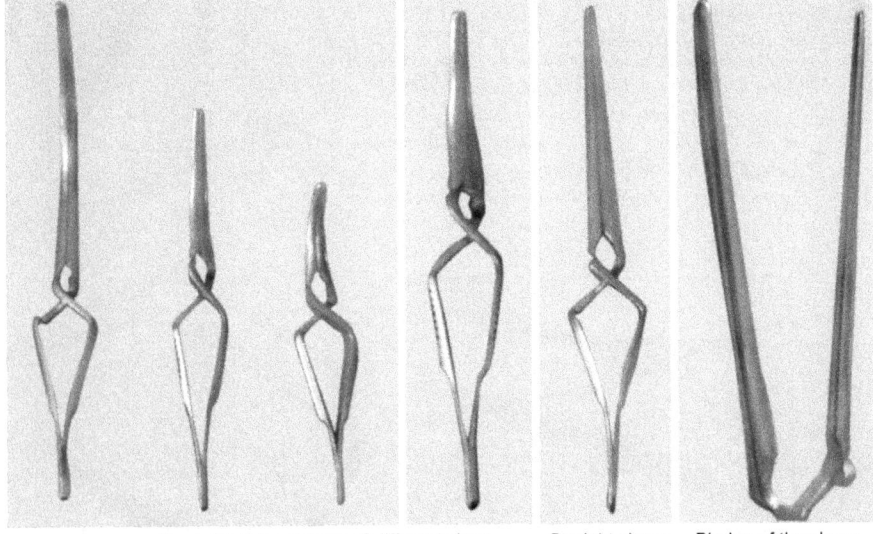

Curved bulldog clamps of different sizes   Straight clamp   Blades of the clamp

Fig. 5: Bulldog vascular clamp.

❖ It is a special type of long vascular clamp, which is curved and having different degrees of angulations at its blades and shaft also, to clamp the vessels in depth and also not to obstruct the vision of the operating surgeon, while applying it
❖ Sterilization by autoclaving (Fig. 6).

Uses

❖ To occlude the large vessels like inferior vena cava, superior vena cava, aorta and its major branches, and other large diameter vessels, while repairing part of that vessel proximally or distally, during repair of their iatrogenic or accidental injury, for bloodless field
❖ During repair of aneurysms, proximal segment of that artery has to be occluded to stop the blood flow in the aneurysm
❖ To arrest the bleeding temporarily during hepatic resections and also during heavy bleeding from liver lacerations or the portal vein, hepatic artery can be occluded in the porta hepatis
❖ Renal or splenic pedicles can also be occluded temporarily, during operating on these organs, and also to arrest the bleeding from their iatrogenic or accidental lacerations due to blunt trauma abdomen.

▪ MAYO'S PEDICLE CLAMP

❖ It is a stout and large forceps (clamp)
❖ Its blades are long and angulated, to provide good view of the operative area even at the depth, without obstructing the operating surgeon's vision.

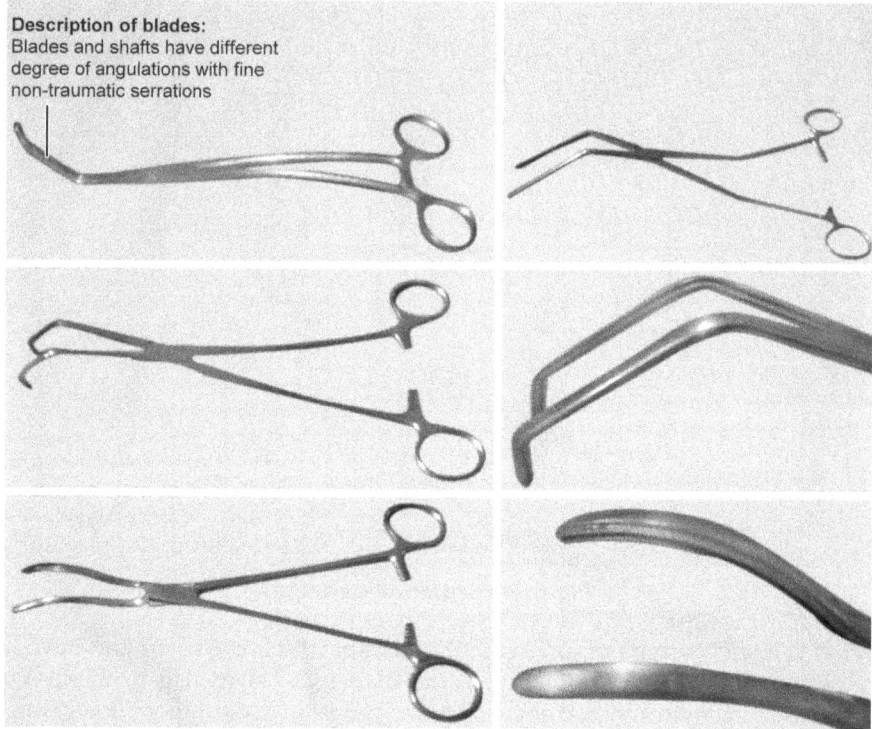

Fig. 6: Satinsky vascular clamps having different angulations.

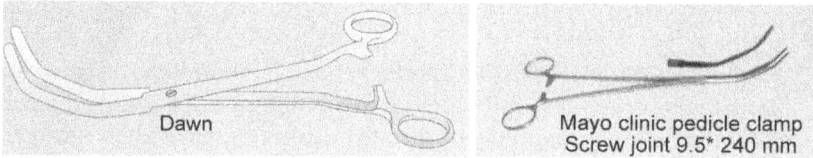

Fig. 7: Mayo's pedicle clamp.

It allows clamping of the pedicle of the organ under direct vision, while avoiding accidental clamping of the adjacent vital structures
- It has vertical serrations on the both the blades
- Sterilization by autoclaving (Fig. 7).

Uses

- During nephrectomy, to clamp the renal pedicle before cutting it, to prevent bleeding from the vessels in the pedicle. Pedicle should be doubly ligated with ligatures before removing the clamp
- During splenectomy, to clamp the splenic pedicle.

CHAPTER 12

Miscellaneous Instruments in General Surgery

KELLY'S RECTAL SPECULUM (PROCTOSCOPE) OR ANAL SPECULUM

- As this instrument mainly visualizes the anal canal and only lower 1/3rd of the rectum, the term 'proctoscope' is misnomer, and students should better use the term 'anal speculum' or anoscope'
- It is '3 or 4' inches long instrument
- Its diameter varies from one end to another, as the sheath is conical in shape, with smaller diameter at the end which has to introduced in the anal canal, and larger at the outer end, which is outside the anal canal at the anal verge
- It has two parts. The hollow outer sheath with a handle, attached somewhat perpendicular to the sheath. The terminal end (inner) of the sheath is either circular or obliquely cut
- The inner rod is called 'obturator'. Its terminal part is smooth and rounded and fits well within the outer sheath and projects out from the sheath, when it is inserted inside the sheath while introducing it in the anal canal, for easy insertion of it in the anal canal without injuring the anal mucosa
- Most of the anoscopes are blind and artificial light source is required during examination. There may be attachment for light in some of the anoscopes, to make them self illuminating
- Sterilization by autoclaving (Fig. 1).

How to do the Proctoscopy or Anoscopy?

Refer Section 9, Chapter 36.

Uses

- For various diagnostic and therapeutic purposes, affecting the anal canal and lower rectum

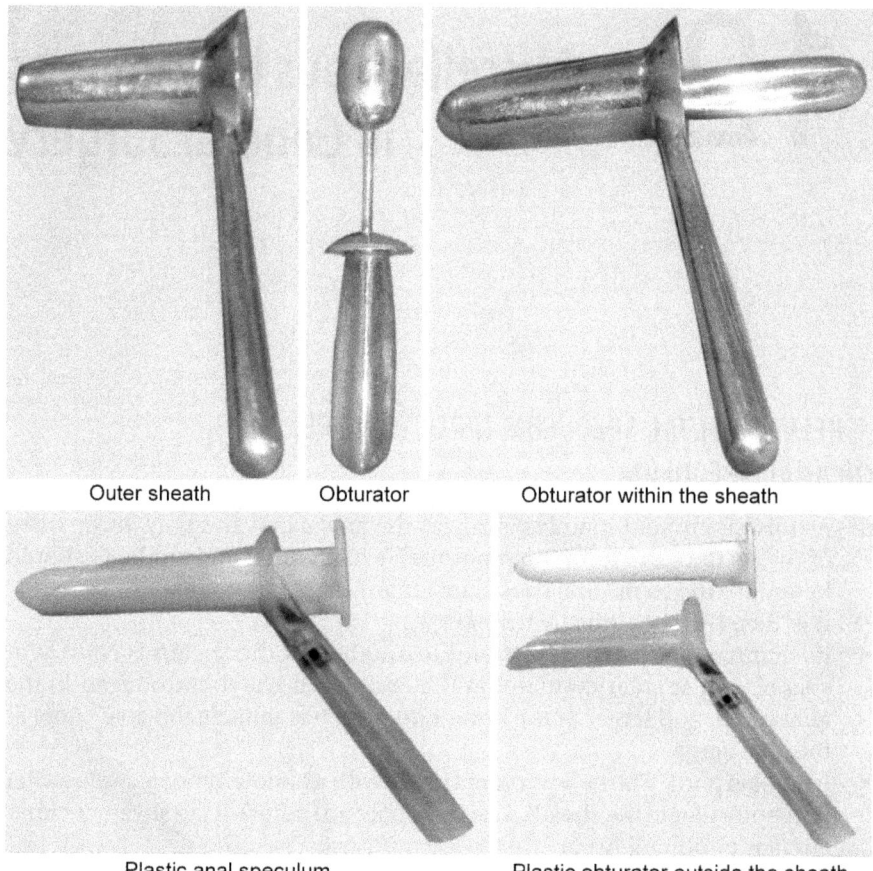

Outer sheath Obturator Obturator within the sheath

Plastic anal speculum Plastic obturator outside the sheath

Fig. 1: Kelly's anal speculum.

- For diagnosis of piles (hemorrhoids), rectal polyps, rectal ulcer, carcinoma of the anal canal or lower rectum, for locating internal opening of the perianal fistula, etc.
- For therapeutic uses like injection of sclerosant in the piles, during excision of polyp, anal dilatation, drainage of pelvic and prostatic abscesses in males, etc.
- For taking biopsy from anal or rectal growth, to rule out malignancy.

BRODIE'S OLIVE POINTED FISTULA DIRECTOR WITH FRENULUM SLIT

- It is a metallic probe with an olive at the tip (narrow, blunt pointed tip)
- There is a groove or tunnel on whole of its length from the tip to the base, along which knife (surgical blade) can be directed, preventing injury to

Chapter 12: Miscellaneous Instruments in General Surgery

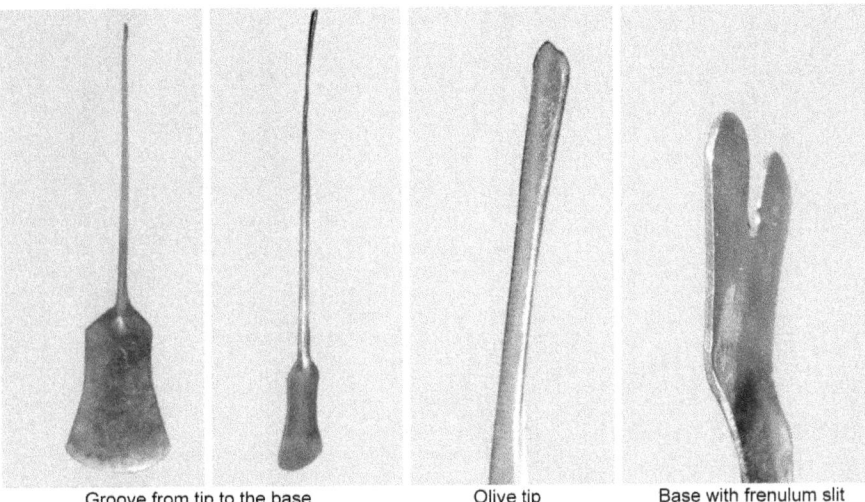

| Groove from tip to the base | Olive tip | Base with frenulum slit |

Fig. 2: Brodie's olive pointed fistula director.

the adjacent structures. It also facilitates control of length and direction of the incision
* The other end (base) is broad, flat, wing shaped and expands into a frenulum slit
* Sterilization by autoclaving (Fig. 2).

Uses

Mainly Used

During fistulotomy, it is passed through the fistulous tract from the external to the internal fistulous opening and the fistulous tract is incised (laid open) over the groove in the probe, to avoid injury to the adjacent important structures like anal sphincters.

May be Used

* As a probe or director to assess the depth, length, direction and number of communications in a fistulous or sinus tract
* During urethroplasty, for stricture urethra, stricturous segment of the urethra is slit open over this probe
* During tongue tie release operation, the frenulum is released (cut) over the wing shaped part
* To lay open the tract of the sinus.

MALLEABLE OLIVE POINTED PROBE

* It is a metallic probe, with an olive at the tip and there is an eye at the other end

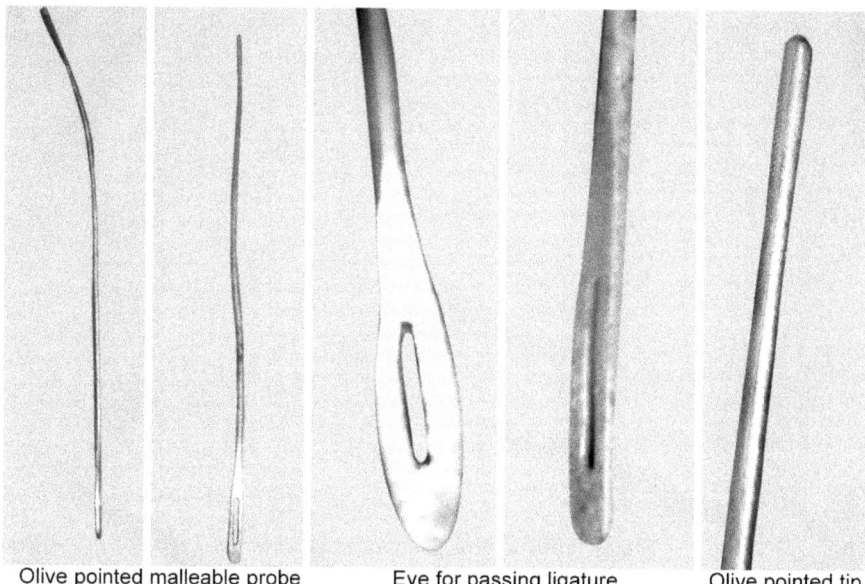

Olive pointed malleable probe   Eye for passing ligature   Olive pointed tip

Fig. 3: Malleable olive pointed probe.

- The probe is malleable, so it can be bent to take different shapes
- The olive point minimizes trauma to the adjacent tissue in the tract and reduces chances of false passage, while it passes through the tract from the external to the internal opening
- The eye is meant for passing a ligature which may be passed around a high fistulous tract
- Sterilization by autoclaving (Fig. 3).

Uses

Mainly Used

During fistulectomy, the probe is passed from the external opening to emerge from the internal opening. It is then bent and an incision around the probe helps in complete excision of the fistulous tract around the probe (fistulectomy).

May be Used

- To pass a ligature through a high fistula in ano, for Seton treatment
- During fistulotomy or while opening the sinus tract, the probe is introduced into the fistula or the sinus tract and the fistula or sinus is laid open over this probe
- To assess the length, depth and direction of a sinus or fistulous tract
- Acts as a guide during excision of a sinus tract

- ❖ To assess the depth and direction of a penetrating wound, in case of penetrating injury of the abdomen, and to assess whether the injuring object has penetrated the peritoneum or not, as if it has penetrated the peritoneum, it is an indication for emergency laparotomy.

TROCAR AND CANNULA

- ❖ A cannula is a hollow tube, open at the both ends for aspirating fluid from body cavities or from an organ
- ❖ A trocar is a sharp pointed stylet which fits closely into the cannula, with a sharp pointing tip projecting beyond the cannula, when the trocar completely fits or is inserted in the cannula, which permits thrusting of the cannula into the cavity
- ❖ Trocar has to be withdrawn by its handle, as soon as it enters in the desired space or cavity and the cannula has to be left in situ, for drainage.
- ❖ Before removing the cannula, trocar should be reinserted and then both are removed, to empty the cannula and also to prevent entry of any adjacent tissue in the cannula
- ❖ Sterilization by autoclaving.

Uses

- ❖ In repair of hydrocele, to drain the hydrocele fluid
- ❖ For suprapubic drainage of bladder (suprapubic cystostomy)
- ❖ To drain pleural effusion, empyema and hemothorax
- ❖ To drain ascities. Rarely used for this purpose due to fear of perforation of the bowel
- ❖ To puncture anterior abdominal wall to insert the camera and laparoscopic instruments during laparascopic procedures
- ❖ To puncture the ovarian cyst, to reduce its size before its removal
- ❖ To empty the gallbladder, before its removal if distended.

SUPRAPUBIC TROCAR AND CANNULA

- ❖ Its external diameter is 10–12 mm
- ❖ It has to be inserted through the small suprapubic incision over the anterior abdominal wall in midline, which passes through the bladder wall in a distended bladder
- ❖ Bladder should be fully distended before insertion of the trocar and cannula, to prevent injury to the intra-abdominal viscera, mostly intestine
- ❖ As it is a blind method of insertion, bleeding due to injury to large vessels and injury to the intra-abdominal viscera, mostly intestine are its common complications
- ❖ Sterilization by autoclaving (Fig. 4).

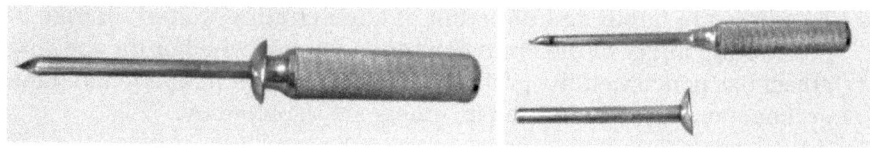

Trocar and cannula   Trocar (up) outside the cannula (below)

Fig. 4: Suprapubic trocar and cannula.

Uses

To drain the bladder suprapubically, in case of acute retention of urine due to stricture urethra or benign hypertrophy of the prostate and also where the perurethral catheter drainage is contraindicated, as in case of rupture urethra.

HYDROCELE, TROCAR AND CANNULA

- It is of small size as compared to the suprapubic trocar and cannula
- Sterilization by autoclaving (Fig. 5).

Uses

In repair of hydrocele, after separation of the overlying layers of the sac, sac filled with the fluid is delivered out of the wound and it is emptied by inserting the trocar and cannula, before opening the sac for eversion or plication.

YANKAUER SUCTION CANNULA

- It has a handle, body and tip
- Tip is blunt, smooth and rounded, and has 2 side holes, along with a main hole at the tip
- Its body is angulated or curved at 2 points, not to obstruct the vision of the operating surgeon while using it and also allows to suck the fluid

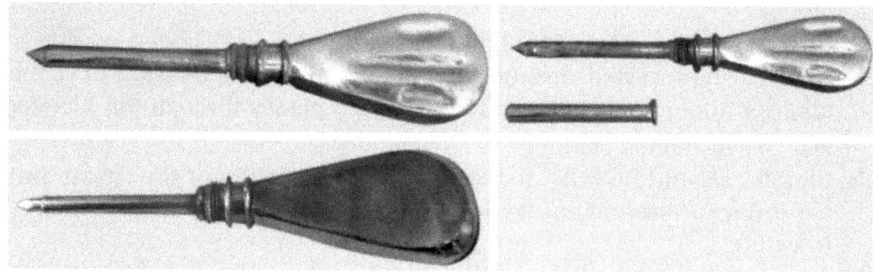

Trocar and cannula   Trocar (up) outside the cannula (below)

Fig. 5: Hydrocele, trocar and cannula

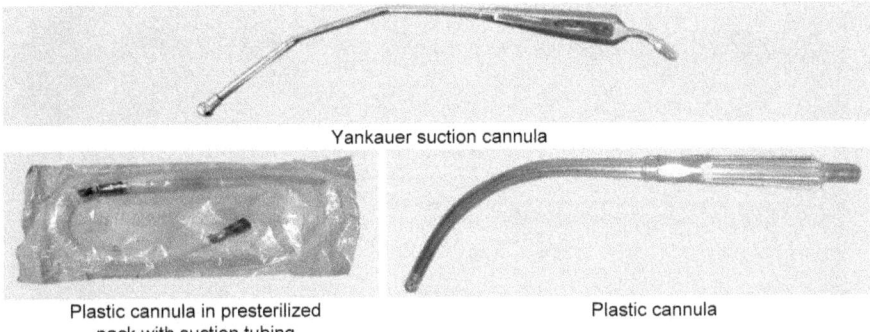

Fig. 6: Suction cannulas.

from deep cavities which are not visible or accessible directly, while operating
- Made up of stainless steel and sterilized by autoclaving
- Plastic suction cannula are also available, and same as the Yankauer suction cannula, except that it is disposable, and provided in pre-sterilized pack (Fig. 6).

Uses

- To suck the fluid, pus, blood from body cavities
- To suck the blood from the operative area, to make the operative field clear for the ongoing surgery
- Especially used to suck the blood, pus from the abdominal cavity during laparotomy
- To suck the urine from the bladder, after opening it during suprapubic cystolithotomy, or open prostatectomy.

MULTIHOLE SUCTION CANNULA

- It is a cylindrical hollow tube with multiple holes on half of the distal tube
- The purpose of the multiple holes is that, all the holes will not block simultaneously, and the suction work and will never be blocked even though the secretions are thick
- Sterilization by autoclaving (Fig. 7).

Uses

For suction of thick secretions like bilious and fecal contents of the intestine during resection of the small bowel, where chances of blockage of 2–3 holes in Yankauer suction or plastic disposable cannula are more.

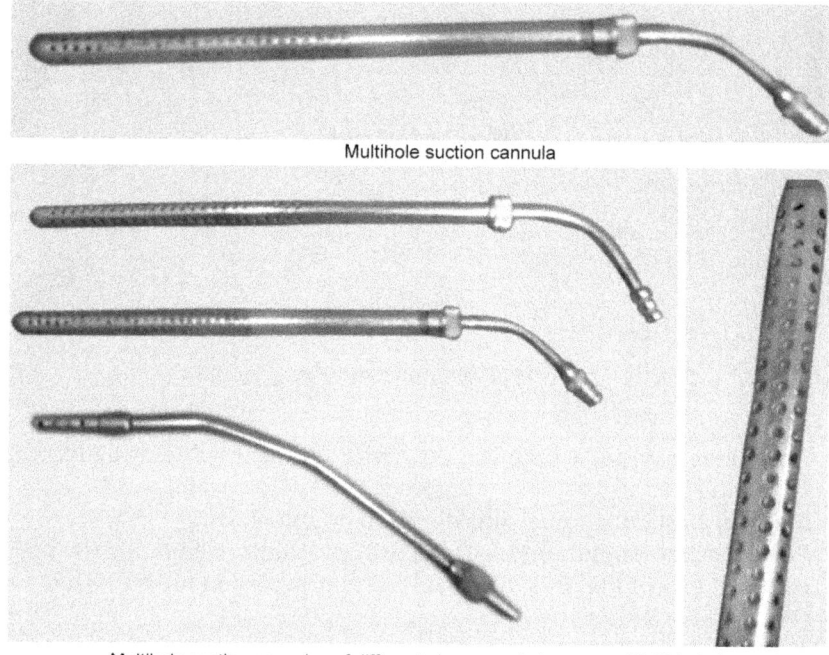

Multihole suction cannula

Multihole suction cannulas of different shapes and sizes

Multiple holes at the tip

Fig. 7: Multihole suction cannulas.

KIDNEY TRAY

- It is kidney shaped, so called as 'kidney tray'
- Sterilization by autoclaving (Fig. 8).

Uses

- To collect hydrocele fluid in operations of hydrocele repair like eversion of the sac

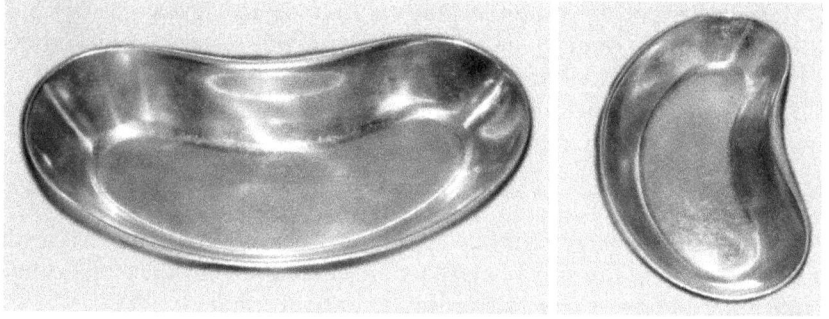

Fig. 8: Kidney tray.

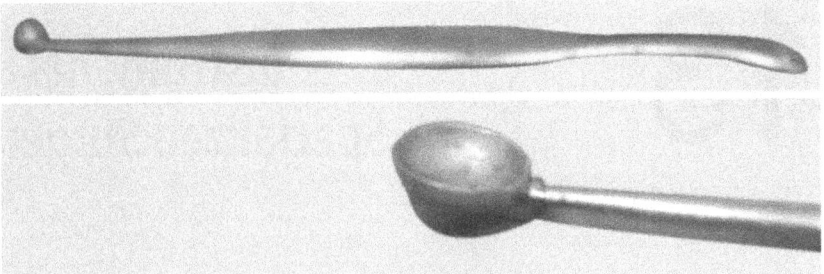

Fig. 9: Volkmann's scoop.

- To collect pus during incision and drainage of an abscess
- To collect daughter cysts and hydatid fluid during operation for hydatid cyst removal.

VOLKMANN'S SPOON OR SCOOP

- It is a long metallic instrument, with spoon like end with sharp edges
- Sterilization by autoclaving (Fig. 9).

Uses

- To curette a chronic abscess cavity, either in the bone or in the soft tissue
- To curette a sinus or fistulous tract, during their excision
- To curette an ulcer, to remove the excess granulation tissue before skin grafting.

CHAPTER 13

Instruments in Specialized Surgery

INSTRUMENTS USED IN THORACOTOMY

DOYEN RIB RASPATORY

- It has polygonal handle for better grip
- Its blades end in a curved fashion, like a hook and the edges are sharp for separating the periosteum from the undersurface of the rib
- For right and left side, they are different, but common for 3rd to 12th ribs
- To determine the side of the rib raspatory, its handle should face laterally, convexity above hook and the tip pointing downwards and away from the surgeon
- Sterilization by autoclaving (Fig. 1).

Uses

It is a blunt elevator. To separate the periosteum from the under surface of the rib, after elevating it by the periosteum elevator during thoracotomies.

Advantages of Separating the Periosteum by Rib Raspatory

- Underlying intercostals artery, vein and nerve will be reflected and protected
- The muscular attachments are reflected and not lacerated
- Avoids injury to the parietal pleura.

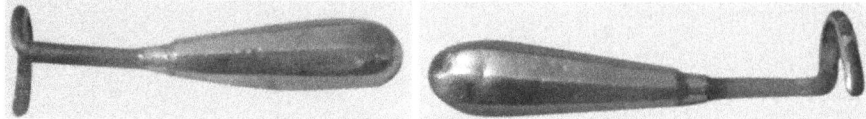

Fig. 1: Rib raspatory.

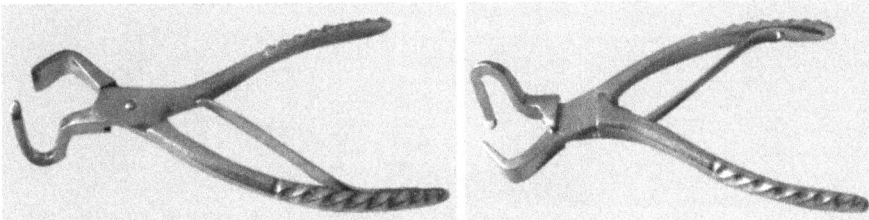

Fig. 2: Schoemaker rib shear.

SCHOEMAKER RIB SHEAR

- Visceral blade is blunt, has serrations and deep grove which is introduced beneath the rib to support the rib while cutting
- The other blade is parietal and is sharp with cutting edge to cut the ribs
- Lever may or may not be present
- The handle is ridged, for firm grip while cutting the rib without slipping it
- Sterilization by autoclaving (Fig. 2).

Uses

To cut the ribs during thoracotomies.

INSTRUMENTS USED IN TRACHEOSTOMY

TRACHEAL DILATORS

- It has finger bows, screw type of joint, pair of shafts and blades. No catch
- Tips of the blades are olive pointed, blunt, smooth, to prevent trauma to the mucosa of the trachea, during its insertion. Blades are gently curved
- When the finger bows are apart the blades are closed, when the finger bows are pressed and brought closed (approximated) to each other, the blades get separated
- Sterilization by autoclaving (Fig. 3).

Uses

- During tracheostomy, it is introduced through the incision over the trachea, in closed position and then it is opened up by pressing the finger bows. The tracheostomy tube is inserted through the gap between the tips of the blades. Then the dilator is closed and withdrawn from the trachea
- It also helps in reinsertion of tracheostomy tube, if it slips out
- It can be used as a laryngotomy dilator, during laryngotomy.

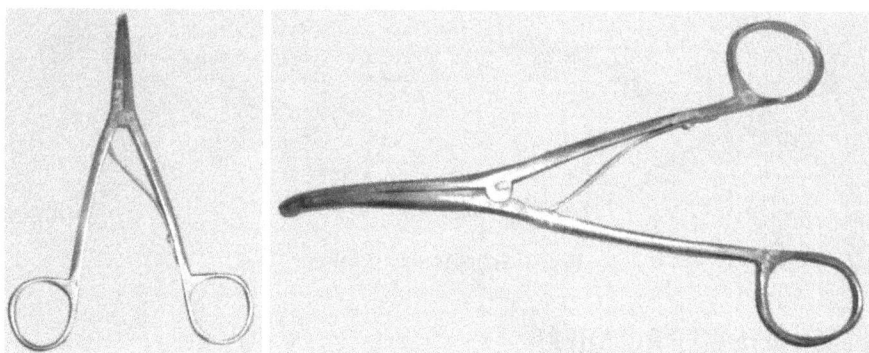

Fig. 3: Tracheal dilator.

INSTRUMENTS USED IN NEUROSURGERY (CRANIOTOMY)

HUDSON'S BRACE/BURR/PERFORATOR

- **Hudson's brace:** It has strong, heavy frame
- **Burr:** Groove with cutting edges and is available in different sizes
- **Perforator:** Initial groove established with the perforator, after which it is replaced by the burr, to make the burr hole
  - Sterilization by autoclaving
  - Nowadays all the above instruments are replaced by electrically driven cutting saw (Fig. 4).

Uses

To make a burr hole for craniectomy, for evacuation of the extradural hematoma, subdural hematoma or to decrease the intracranial tension (ICT), by decompressing the cranial cavity by making a burr hole.

BONE CUTTER AND BONE NIBBLER

Used in neurosurgery, are described in orthopedic section.

HORSLEY'S DURA MATER SEPARATOR AND SKULL ELEVATOR

- It has a 'zigzag' shape
- It has two ends, one is flat and blunt, while other is rounded, olive tipped
- In between the two ends, there is a handle which is grooved for providing better grip
- Sterilization by autoclaving (Fig. 5).

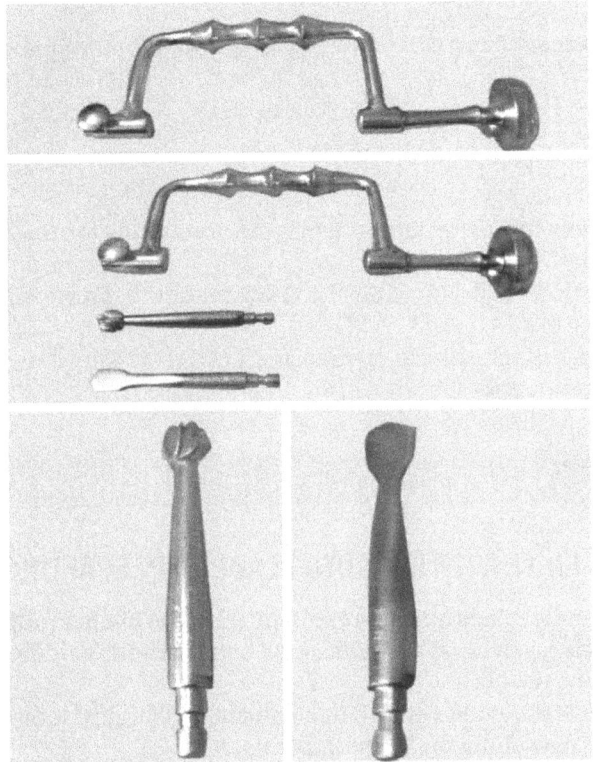

Fig. 4: Hudson's brace with burr and perforator.

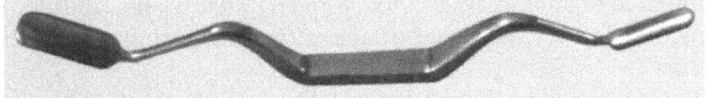

Fig. 5: Horsley's dura mater separator and skull elevator.

Uses

- To separate the dura mater, from inner side of the skull during craniotomy.
- As a director while incising the dura mater, to prevent injury to the underlying brain
- As a elevator, while elevating depressed fracture of the skull bones.

DURA SEPARATOR

- It has handle, with two ends. One end is flat, while the other one is curved
- Sterilization by autoclaving (Fig. 6).

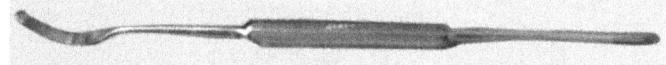

Fig. 6: Dura separator.

Uses

- To separate the dura mater, from the inner side of the skull during craniotomy
- As a director, while incising the dura mater, to prevent injury to the underlying brain
- Exploring the extradural hematoma (EDH), if found away from the burr hole.

INSTRUMENTS USED IN PLASTIC SURGERY

HUMBY'S KNIFE WITH GUARDED BLADE (SKIN GRAFTING KNIFE)

- It has a handle, blade and a screw at the tip of the blade to adjust the blade
- Handle has grooves on its surface for better gripping of the instrument, while taking the graft
- The blade is provided with a slot, to attach the surgical long blade, which is fixed by tightening the screw at the tip
- Graft is taken by to and fro movements of the grafting knife, after gently stretching the donor area
- Recipient area should not be avascular, and it should be free from infection
- Recipient area should be washed with soap and water, and then scrape the recipient area to expose the flat healthy granulation tissue, just before grafting
- Donor area should be shaved, before 24 hours of the operation and cleaned it with soap and spirit, and then immediately dressed with sterile gauze and bandage, which has to be opened at time of surgery only
- Grafting is done whenever a large raw area has to be covered
- To increase the surface area of the taken graft, it can be meshed by cutting it at regular slits and allowing it to expand
- Slits allows blood or serous exudates to escape to the surface of grafted wound, reducing chances of hematoma underneath the graft and improving the graft take
- Valuable in burn patients where large areas of skin has to be grafted (Fig. 7).

Uses

To take partial (split thickness or Thiersch graft) or full thickness (Wolfe graft) skin grafts, from the patient's donor site as per requirement of its recipient area.

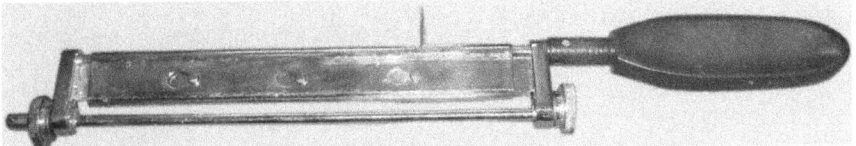

Fig. 7: Humby's skin grafting knife.

UROLOGY INSTRUMENTS

METALLIC URETHRAL BOUGIE

Lister's Metallic Bougie

- This is a solid, metallic curved rod having handle, body (shaft), shoulder and tip
- The handle is cylindrical (rounded)
- It has a long shaft tapering towards the tip and the terminal end has a smooth curve with olive pointed tip, to prevent injury to the urethra and the bladder, and also avoids false passage by the bougie
- The shoulder has a gentle curve, and is the dilating part as it corresponds with the bulbar urethra, which is the common site of the urethral stricture
- Tip narrows at the neck and widens at the shoulder
- They are available in a set of 12 with graduated thickness, and diameter increases as the number of the bougie increases
- Size is written on the handle. The upper and lower number written on the handle has a difference of 3. The denominator number (lower figure) denotes the diameter in milimeters at the base of the bougie, and the numerator (upper figure) indicates the diameter of the bougie in milimeters at the tip
- Female metallic bougies are also available, which are more curved at the shoulder than the male bougies
- Other metallic bougies are Clutton's metallic bougie, Miller's bougie, etc.
- Clutton's metallic bougie is same as Lister's metallic bougie, except handle is violin shaped, and the number written on the handle has a difference of 4, in denominator and numerator
- Miller's bougie is available in one size only
- Nowadays these bougies are routinely not used and are replaced by flexible gum elastic bougie, as chances of mucosal trauma to the urethra and bladder are less with gum elastic bougie. Also complications like false passage, bleeding, fistula formation are negligible as compared to the metallic bougie
- Sterilization by autoclaving (Fig. 8).

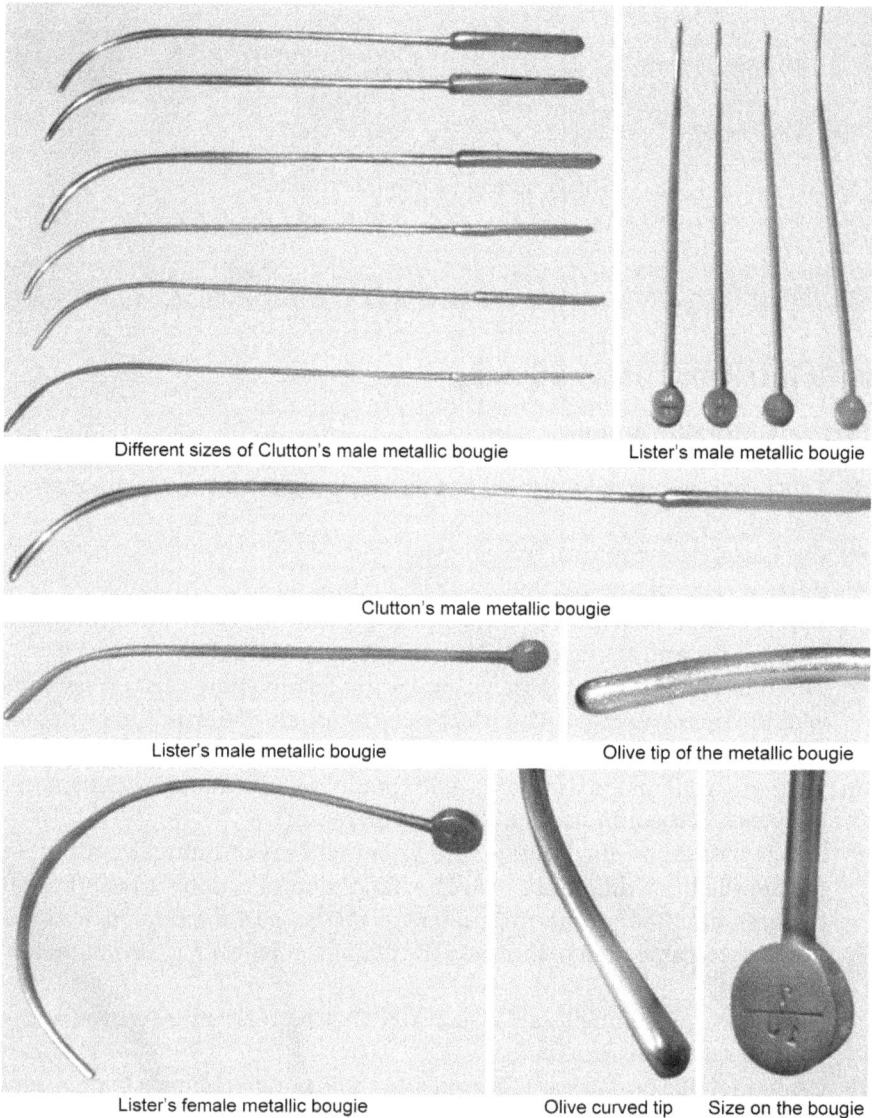

Fig. 8: Metallic urethral bougies.

Uses

- For dilatation of urethra in stricture urethra
- During repair of rupture urethra by 'Railroad technique'
- Dilatation of the urethra prior to urethrocystoscopy.

Section 3

Catheters, Tubes and Drains

Section Outline

14. Catheters
15. Trocar and Cannula
16. Tubes
17. Drains

CHAPTER 14

Catheters

■ INTRODUCTION

- It is a hollow tube to drain or withdraw the fluid from the body cavities.
- Most of them are kept postoperatively in the dependent abdominal cavities and also in the pleural cavity to drain the pleural cavity.
- Perurethral catheters are also used routinely for draining the bladder
- It can also be used, to introduce fluid in the body cavities or organs for washing the cavities as in case of intra-abdominal or liver abscess.

■ METALLIC URETHRAL CATHETER FOR MALE

- It is a long metallic catheter having body, shoulder and tip
- The terminal part of the catheter is curved like urethral dilator
- The tip is rounded and there are side holes near the tip on either side of it, situated at different levels, for free drainage of urine, so that both of them will not get simultaneously blocked
- There are two rings near its base or handle for holding the catheter and also gauze tape can be passed through it and tied to the thigh or waist to make it, self-retaining
- It has a shield at the other end of the catheter, to keep the drainage lumen occluded till the collecting device like kidney tray is made available
- It can cause urethral injury, false passage, and difficulty in retaining it for long time, makes its use less common
- Female metallic catheter is also available, which is short and slightly more bent as compared to male metallic catheter and having multiple side holes near the tip
- Sterilization by autoclaving (Fig. 1).

Uses

To relieve acute retention of urine when soft catheters like simple rubber catheter, Foley's catheter, etc. cannot be passed through the urethra.

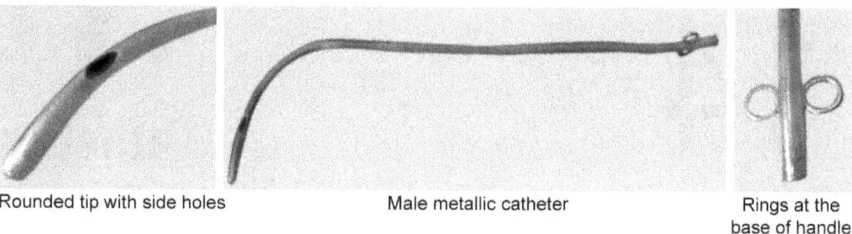

Rounded tip with side holes · Male metallic catheter · Rings at the base of handle

Fig. 1: Male metallic urethral catheter.

SIMPLE OR PLAIN RUBBER CATHETER

- It is made up of Indian red rubber
- Its tip is smooth, rounded and there is an opening near its tip, while the other end is open for drainage
- Sizes ranges from 6, 8, 10, etc.
- They are always preferred over the metallic urethral catheter for perurethral insertion, as they are soft, less rigid, easy for introduction, without risk of false passage
- Disadvantage of this catheter is that, it is not self-retaining, so used only for emergency and postoperatively for temporary perurethral catheterization
- Sterilization by autoclaving for 15 minutes (Fig. 2).

Uses

Urological Uses

- To relive acute retention of urine, by perurethral catheterization
- To diagnose the urinary tract injuries, upper and mid tract injuries. If catheterization of the bladder reveals hematuria, it indicates injury to the kidney, ureter or bladder
- To measure bladder pressure by cystometry, and also bladder capacity
- For administration of intravesical chemotherapy, for the treatment of bladder carcinoma
- For cystography and micturating cystourethrogram (MCU). Dye is inserted into the bladder through the perurethral catheter, which is then removed

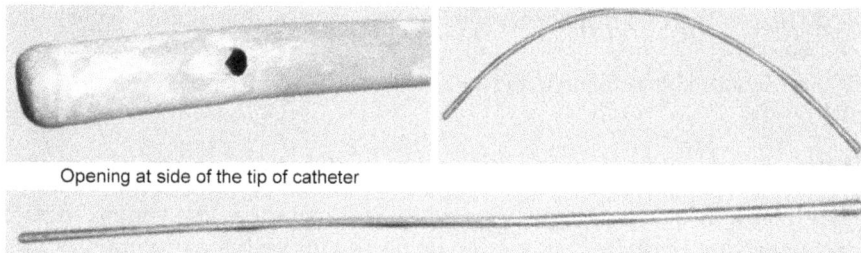

Opening at side of the tip of catheter

Fig. 2: Plain red rubber catheter.

and the patient is asked to pass urine, and radiographs are taken during micturition
- To obtain urine for examination
- To differentiate oliguria/anuria from retention of urine.

Non-Urological Uses

- For diagnosis of esophageal atresia in the newborn. Catheter cannot be passed into the stomach, in such cases and usually get obstructed at a level of 10 cm from the incisors
- To diagnose, posterior choanal atresia
- As a nasal catheter, to deliver oxygen to the patient
- Used during choledocholithotomy, for flushing the common bile duct with normal saline, to remove the sludge and small stones within it
- To encircle the colostomy loop, to prevent its retraction into the peritoneal cavity, for initial 10–14 days, till adhesions between it and the peritoneum and skin of anterior abdominal wall are formed
- During vagotomy, to encircle the lower esophagus for traction, to identify the vagus nerve
- As a suction catheter in emergency
- As a tourniquet to the upper arm, to make the veins prominent, while withdrawing blood for blood investigations
- Can replace hernia ring to retract the cord away from the site of hernia repair.

FOLEY'S SELF-RETAINING BALLOON CATHETER

- It is made up of latex (latex-siliconized), so less irritating and causes less crust formation with its use, so preferred for prolong use
- It may be 2-way or 3-way catheter, mostly 2-way catheter is routinely used in clinical practice
- In 2-way catheter, there are 2 channels. Main big channel is for free drainage of urine from the bladder and small channel which is having a valve, is connected to the balloon for inflating the balloon, to make it self-retaining or indwelling
- In 3-way catheter, there is an additional 3rd channel for irrigation of the bladder
- Catheter number and capacity of balloon is mentioned on the main or side channel
- Capacity of balloon varies from 5–50 mL. It has to be inflated with sterile water. Mostly, it is inflated with 10 mL of sterile water to make it self retaining. For its hemostatic compression effect, after transurethral resection of the prostate, it can be inflated with 30–50 mL of sterile water, and traction given to it by adhering it to the thigh, to occlude the balloon at the bladder neck in the prostatic bed to stop bleeding from the prostatic fossa

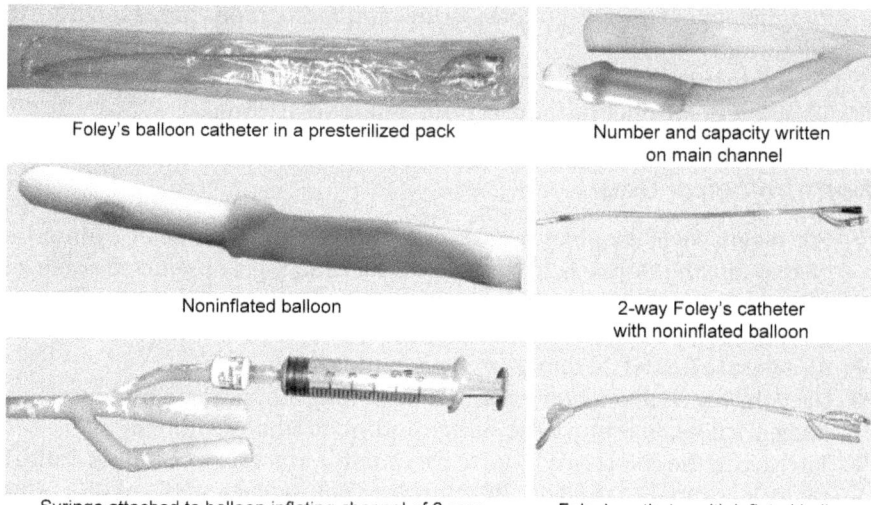

Fig. 3: Foley's self-retaining balloon catheter.

- ❖ They are available in various sizes according to French scale from 4, 6, 8, 10, 12, 14, 16, 18, 20, 22, 24, 26 Fr
- ❖ As the number increases the diameter of the catheter increases
- ❖ Diameter of catheter in millimetres = Number of catheter in Fr/3. Ex.:18 Fr catheters mean its diameter in French scale, i.e.18 Fr/3 = 6 mm
- ❖ Number 4, 6, 8, 10 Fr are used in the pediatric patients, and having a plastic wire like stylet, to keep the catheter straight and does not allow it to bend in the presterilized pack. As the catheter is flexible, it may bend if not provided with stylet, which may cause difficulty in its insertion, if it is bend before its use
- ❖ Number 12, 14, 16, 18 Fr are routinely used in adults. Number 14 is mostly used in adult females and number 16 is preferred in adult males
- ❖ In patients with benign prostatic hyperplasia number 12 or 14 Fr catheter is preferred, due to decrease in the caliber of urethra, because of compression of the prostatic urethra by median lobes of the prostate
- ❖ Number 20, 22, 24 Fr are mostly used as 3-way catheter, for postoperative irrigation of the bladder after transurethral resection of the prostate or in case of hematuria
- ❖ Perurethral or suprapubic catheter in the bladder should be changed every 3 weekly to prevent infection of the bladder, and also crust formations over the Foley's balloon, which causes difficulty in removing the catheter
- ❖ Supplied in presterilized pack which is sterilized by gamma irradiation (Fig. 3).

Uses

Urological Uses

- ❖ To relieve retention of urine by catheterization, in case of benign hyperplasia of the prostate, unconscious or comatose patient unable to pass urine

- To measure the urine output, in the postoperative patient or patient of renal failure
- To diagnose upper and mid-urinary tract injuries. If catheterization of the bladder reveals hematuria, it indicates presence of injury to the kidney, ureter, or bladder
- For the administration of intravesical chemotherapy, for treatment of bladder carcinoma
- 3-way Foley's catheter, is used after open prostatectomy or transurethral resection of the prostate for benign prostatic hyperplasia, for postoperative irrigation of the bladder
- 3-way catheter is also used for irrigation, in case of hematuria due to injury to the upper- and mid-urinary tract or in case of hematuria, due to malignant growth of the bladder, to prevent formation of clots in the bladder, which may block the catheter and subsequently its drainage
- May be used for suprapubic cystostomy, in case of benign hypertrophy of the prostate, stricture or rupture urethra, where perurethral catheterization is not possible or contraindicated
- For tube nephrostomy, in case of obstructed or pyonephrotic kidney.

Non-Urological Uses

- For postoperative drainage of the peritoneal cavity, after laparotomy
- May be used as an intercostal drain for tube thoracostomy for drainage of empyema, pleural effusion, hemothorax, pneumothorax, etc.
- May be used for feeding gastrostomy or jejunostomy in case of nonoperable obstructive carcinoma of stomach or esophagus or in case of comatose patient for giving enteral feeding
- May be used for tube cecostomy, in case of perforation of the cecum
- For control of epistaxis through posterior nares

SILICONE SELF-RETAINING CATHETER

- It is made up of 100% silicone
- Description and uses are same as the Foley's catheter
- Supplied in presterilized pack which is sterilized by gamma irradiation (Fig. 4).

Uses

Uses are same as like that of Foley's catheter, except that it can be kept for longer time than the Foley's catheter.

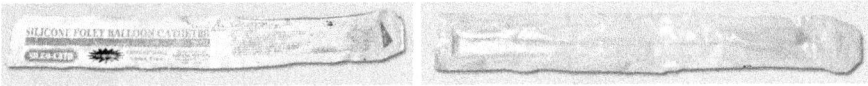

Fig. 4: Silicone self-retaining balloon catheter.

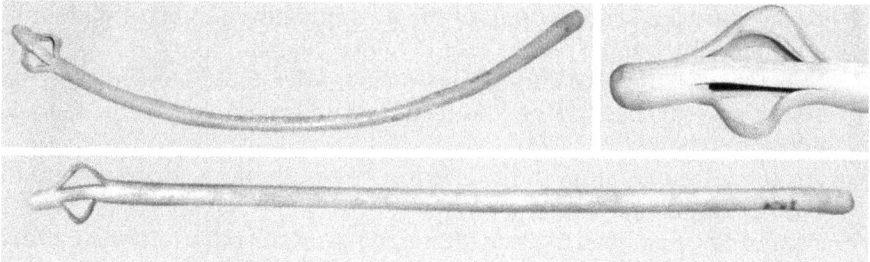

Fig. 5: Malecot's self-retaining rubber catheter.

MALECOT'S CATHETER

- It is a type of self-retaining catheter, but having only one channel for drainage like simple rubber catheter
- It is made up of Indian red rubber
- Tip of the catheter is made like a flower or having dilated winged end which makes it 'self-retaining'
- To introduce it in the cavity, the dilated winged end has to be made straight by inserting a hemostatic forceps into the dilated end, straighten it over the hemostatic forceps and insert along with it in the cavity and then remove the forceps. The dilated winged end takes its normal shape and will not allow the catheter to come outside the cavity, where it is introduced (pleural, peritoneal cavity) (Fig. 5).

Uses

- Same as Foley's catheter, except for perurethral catheterization
- Mainly used for tube thoracostomy, suprapubic cystostomy, postoperative drainage of the peritoneal cavity (one in Morrison's or hepatorenal pouch and another one in the pelvis, as these two are the dependent cavities in supine and standing position).

CHAPTER 15

Trocar and Cannula

■ SUPRAPUBIC TROCAR CANNULA (SUPRACATH)

- ❖ It consists of trocar and cannula
- ❖ Trocar is made up of steel and one of its end is pointed for piercing the skin, subcutaneous tissue, to reach and pierce the bladder wall
- ❖ Cannula is made up of plastic
- ❖ Trocar is inserted into the cannula, which comes out of the terminal end of the cannula, when it is inserted and fixed inside the cannula
- ❖ After piercing it from the skin up to the inside of the bladder and urine is seen flowing through the cannula, the trocar should not be advanced further and withdrawn quickly inside the cannula to prevent injury to the mucosa of the posterior wall of the bladder
- ❖ After completely withdrawing the trocar from the cannula, cannula is fixed to the overlying skin with the help of skin sutures, and then outer end of the cannula is attached to the collecting (urosac) bag to drain the urine from the bladder
- ❖ Supplied in presterilized pack.

Uses

To drain the bladder by suprapubic route (suprapubic cystostomy), when the periurethral cauterization has failed as in severe cases of benign hypertrophy of prostate or stricture urethra or when periurethral catheterization is contraindicated like in suspected cases of rupture urethra.

■ INTERCOSTAL TROCAR CANNULA

- ❖ It consist of trocar and cannula
- ❖ Trocar is made up of steel and one of its end is pointed for piercing the skin, subcutaneous tissue, intercostals muscles to reach and pierce the parietal pleura

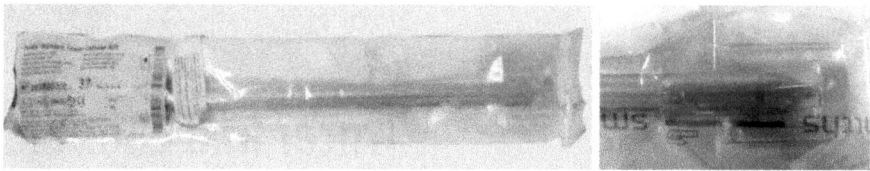

Fig. 1: Intercostal drainage trocar and cannula.

- Cannula is made up of plastic and is having multiple holes at the tip with markings
- Trocar is inserted into the cannula, which comes out of the terminal end of the cannula, when it is inserted and fixed inside the cannula
- After piercing it from the skin through the intercostals muscles to the pleural cavity, and blood or pleural fluid is seen flowing through the cannula, the trocar should not be advanced further and withdrawn quickly inside the cannula, to prevent injury to the underlying lung
- After completely withdrawing the trocar from the cannula, cannula is fixed to the overlying skin with the help of skin sutures, and then outer end of the cannula is attached to the underwater seal bag to drain the blood or pleural fluid from the pleura cavity
- Supplied in presterilized pack (Fig. 1).

Uses

- To drain air from the pleural cavity in case of pneumothorax
- To drain fluid from the pleural cavity in case of pleural effusion
- To drain air and blood from the pleural cavity in case of hemopneumothorax
- To drain blood from the pleural cavity in case of hemothorax
- To drain pus from the pleural cavity in case of empyema.

CHAPTER 16

Tubes

NASOGASTRIC TUBE (RYLE'S TUBE)

- 1 m or 100 cm long, made up of transparent plastic tubing or polyvinyl chloride (PVC)
- Number 10, 12, 14, 16, 18 are commonly used in clinical practice. As the number increases the diameter of the tube increases
- Few lead shots are there near the rounded tip of the tube at its closed end or in some tubes tip may be painted with lead. Lead shots make them radio-opaque, to show the position of the tip of the tube in the stomach on plain X-ray
- There are multiple side holes near the tip of the tube for drainage
- Lead (blue) line may be present on the entire tube, to make the tube radio-opaque in its entire length
- Number of markings on the tube are mostly 3 or 4 in number and markings are at 40, 50, 60 and 70 cm from the incisor teeth
- First single line or circular marking is at 40 cm from the tip, and when the nasogastric tube is inserted in the stomach up to this mark, tip of the tube is at gastroesophageal (GE) junction or at cardiac end of the stomach
- Second circular marking or 2 lines is situated at 50 cm from the tip of the tube, and when the nasogastric tube is inserted up to this mark, tip of the tube is lying in the body of the stomach
- Third circular marking or 3 lines, is at 60 cm from the tip, and when the nasogastric tube is inserted up to this mark, tip is lying in the pyloric region of the stomach
- Fourth circular marking or 4 lines, is at 70 cm from the tip, and when the nasogastric tube is inserted up to this mark, tip is lying in the 1st part of the duodenum
- Supplied in a presterilized pack (Fig. 1).

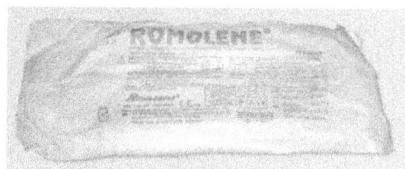 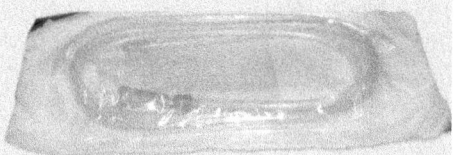

Fig. 1: Nasogastric tube.

Uses

- To decompress the stomach in intestinal obstruction, gastric outlet obstruction (GOO)
- To decompress the stomach in perforation peritonitis, to limit the peritoneal contamination by aspirating gastric contents through the nasogastric tube
- Preoperative decompression of the stomach in surgeries of upper gastrointestinal tract, to prevent intraoperative contamination from the gastric or intestinal contents
- Decompression of the stomach in comatose patient of head injury, to avoid aspiration of the gastric contents into the trachea leading to aspiration pneumonitis
- To monitor gastric bleeding and to give stomach wash, in case of bleeding peptic or malignant ulcer
- To aspirate the gastric contents and for giving gastric lavage, in case of suspected oral poisoning, drug overdose, etc.
- For giving nasogastric feeding to the comatose patients, who are on intravenous fluids and parental nutrition for long time or patients who are not able to feed themselves properly.

FLATUS TUBE

- It is a thick rubber tube, made up of Indian red rubber
- Tip is rounded and smooth like simple rubber catheter, but there is a large opening at the tip
- In addition to that, there are two side openings
- Other end of the tube is for release of flatus and feces
- Sterilization by autoclaving for 15 minutes (Fig. 2).

Uses

- For non-operative decompression of the sigmoid volvulus
- To relieve gaseous distension of large intestine due to paralytic ileus.

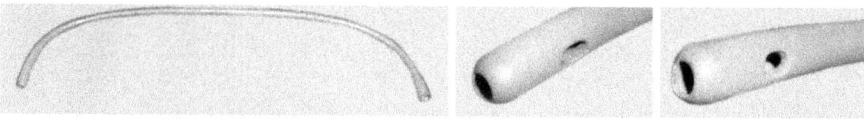

Flatus tube   Tip with large opening at the tip and 2 side holes

Fig. 2: Flatus tube.

TRACHEOSTOMY TUBES

- Gently curved tubes
- Different sizes as per the diameter of the tubes ranging from No. 30 to 37
- Usually inserted through the 2nd, 3rd and 4th tracheal cartilage rings
- It consists of outer tube, inner tube and obturator (pilot), also called 'introducer' for insertion
- Outer tube has flangs (wings) with holes on either sides, to secure the tube to the skin with sutures or tape may pass through the holes and tied around the neck. It always remains in the trachea. It has a lock which locks the inner tube with the outer tube
- Inner tube is little longer than the outer, so that both the tubes do not get blocked simultaneously. It is removed regularly for cleaning, and also when it gets blocked by the secretions
- Obturator or pilot has a smooth, bulbous tip which helps in the introduction of the outer tube
- First outer tube with obturator is introduced, and then the obturator is removed immediately and replaced by the inner tube
- It may be metallic made up of silver or aluminum or nonmetallic made up of red rubber or polyvinyl chloride (PVC)
- PVC tubes may be cuffed or uncuffed
- Cuffed tubes are self-retaining, so no need to strap or suture the tube
- at the neck. Also having less chances of pressure necrosis of the trachea
- PVC tubes are inert and less traumatic than metallic tubes (Fig. 3).

Uses

- For long-term intermittent positive pressure ventilation
- When the patient is having upper airway obstruction or spasm as in case of tetanus, that cannot be relived with the passage of an oral/nasal tube
- Maintenance of an airway and to protect the lungs in patients with impaired pharyngeal or laryngeal reflexes, and after major head and neck surgeries
- Long-term control of excessive bronchial secretions especially in patients with reduced level of consciousness like in a comatose patient of head injury, after 4–5 days of endotracheal intubation (ETT) insertion
- Patient of orofaciomaxillary injuries, in which endotracheal intubation is not possible
- Facilitating weaning from a ventilator, as the patients tolerate tracheostomy tubes better than endotracheal tubes.

Complications of Tracheostomy

- Hemorrhage
- Tube misplacement
- Occlusion of the tube by cuff herniation
- Occlusion of the tip of the tube against carina or tracheal wall

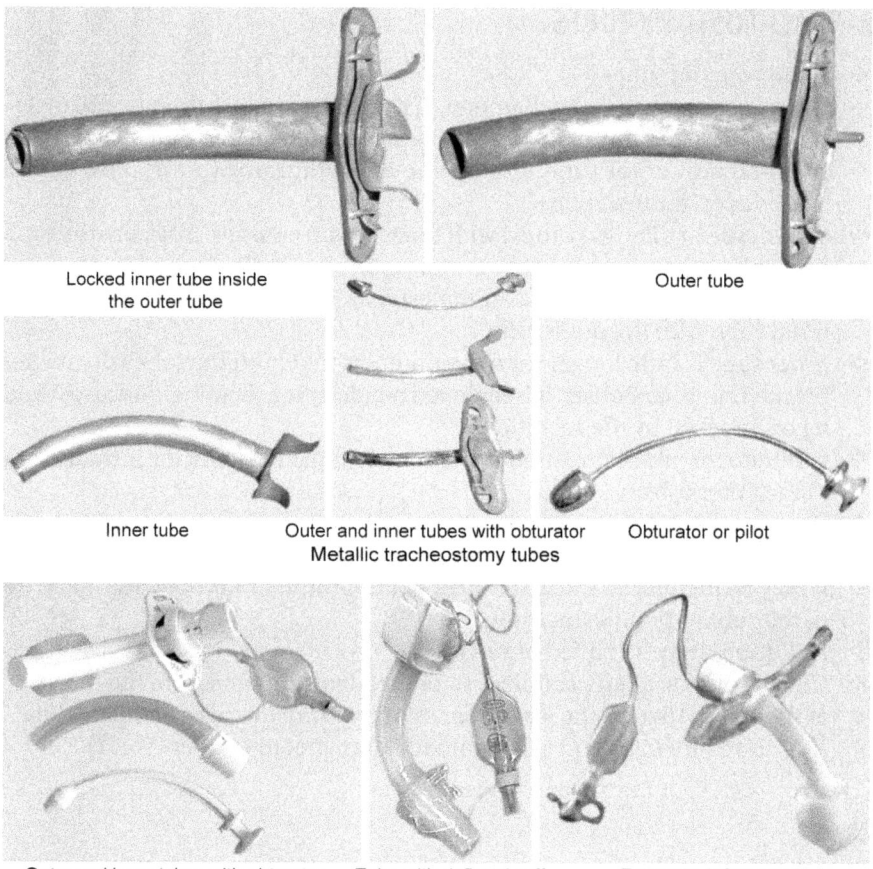

Fig. 3: Tracheostomy tubes.

- Blockage of the tube by secretions
- Infection of the stoma
- Over inflation of the cuff may lead to ulceration and distension of the trachea
- Persistent sinus at the tracheostomy site
- Tracheal stenosis at the cuff site.

SUCTION TUBINGS

- It is made up of plastic and having two open ends
- Sterilization by boiling or keeping it in the formalin chamber (Fig. 4).

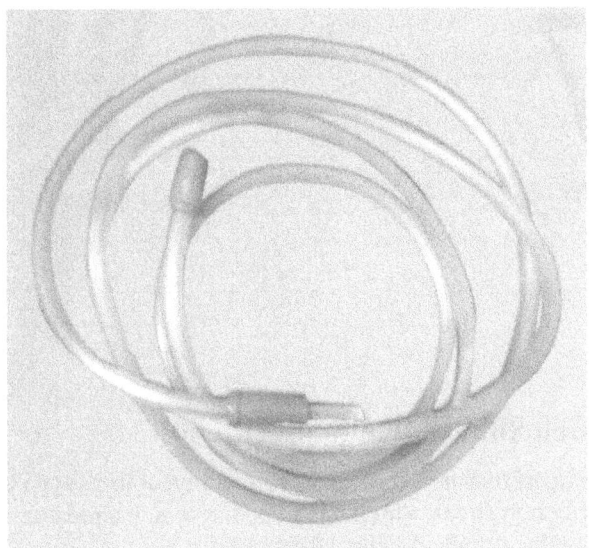

Fig. 4: Suction tubings.

Uses

Its one end is attached to the suction cannula and other end is attached to the suction bottle to drain fluid, blood, pus during any operative procedure.

CHAPTER 17

Drains

CORRUGATED RUBBER DRAIN/SHEET (CRD)

- ❖ It is made up of Indian red rubber or polyvinyl chloride (PVC)
- ❖ It is a corrugated sheet, which has to be cut to a desired size as required
- ❖ Sterilization by autoclaving for 15 minutes
- ❖ Now manufactured in a presterilized pack made up of PVC
- ❖ Nowadays mostly closed suction drain is used instead of CRD (Fig. 1).

Uses

- ❖ To drain the blood, pus, serous collections, etc. postoperatively from the cavities
- ❖ Postoperatively after eversion of the sac for hydrocele repair, to drain postoperative hemorrhage or serous collection. It is kept in the scrotum deep to the dartos muscle
- ❖ Following modified radical mastectomy, drain is kept in the axilla and under the skin flaps

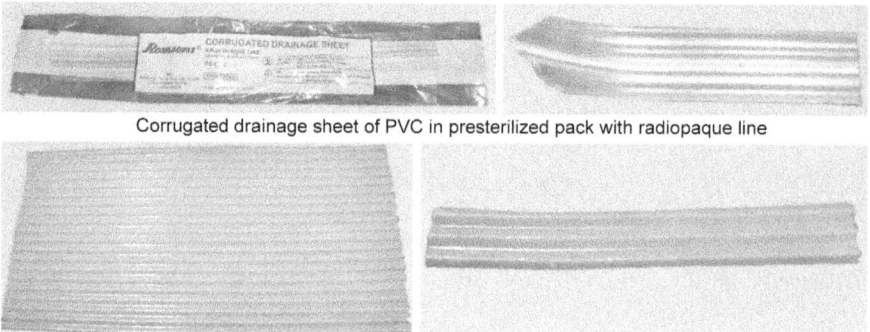

Corrugated drainage sheet of PVC in presterilized pack with radiopaque line

Corrugated rubber drainage sheet of Indian red rubber cut to different sizes

Fig. 1: Corrugated drainage sheet.

- Following repair of incisional hernia, one CRD is kept in preperitoneal space and other in the subcutaneous space below the skin
- To drain the pus and to keep the track patent in case of counter incision given in the breast abscess. Drain inserted from incision given through the most prominent part and brought out through the incision given in the most dependent part.

SUCTION DRAIN

- It has pinch cap, connecting tube, connector, below unit container, tie band, U connector, curved needle (trocar) and redon drain (radiopaque)
- It is called as 'suction drain', as it drains the fluid in the cavity where it is kept by negative suction, which is created in the below unit container by making it air tight
- Pinch cap is used to open or close the drain tubing which clamps the tubing completely and occludes its lumen when pinched (closed)
- The connecting tube connects the below unit container to the 'U' connector, which is connecting the redon drains
- The connector connects the connecting tube to the below unit container
- 'U' connector connects the connecting tube to the redon drains kept in the cavity
- Tie band is to tie the below unit container to the side of the bed
- Curved needle or pointed trocar is there to pierce the skin from inside the cavity to pass the redon drains
- Redon drains are 2 in number and having multiple holes on their tip for free drainage of fluid without getting blocked. They are radiopaque to make them visible on X-rays
- It has the advantage that, as being closed at the outer end, chances of infection from the atmosphere and surrounding will be less or negligible as compared to the corrugated rubber drain, which are open at the outer end
- The other advantage of this drain is that, even though the tip of the tubes are nondependent in the cavity to be drained, fluid will be drained or sucked by negative suction in the container
- Negative suction in the below unit container is created by compressing or pressing the container and applying (closing) the tube connecter by rotating movements with pinch clamp closed
- A modification of the suction drain in small size, is called as 'Mini Vac suction drain', which has a single draining tube and does not have pinch and tie band (Fig. 2).

Uses

- Postoperatively to drain the cavities (dead space) where fluid like blood, serous collection may get collected. As if the fluid gets collected, it may cause postoperative hematoma, or seroma which may get infected later on

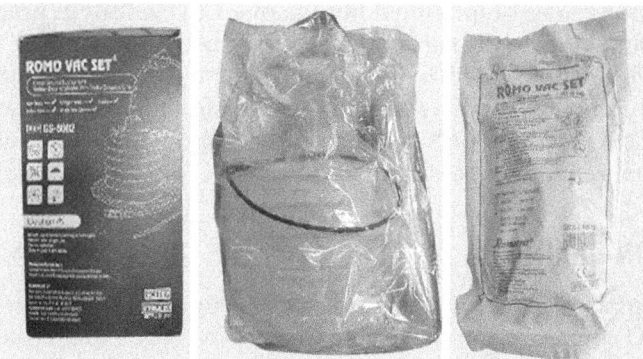

Fig. 2: Suction drain.

- Most commonly kept in the subcutaneous plane and in the axilla after modified radical mastectomy, below the sternohyoid and sternothyroid muscles after thyroid surgeries, in the preperitoneal fat and the subcutaneous fat, after repair of the incisional area
- Mini Vac suction drain is kept commonly in the breast tissue after excision of the fibroadenoma and also in the subcutaneous plane after excision of a large subcutaneous lipoma or cyst.

ABDOMINAL DRAIN

- It is made up of plastic or polyvinyl chloride (PVC)
- It has multiple holes at one end (inner) for free drainage of the space or cavity where it is kept
- The other end (outer) is attached to the collecting bag (urosac bag)
- Usually the drains are kept in the most dependent spaces of the abdominal cavity in supine position, which are Morrison's pouch (hepatorenal space) and pelvis (pelvic cavity)
- Supplied in a presterilized pack
- Simple plain red rubber or Malecot's catheter, can be cut from their tip, and 3–4 side holes are made in that at different levels for free drainage, can also be used as a abdominal drain (Fig. 3).

Uses

- Postoperatively to drain the dependent spaces of the abdominal cavity for draining blood, serous fluid, etc. which gets collected if not drained and later on may get infected
- To drain pus in case of appendicular abscess, perforation peritonitis, if general condition of the patient is not allowing the definitive operative procedure to be undertaken.

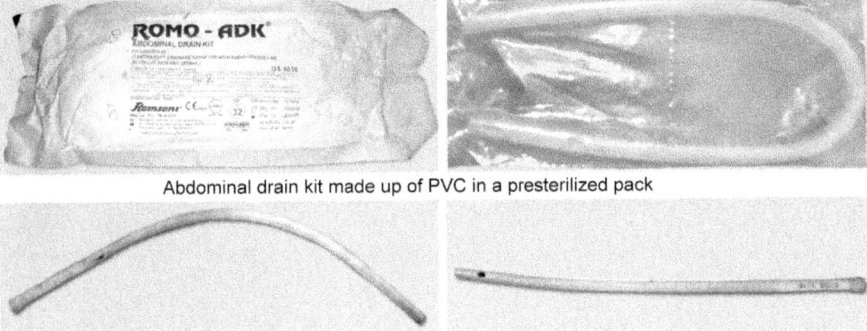

Fig. 3: Abdominal drain.

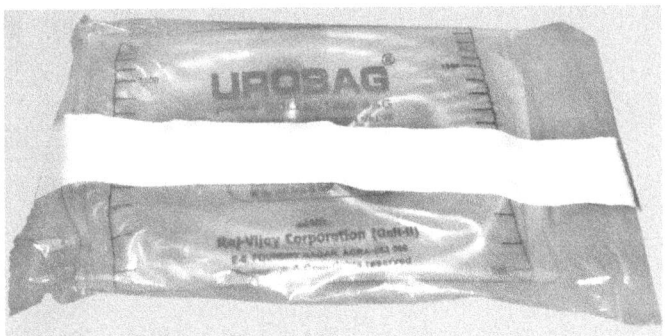

Fig. 4: Urosac bag.

UROSAC BAG

- This is a collecting bag attached to the outer end of the Foley's catheter or drainage tube kept in the peritoneal cavity
- Made up of plastic and supplied in a presterilized pack (Fig. 4).

Uses

- To collect urine from the bladder via per urethral or suprapubic catheter
- It is attached to the drain to collect fluids like blood, serous fluid, pus from the peritoneal cavity.

Section 4

Intravenous Cannulas, Intravenous and Blood Sets, Intravenous Fluids

Section Outline

18. Intravenous Cannulas and Sets
19. Intravenous Fluid Bottles (Crystalloid Bottles)
20. Syringes and Needles

CHAPTER 18

Intravenous Cannulas and Sets

INTRAVENOUS CANNULA (INTRACATH/VASOFIX)

- It has an outer plastic cannula along with the inner long needle or stylet, which comes out of the terminal end (proximal) of the outer cannula, when it is inserted and fixed within the cannula
- It has two wings near the outer end (distal), which has to be flattened before insertion of the cannula, which makes it easy to hold during its insertion. They have to be fixed to the skin with adhesive tape after proper positioning of the cannula in the selected vein
- Its outer (distal) end has two outlets. One in the continuity with the cannula for attaching infusion set tubing and other one at right angle to the cannula (facing towards the ceiling), for giving drugs like anesthesia drugs or antibiotics
- They are provided in different sizes and color codes, according to the diameter of the cannula
- As the number of the cannula increases its diameter decreases
- Provided in a presterilized pack (Fig. 1).

Uses

- For giving intravenous fluids and drugs like antibiotics, analgesics, antacids, etc.
- For giving intravenous fluids preoperatively, intraoperatively as well as postoperatively for volume replacement of the patient, which has been lost intraoperatively during surgeries and also till the patient is allowed to take the oral feeds
- In case of trauma, burns, dehydrated patients to treat the hypovolemia, for volume replacement to maintain the blood pressure.

Section 4: Intravenous Cannulas, Intravenous and Blood Sets, Intravenous Fluids

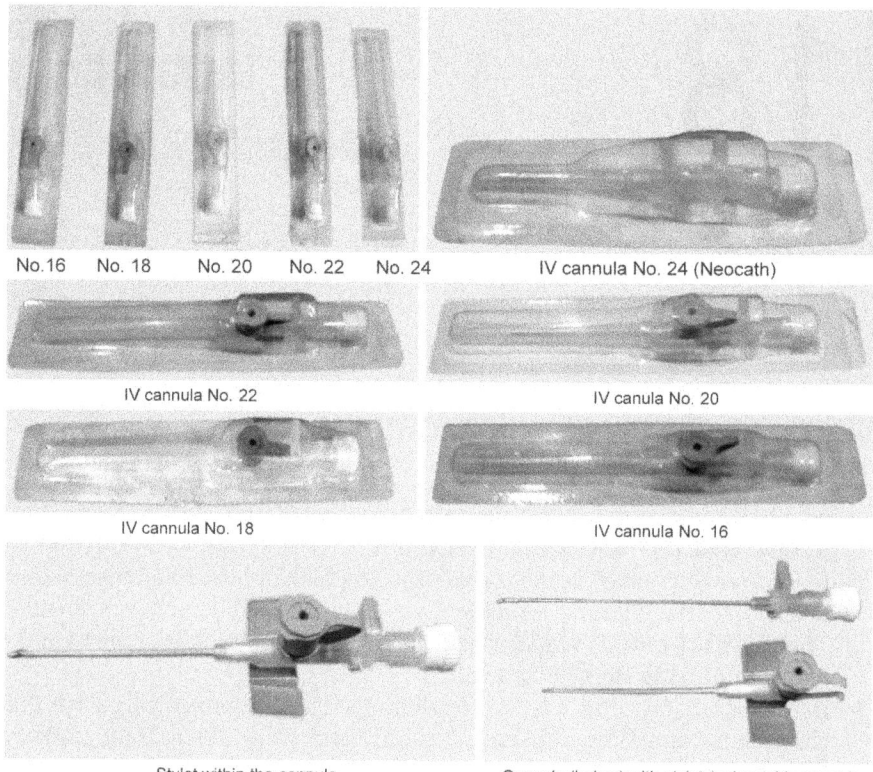

Fig. 1: Intravenous cannula of different sizes.

Number	Color	Diameter (mm)	Length (mm)	Max flow (mL/min)
16 gauge (G)	Gray	1.8	45	200
18 G	Green	1.3	45	80
20 G	Pink	1.10	32	55
22 G	Blue	0.90	25	31
24 G (Neocath)	Yellow	0.70	19	15

SCALP VEIN SET

- It is also called 'butterfly cannula', as after flattening its wings it looks like butterfly
- It has a small needle with wings, and a short length of infusion tubing for attaching it to the infusion set
- Needle has to be pierced in the selected vein and the wings adhered to the skin with adhesive tape to fix it to the skin
- As it does not have the outer plastic cannula like the intravenous cannula, counter puncture of the vein can occur during its insertion and also after

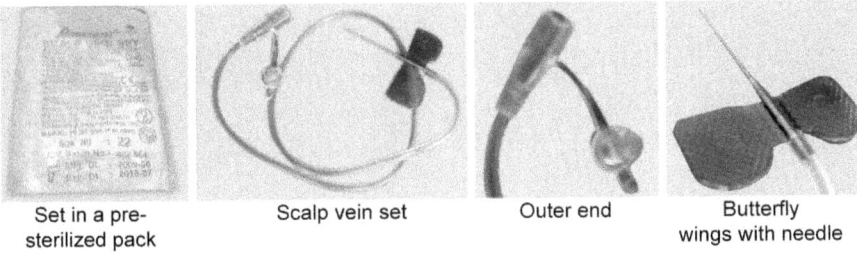

| Set in a pre-sterilized pack | Scalp vein set | Outer end | Butterfly wings with needle |

Fig. 2: Scalp vein set in a presterilized pack.

that if the patient moves that limb, where it is inserted. It leads to counter puncture or removal of the needle from the vein, and accumulation of fluid in the subcutaneous tissue. Because of this disadvantage, it is not routinely used whenever intravenous cannulation required for long period (more than a day)
- It has different numbers and color of the wings as per its diameter, from No. 16 to 24
- As the number increases, its diameter decreases like intravenous cannula
- Provided in a presterilized pack
- Advantage over the intravenous cannula is that, cost wise, it is a much cheaper option than an intravenous cannula (Fig. 2).

Uses

For giving intravenous fluids and antibiotics in emergency, if intravenous cannula is not available or if it has to be given for short span (not more than 24 hours).

INTRAVENOUS INFUSION SET

It has following parts:
- **Spike or pivot:** To penetrate the intravenous fluid or antibiotic bottle. It drains the fluid from the bottle to the infusion tube.
- **Drip chamber:** It has to be filled to the half level of the chamber with the intravenous fluid from the bottle, before opening the regulator. It prevents flow of air present in the infusion set from going in the general venous circulation.
- **Fluid filter:** It is present just below the drip chamber. It removes the impurities present in the intravenous fluid bottle, if any.
- **Infusion tubing:** It is a long connecting plastic tube from the drip chamber up to the injection site. It provides necessary length to the infusion set from the intravenous fluid bottle, where it is anchored to the intravenous stand up to the patient's intravenous cannula, which allows free movements of the limb, where the cannula is inserted without accidental removal of the cannula.

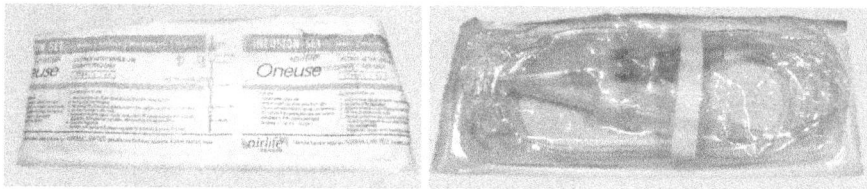

Intravenous set in a presterilized pack

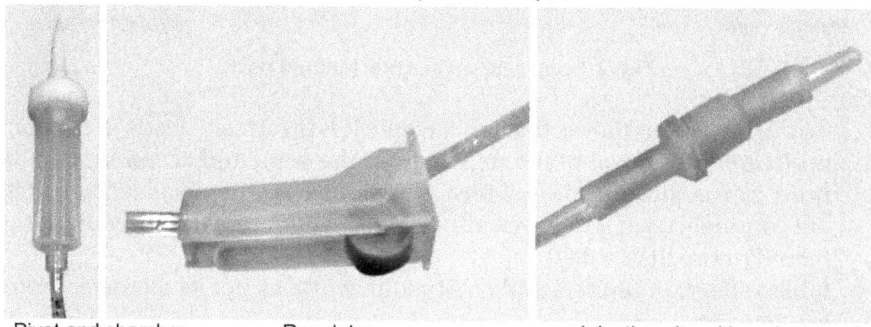

Pivot and chamber Regulator Injection site with patients end

Fig. 3: Intravenous infusion set.

Regulator: It regulates the flow of intravenous fluid to be given to the patient as per patient's requirement.

Injection site: It is a soft tubing of short length near the patient's end of the infusion set, just near where it is attached to the patient's intravenous cannula. Through this tubing, injections can be given to the patient along with or without interrupting the ongoing fluid by piercing the tubing.

Needle with needle protector (plastic cap): It is attached to the terminal end (towards patient's side) of the infusion set. It is pierced in the fluid bottle when the intravenous fluid is being made ready for infusion, to prevent contamination of the patient's end of the infusion set. Later on the needle is removed and the terminal end of the infusion set is attached to the patients' intravenous cannula.

Provided in a presterilized pack (Fig. 3).

Uses

To give intravenous fluids, antibiotics in the bottles to the patient.

■ BLOOD TRANSFUSION SET

- ❖ It has same parts like that of infusion set except the drip chamber larger with a filter
- ❖ Its drip chamber is larger than the infusion set
- ❖ The filter is within the drip chamber and is long and compromising the whole circumference of the chamber and about 3/4th of the length of the chamber to filter the blood properly
- ❖ Provided in a presterilized pack (Fig. 4).

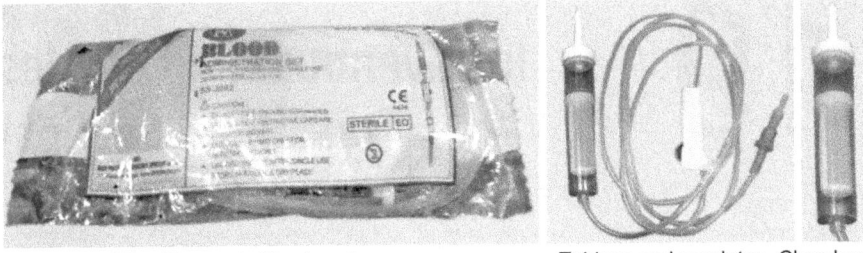

BT set in presterilized pack   Tubings and regulator   Chamber and filter

Fig. 4: Blood transfusion set.

Uses

To give the whole blood and its components like packed cell volume, fresh frozen plasma, etc. to the patient.

THREE-WAY CANNULA

- It has three ways or channels
- It has a marker with three arrows over it, which indicates the channels in working
- All the three channels can be working at the same time or alternatively two channels can work at one time with blocking of one channel
- All the three channels can also be blocked, to block the intravenous cannula
- It can be converted to four-way cannula, if another three way cannula is attached to one of its channel
- Made up of plastic and provided in a presterilized pack (Fig. 5).

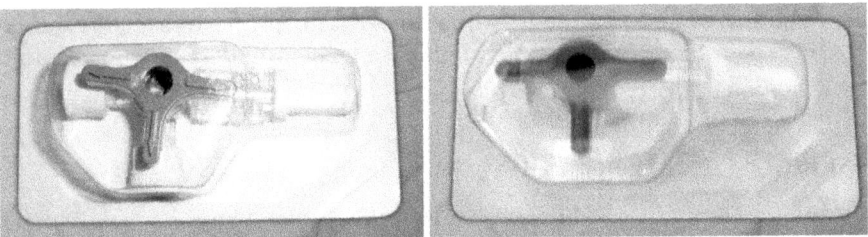

Fig. 5: Three-way cannula.

Uses

- To give the drug or additional intravenous fluid along with the ongoing fluid in the same vein
- To infuse blood or other intravenous fluid like colloids in patients of hypovolemic shock, who need rapid volume replacement within short period of time using large syringe.

CHAPTER 19

Intravenous Fluid Bottles (Crystalloid Bottles)

■ INTRODUCTION

Mostly provided in 500 mL bottles, but can also be provided in 100 mL or 1 L (1000 mL) bottles (Fig. 1).

■ 5% DEXTROSE INJECTION

- ❖ It contains dextrose injection IP (5% W/V)
- ❖ Each 100 mL contains dextrose anhydrous IP 5 g qs
- ❖ It contains 170 Kcal/L with osmolarity of 277 mOsmol/L
- ❖ It should be cautiously used in a known diabetic patient, and otherwise also whose blood sugar status is not known (Fig. 2).

Uses

- ❖ As a daily intravenous fluid supplement to a nil by mouth (fasting) patient or otherwise also to a patient whose intake is not proper as a energy source
- ❖ It is given to increase the blood glucose level rapidly in a hypoglycemic patient.

■ RINGER LACTATE INJECTION

It contains compound sodium lactate injection Indian Pharmacopeia (Ringer lactate solution for injection IP).

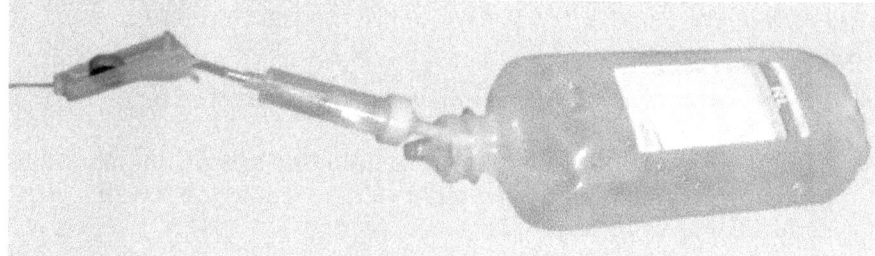

Fig. 1: Intravenous set attached to an intravenous fluid bottle.

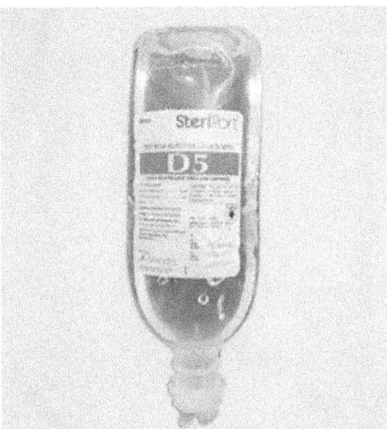

Fig. 2: Dextrose injection IP (5% W/V).

Each 100 mL contains:
- Sodium lactate solution USP (United States Pharmacopeia) equivalent to sodium lactate: 0.320 g
- Sodium chloride IP: 0.60 g
- Potassium chloride: 0.40 g
- Calcium chloride: 0.027 g
- It contains Na^+: 131 mmol/L, K^+: 5 mmol/L, Ca^{++}: 2, bicarbonate as lactate: 29 mmol/L, close to Cl^- 111 mmol/L
- Its osmolarity is 308 mOsmol/L
- It should be cautiously used or better not be given to a patient of acute or chronic renal failure (Fig. 3).

Uses

- It contains all the ions and electrolytes in the body so it is a life-saving fluid in a patient of electrolyte imbalance due to severe fluid loss because of repeated vomiting, diarrhea, hypovolemia due to blood loss
- As a daily intravenous fluid supplement to nil by mouth patient to provides ions and electrolytes.

SODIUM CHLORIDE SOLUTION

- It contains sodium chloride injection IP (0.9% W/V)
- Each 100 mL contains sodium chloride IP 0.9 g
- It contains Na^+:150 mmol/L and Cl^-:150 mmol/L
- Its osmolarity is 308 mOsmol/L (Fig. 4).

Uses

- As a daily intravenous fluid supplement to a nil by mouth patient, to provide sodium chloride

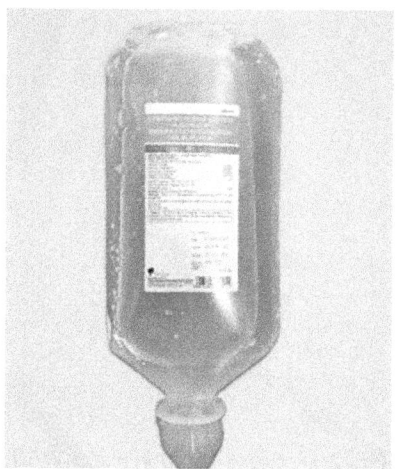

Fig. 3: Ringer lactate solution for injection IP.

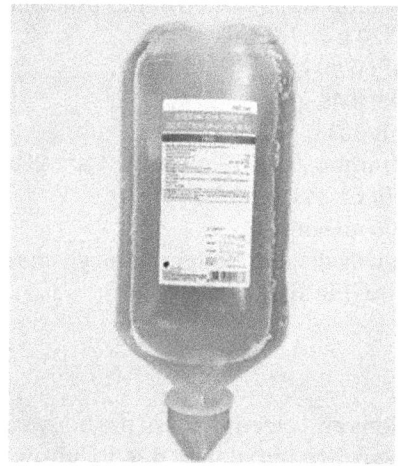

Fig. 4: Sodium chloride injection (0.9% W/V).

- To give peritoneal wash to remove all the peritoneal contaminants in case of perforation peritonitis
- For cleaning and dressing of the wound.

DEXTROSE NORMAL SALINE

- It contains sodium chloride injection IP (0.9% W/V) and dextrose (5% W/V)
- Each 100 mL contains dextrose anhydrous 5.00 g and sodium chloride IP 0.9 g
- It contains Na^+:150 mmol/L and Cl^-:150 mmol/L
- It contains 170 Kcal/L, dextrose 50 g/L (Fig. 5).

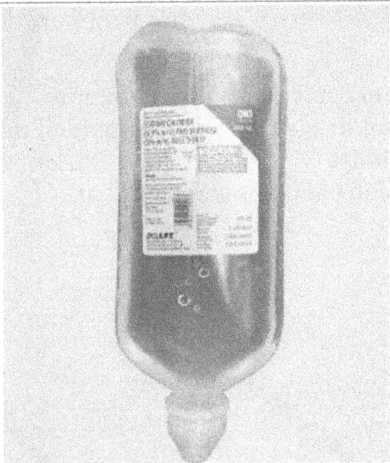

Fig. 5: Sodium chloride (0.9% W/V) and dextrose (5% W/V) injection.

Uses

As a daily intravenous fluid supplement to a nil by mouth patient (fasting), to provide sodium chloride as well as dextrose as it contains both.

■ STERILE WATER VIAL
- It contains sterile water
- Provided in 5 or 10 mL presterilized plastic bottle (Fig. 6).

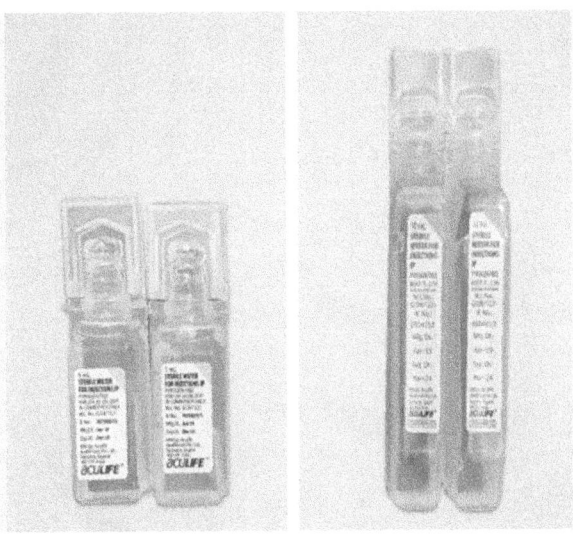

Fig. 6: Sterile water for injection.

Uses

- To dilute the drug to decrease its concentration
- To reconstitute the drugs, which are provided in powdered form like intravenous antibiotics
- To inflate the balloon of Foley's catheter.

CHAPTER 20

Syringes and Needles

■ SYRINGES

- It may be made up of plastic or glass
- It has different sizes as per capacity of the syringe like 2 mL, 5 mL, 10 mL, 20 mL, 50 mL etc.
- It has piston, outer sheath, and a nozzle
- Piston creates negative pressure in the syringe, when it is withdrawn from the syringe
- Nozzle of the syringe is universal to fit properly in any tube channel like intravenous cannula, spinal needle, balloon channel of the Foley's catheter, balloon channel of the endotracheal tube, and all routinely used tube channels, as it is of same diameter in all syringes even though the capacity of the syringe differs
- Syringe fills-up with the fluid which is aspirated by creating negative pressure within it. According to the capacity of outer sheath, capacity of the syringe is labeled.
- When the nozzle is fixed to the intravenous cannula, and piston is pushed inside the outer sheath, fluid in the syringe flows to the cannula
- Plastic syringes are provided in a presterilized pack, while glass syringes are sterilized by boiling for 3 minutes (Fig. 1).

Uses

Mainly Used

For giving the drugs intravenously or intramuscularly.

Additional Uses

- For dilution of the drugs, to decrease its concentration
- For dissolution of the antibiotic with distilled water which are in the powdered form

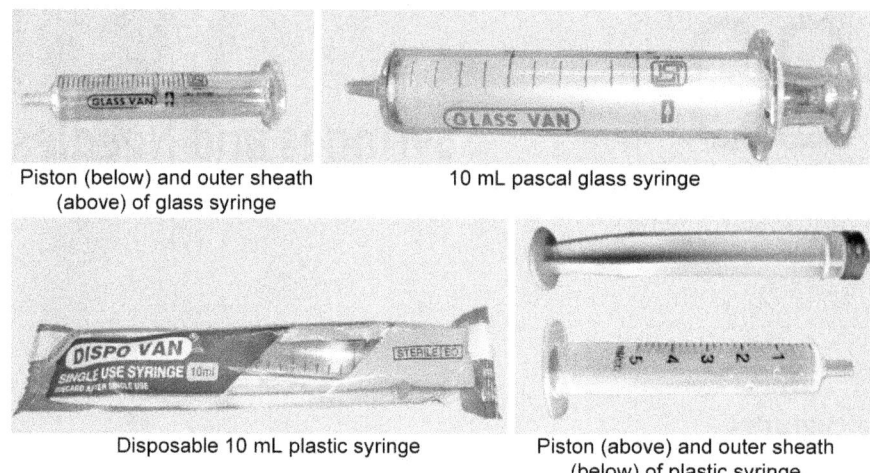

Fig. 1: Syringes.

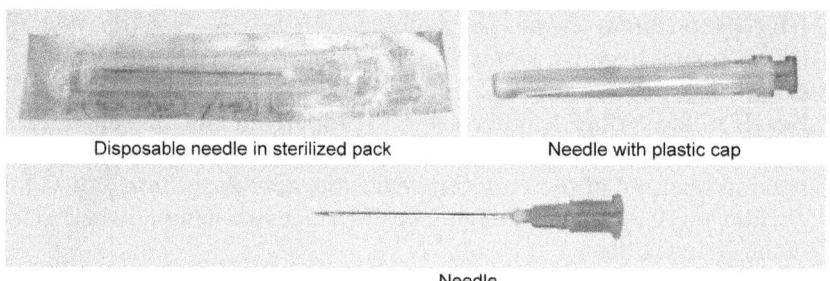

Fig. 2: Hypodermic needle.

- For infiltrating local anesthetic drug in the procedures which has to be done under local anesthesia, also in case of suturing of the wound
- For diagnostic tapping in case of hemoperitoneum, ascites, hemothorax, pneumothorax, etc.
- For inflating the balloon of the self-retaining Foley's catheter, endotracheal tube, etc.

HYPODERMIC NEEDLE

- It is made up of stainless steel
- One end is beveled, sharp, pointed while other end is dilated and universal to get connected to the syringe of any capacity (Fig. 2).

Section 5

Orthopedics Instruments and Implants

Section Outline

21. Orthopedics Instruments
22. Orthopedics Implants
23. Bandages, Crepe Bandages and Plaster of Paris Bandages

CHAPTER 21

Orthopedics Instruments

▮ FARABEUF'S RASPATORY OR PERIOSTEUM ELEVATOR

- ❖ It has a handle, thumb rest and a blade
- ❖ Its handle is flat, long for gripping the instrument, may be grooved on both the surfaces, for better grip of the instrument, while using it during surgeries
- ❖ Its upper surface is provided with a thumb rest, which is transversely serrated, corrugated and concave. It gives better grip to the thumb when placed over it, and also provides better control over the instrument and avoids slipping of the instrument, while working with it
- ❖ Handle has to be held (to be gripped) with rest of the fingers from below with the thumb kept over the thumb rest from above
- ❖ Ideally the ratio of the handle with the thumb rest to the sharp tip of the blade is 3:1
- ❖ Its blade may be straight or curved. It is rectangular, broad or narrow, with a sharp beveled edge, which has to be closely applied to the bone, to strip the periosteum by sliding movements, taking care not to injure the neurovascular bundle of the bone, while stripping the periosteum
- ❖ Scalpel or the surgical blade is used to cut the periosteum, before the periosteum elevator is insinuated, in between the bone and its periosteum
- ❖ Periosteum is not elevated in case of cervical rib, which has to be excised extraperiosteally to avoid regeneration and is also not elevated in case of tuberculosis and malignant bone tumors
- ❖ Sterilization by autoclaving (Fig. 1).

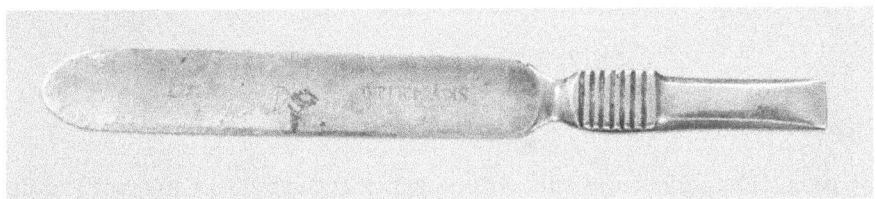

Fig. 1: Periosteum elevator.

Uses

As the periosteum is tough and slippery, cutting instruments cannot be steadied to cut the bone and slips easily, making bone cutting, drilling, etc. difficult, so the periosteum has to be elevated before cutting the bone.

❖ To elevate the periosteum from the surface of the bone during removal of the periosteum from the undersurface of the rib in thoracotomies, resecting 11th or 12th rib in case of pyelolithotomy or nephrolithotomy through 12th rib approach (rib cutting incisions)
❖ For stripping periosteum from the bone, in case of amputation of the extremity (long bones) and while internal fixation of the fracture
❖ To strip the pericranium from the skull while performing craniotomy, mastoidectomy, etc.
❖ To strip the periosteum, during saucerization and sequestrectomy for chronic osteomyelitis
❖ For stripping the muscular attachments from the bone.

▮ LANE'S BONE LEVERS

❖ It has a blade, handle and a single finger bow
❖ It has to be held by putting a thumb in the finger bow and grasping the handle with the rest of the fingers
❖ Sterilization by autoclaving (Fig. 2).

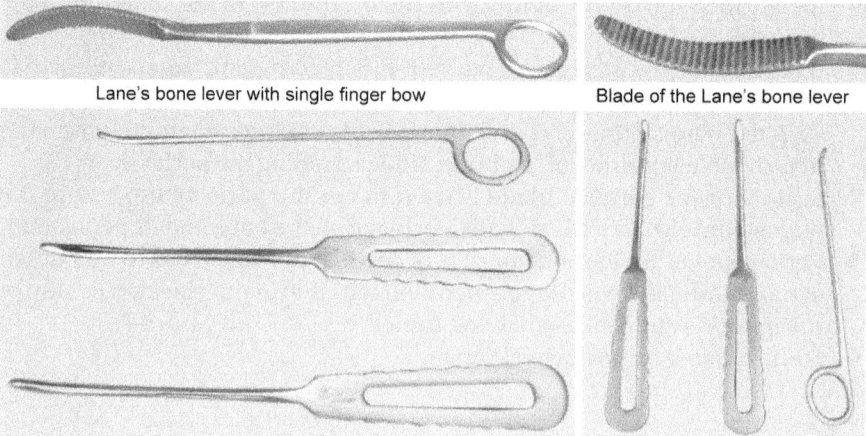

Fig. 2: Different types of bone levers.

Uses

To retract the periosteum after stripping it from the bone by the periosteum elevator along with its soft tissue attachments away from the bone (operative zone), to prevent trauma to the adjacent soft tissue like blood vessels, nerves, muscles, tendons, etc. Muscles and neurovascular bundle of the bone should be retracted, along with the periosteum to avoid injury to them, while cutting the bone.

■ OSTEOTOME (Osteo = Bone, Tomy = Cutting)

- ❖ It has a head, shaft and blade
- ❖ Head is rounded, smooth, blunt and projecting to receive the blows of the mallet
- ❖ Shaft or handle is octagonal in shape, for convenience while holding it firmly with nondominant hand, which prevents rotating of the instrument, while mallet blows are received on its head
- ❖ The blade is quadrangular (square) and flattened, gradually tapering towards the sharp end of the tip, which is equally beveled on the both sides to cut the bone
- ❖ It may be curved or straight
- ❖ Sterilization by autoclaving (Fig. 3).

How to Differentiate Chisel from an Osteotome?

Osteotome is beveled on both sides at sharp end of its blade, while chisel is beveled on one side only.

Uses

- ❖ During osteotomies for dividing (cutting) the bones like French osteotomy, McMurray's osteotomy, etc.
- ❖ While talking the bone graft, excision of exostosis, etc.
- ❖ For breaking the malunited fracture, before internal fixation
- ❖ During saucerization operation
- ❖ During fish-scaling of the bone surfaces, before bone grafting.

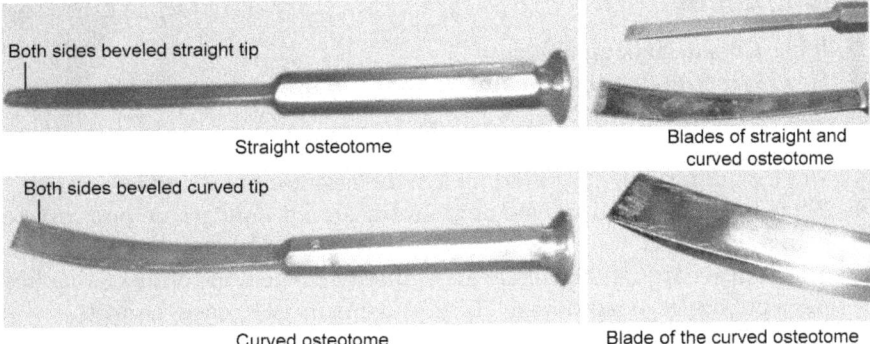

Fig. 3: Osteotomes.

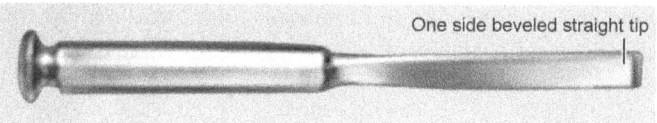

Fig. 4: Chisel.

CHISEL

- It has a head, shaft and blade
- Head and shaft or handle is similar to the osteotome and the only difference being at the tip of its blade, which is beveled on one side only while the other side is flat
- Beveled flat surface of the blade is in contact with the bone and the cutting edge is held obliquely, and the mallet is stuck on the head to remove a thick chunk of bone
- If the beveled surface is in contact with the bone while cutting, a thin slice of bone is removed
- Sterilization by autoclaving (Fig. 4).

Uses

- Used for cutting or shaping the bones
- To remove sleeves of bone for bone grafting
- During sequestrectomy, to enlarge the opening in the involucrum to reach the sequestrum
- Excision of exostosis, bony spur, osteomas, ossifying fibroma of maxilla, etc.
- Removing bone chips around screws and plates before removing them
- While removing excess callus in malunited fractures
- In chronic osteomyelitis for saucerization of the bone
- It can be used as an osteotome.

BONE GOUGE

- It has a head, shaft and blade
- Head is rounded, smooth, blunt and projecting to receive the blows of the mallet
- Shaft or handle is cylindrical and ridged for better grip of the instrument while working with it, by holding it in the nondominant hand
- Blade is trough like tunneled or grooved, curved, concave on one surface with a sharp end
- The concave trough like blade accommodates the bone chunks, that has been cut by the osteotome or chisel and ensure their easy removal
- Edge or tip of the blade is cutting and rounded
- Sterilization by autoclaving (Fig. 5).

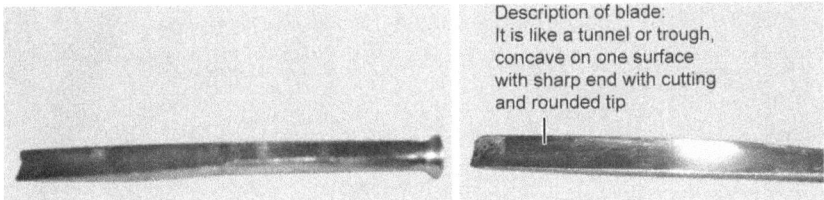

Description of blade:
It is like a tunnel or trough, concave on one surface with sharp end with cutting and rounded tip

Fig. 5: Bone gouge.

Uses

- For cutting out a gutter or hollow in the bone
- In chronic osteomyelitis for saucerization of the bone
- For drainage of the mastoid antrum
- To take out bone chips for bone grafting
- In orthoplasty and orthodesis
- In maxillary antrostomy
- In rhinoplasty
- While taking bone biopsy usually from the iliac crest
- To take out cortical bone just below the greater trochanter before guide wire is passed
- Drilling a bone in osteomyelitis for drainage of medullary cavity
- During hemiarthroplasty of the hip, it may be used to open the femoral medullary canal before starting of reaming.

BONE AWL OR BRADAWL

- It has a handle and blade
- The tip of the blade is sharp, pointed arrow head with a small eye or hole at its tip
- Through the eye wire or suture material can be threaded and drawn back
- Sterilization by autoclaving (Fig. 6).

Uses

- For suturing tendon to bones like patella and patellar tendon, triceps tendon to olecranon, where a wire is passed through the hole and the bone awl is used like a Cobbler's needle
- Before reduction of the malunited or old untreated fractures, medullary cavities of the bones are opened up by the arrow head of the bone awl and the fibrous plug from the fracture ends is removed which helps in healing of the fracture ends.

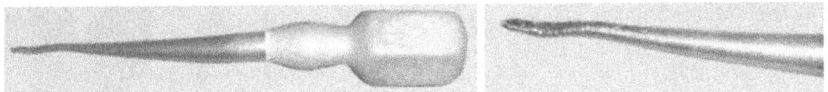

Fig. 6: Bone awl.

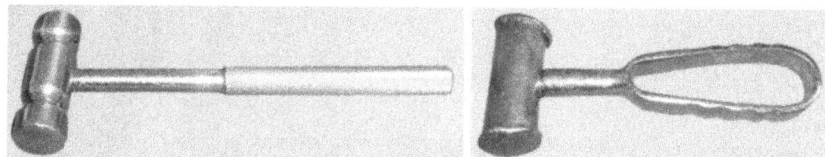

Fig. 7: Mallet.

MALLET

- It has a handle and head
- Handle is grooved or plain for firm holding of the instrument, while giving blows to the chisel or osteotome
- Head is heavy, blunt, cylindrical and flat ended for striking
- It is made up of steel or lead
- It is made up of metal, for sterilization and strength
- It is always held with the dominant hand while striking on the instrument (osteotome, chisel, bone gouge) or implant, which are steadied by the non-dominant hand
- Sterilization by autoclaving (Fig. 7).

Uses

- To strike on the chisel or bone gouge, for removing the bone chips
- To strike the osteotome, while dividing the bone during osteotomies
- To drive or insert guidewire and nail, in internal fixation of the fractures via a punch.

PUNCH

- It has a handle and head
- One end of the punch is kept on the inserted nail and head is stucked by the hammer
- It is cylindrical in shape
- It is cannulated, so that it can be used with guidewire in situ
- Sterilization by autoclaving (Fig. 8).

Uses

To hammer the nail inside the bone through the hole made by the trifin osteotome, while internal fixation of the fractured fragments of the bone.

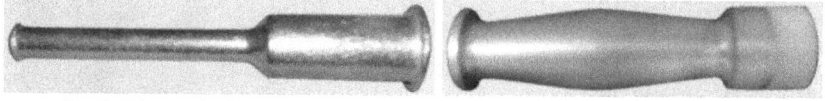

Punch to be stucked by a mallet   Hand punch to be stucked by hand

Fig. 8: Punch.

Chapter 21: Orthopedics Instruments **117**

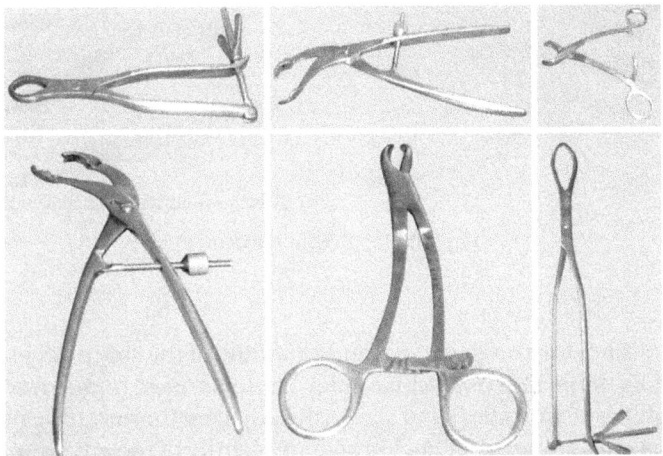

Fig. 9: Various types of bone holding forceps.

BONE HOLDING FORCEPS

- It is strong and stout instrument
- It has handle, pivot type of joint and blades. No catch
- Handle may be serrated for providing firm grip to the instrument while working with it
- Blades are short, hollow and curved and may have sharp teeth at its tip for better grip of the tissue (bone) held in it. They are curved to accommodate the bone in between the blades
- Sterilization by autoclaving (Fig. 9).

Uses

- To hold and fix the bone during open reduction of the fracture, amputation of the extremity, while plating and nailing the bones
- To steady the bone while reaming, cutting, nibbling or drilling a bone
- To fix the maxilla during maxillectomy.

BONE CUTTING FORCEPS OR BONE SHEARS

- It is a strong and stout instrument designed for cutting bone. It has a handle, pivot type of joint and blades
- It may be simple or double action with lever arrangement (single or double fulcrum), which gives mechanical advantage
- Double fulcrum is useful to augment and multiply the force applied (double action)
- Handle is ridged for better grip of the instrument
- Blades are triangular, having sharp edge for cutting the bone
- Blades may be straight or angled (curved)
- Sterilization by autoclaving (Fig. 10).

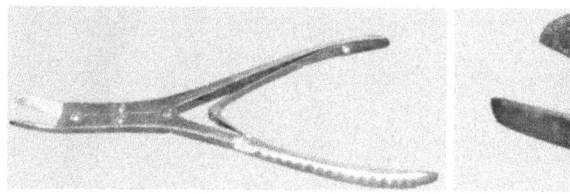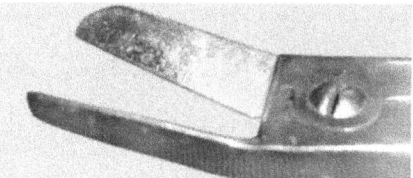

Triangular blades with sharp cutting edges

Fig. 10: Bone cutting forceps.

Uses

- To smoothen the rough surface and rounding of the sharp edges of the cut bones, as projecting bony spikes may cause damage to the overlying skin and soft tissue (muscles) and also to the adjacent important structures like artery, vein and nerve in the immediate vicinity of the cut bone
- To cut through the involucrum during sequestrectomy
- To remove the bony spur
- To remove the styloid process
- To cut the small as well as long thin bones like phalanges, metatarsals, metacarpals, fibula, spinous process of the vertebrae, etc.

BONE NIBBLER OR BONE NIBBLING FORCEPS

- It has a handle, pivot type of joint and blades
- Available in various sizes and lengths and may have single or double fulcrum
- Blades may have straight or curved ends
- Blades are cup shaped, hollow with sharp edges to cut a small regular piece of bone at a time from edge and tip of the blade
- Sterilization by autoclaving (Fig. 11).

Uses

- Primarily designed to enlarge the burr hole, done by Hudson's brace during craniectomy
- Removing or shapping of the bones for any purpose
- To cut the lamina, during laminectomy
- To remove bony spur, after rib resection

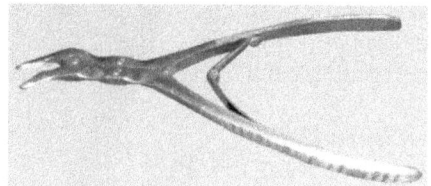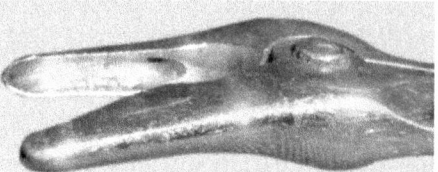

Blades are cup shaped, hollow with sharp edges

Fig. 11: Bone nibbler.

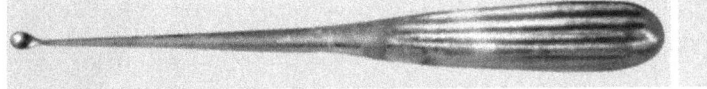
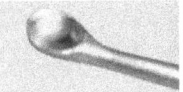

Volkmann's scoop with serrated handle   Spoon like trough end

Fig. 12: Volkmann's scoop.

- To nibble the amputated stump of the bone, to make it smooth, so that it does not injure the surrounding soft tissue
- Removing adherent soft tissues from the removed bone graft pieces, before placing them to the recipient area, to prevent rejection of the graft.

VOLKMANN'S SPOON OR SCOOP

- It is a long metallic instrument
- It has a handle with serrations for better grip and has sharp edged, curved, spoon like trough at its end (Fig. 12).

Uses

- To curette or scrape the wall of the cavities of benign tumors like bone cysts, benign giant cell tumors, aneurysmal bone cysts, etc.
- Scraping osteomyelitic cavities or Brodie's abscess
- To remove the immature callus and fibrous tissue from neglected fracture ends of bone, so as to freshen them before attempting reduction of the fracture
- To curette and freshen a sinus or fistulous tract during their excision
- To curette an ulcer, to remove the excess granulation tissue before skin grafting.

GIGLI'S WIRE SAW

- It has 2–4 strong wires of flexible metal (stainless steel) 15–20 inches long twisted together, which works like a saw
- Two handles with hook, to which ends of wire are anchored
- The introducer is passed through ends of the loop of the wire (Fig. 13).

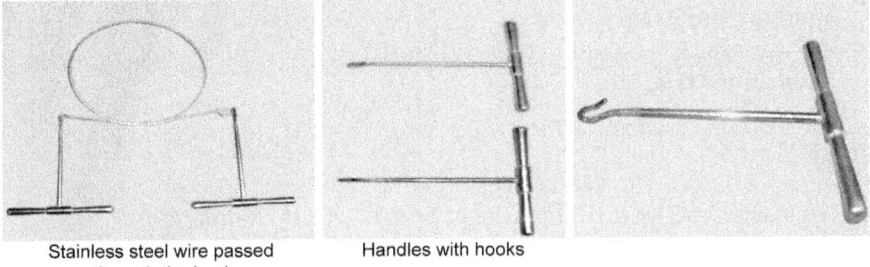

Stainless steel wire passed through the hook   Handles with hooks

Fig. 13: Gigli's wire saw.

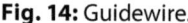

Fig. 14: Guidewire.

Uses

- To cut the bone quickly at a desired level during amputation of extremities with minimum working space, without injuring the adjacent soft tissue
- During hemimandibulectomy
- It also allows division of bones situated at depth.

GUIDEWIRE

- Its one end is sharp trocar pointed, while other end is blunt and has cylindrical shaft in between the ends
- It has sharp tip for its easy introduction, while its other end fits to a metal handle
- It is thin and strong, so that it should not break
- Available in various sizes and graduated in ¼" or centimeters
- It is passed under radiological control (C-arm) through neck of the femur, after reduction of the fracture segments
- Length of the nail is calculated by measuring the length of the guidewire outside (Fig. 14).

Uses

It determines the central position of head and neck, and over it nail is guided and hammered, it means it guides the insertion of the nail.

HAND DRILL

- It has a handle which has finger grip impression and it has to be held with the nondominant hand
- Another rotating handle is present by virtue of its rotatory movements, the bone is drilled for K-wire insertion, to make screw holes, by attaching the guidewire to its tip
- Nowadays, it has been replaced by electrical drill except for certain indications (Fig. 15).

Uses

- To insert the K-wire for internal or percutaneous fixation
- In drilling screw holes, for insertion of screws during fracture fixation
- To drill holes, for Schanz pins for external fixation.

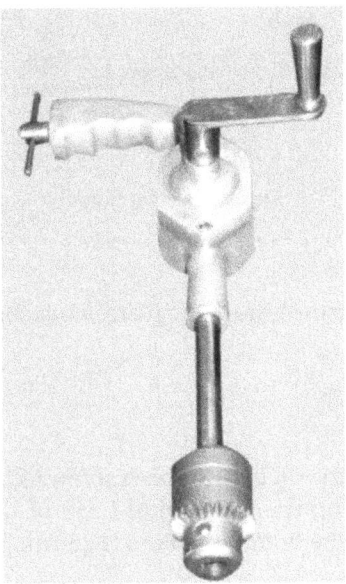

Fig. 15: Hand drill.

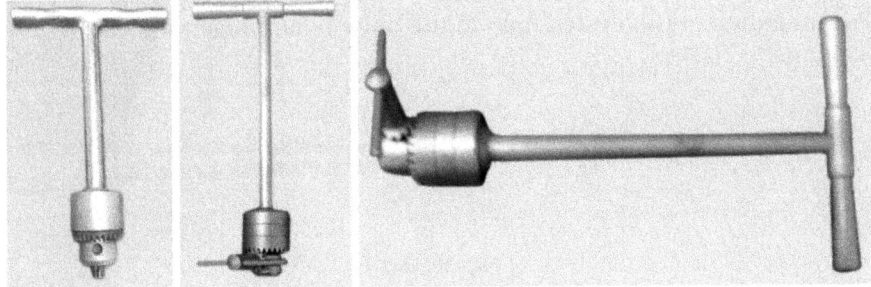

Fig. 16: 'T' handle.

■ 'T' HANDLE OR CHUCK HANDLE FOR INSERTING GUIDEWIRE

❖ Guidewire is inserted through the cannulated 'T' handle
❖ It is provided with a key for tightening, to hold the guidewire (Fig. 16).

Uses

❖ While inserting a guide-wire, K-wire during intramedullary interlock nailing
❖ It can be used to hold the reamer.

■ DRILL BIT GUIDE

❖ It has a handle and a shaft
❖ Shaft is attached to the handle at an angle, and is hollow
❖ Handle is fenestrated to make the instrument light (Fig. 17).

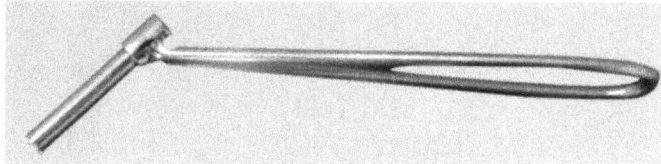

Fig. 17: Drill bit guide.

Uses

To guide the drill bit into the hole of the plate, while making holes in the bone.

■ TAP

- ❖ Its like a 'T'
- ❖ It has a handle and the tip of the limb is screw like
- ❖ It is used by holding the horizontal limb of the 'T' and by rotating movements of it by the dominant hand (Fig. 18).

Uses

For threading of the drilled hole in the bone before inserting a screw for fixation.

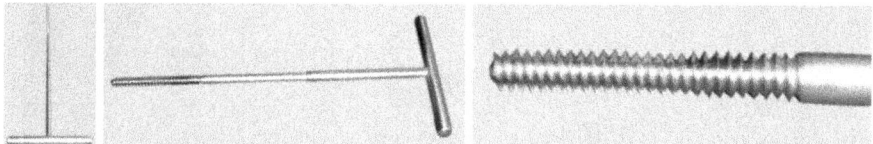

Fig. 18: Tap.

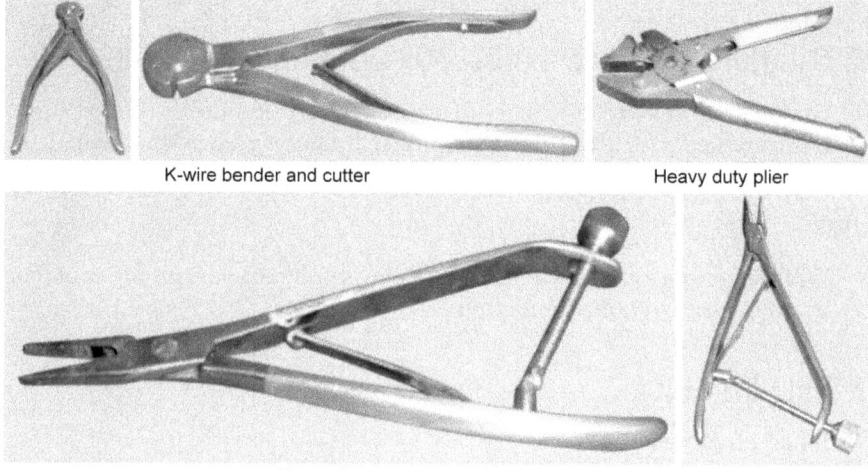

K-wire bender and cutter　　　　　　Heavy duty plier

Nose plier

Fig. 19: K-wire bender and cutter, heavy duty plier and Nose plier.

■ K-WIRE BENDER AND CUTTER HEAVY DUTY PLIER NOSE PLIER

Uses of K-wire Bender and Cutter, Heavy Duty Plier and Nose Plier
- ❖ For extraction of K-wire
- ❖ Prebending and contouring of the plates (Fig. 19).

CHAPTER
22
Orthopedics Implants

■ PLATES

- ❖ Made up of stainless steel, vitallium or titanium
- ❖ They are of different shapes like straight or angled and flat or tubular
- ❖ Holes in the plates may be round or oval and are arranged in rows or staggered
- ❖ Fragments of fractured bone are arranged in correct alignment before fixing the plate
- ❖ Plate of appropriate size is kept on the aligned bone fragments with minimum two holes lying over each fracture fragment
- ❖ Plate is fixed in place by drilling through each hole
- ❖ Screw of correct size should be selected
- ❖ Sterilization by autoclaving.
- ❖ Different varieties of plates are dynamic compression plate, low contact dynamic compression plate, reconstruction plate, locking plate, etc. (Fig. 1).

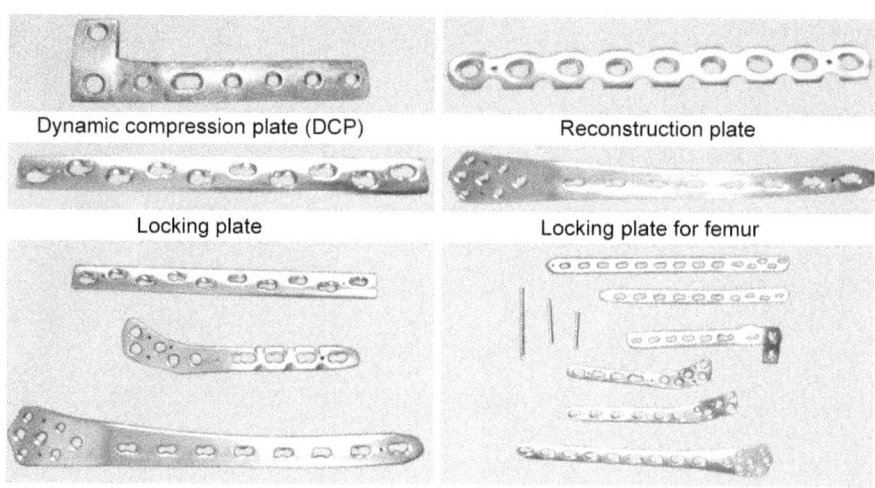

Dynamic compression plate (DCP)　　Reconstruction plate

Locking plate　　Locking plate for femur

Locking plates for different bones　　Locking plates and locking screws

Fig. 1: Plates.

Dynamic Compression Plate (DCP)

Screw holes in this plate are sloped in such a way that screw tightening through the holes causes the plate to move at 90° to the direction of the descending screw, thus effecting compression at the fracture site. Used in fracture shaft of radius, ulna, humerus, and sometimes femur and tibia.

Low Contact Dynamic Compression Plate (LCDCP)

Designed to preserve periosteal vascularity, which is impaired with DCP.

Reconstruction Plate

It can be moulded or bent in all planes. Useful in distal humerus fracture, clavicle fracture, etc.

Locking Plate

It has two conjoined holes—one of which can be used for locking screw insertion. It has advantage of good structural length, even when the screw has uncortical bone purchase making it very useful for osteoporotic bones. Useful in fractures of proximal humerus, distal and proximal tibia, distal femur. Nowadays, these types of plates are commonly used.

Uses

To hold and give mechanical support to the aligned fragments of fractured bone mostly at the ends of the bones, and transmit forces from one end of the bone to the other, protecting and bypassing the fracture site (load bearing implant).

SCREWS

- ❖ Screws are inserted into the predrilled and tapped holes
- ❖ Different varieties of screws are cortical, cancellous, malleolar, herbet (headless) (Fig. 2).

Uses

- ❖ Fixing plates to the correctly aligned fractured segments of the bone, as 'positioning screw'
- ❖ Also as a 'lag screw' for interfragmentary compression.

PROSTHESIS FOR HIP HEMIARTHROPLASTY

Commonly two varieties of prosthesis are used:
1. Austin Moore's prosthesis
2. Thompson's prosthesis

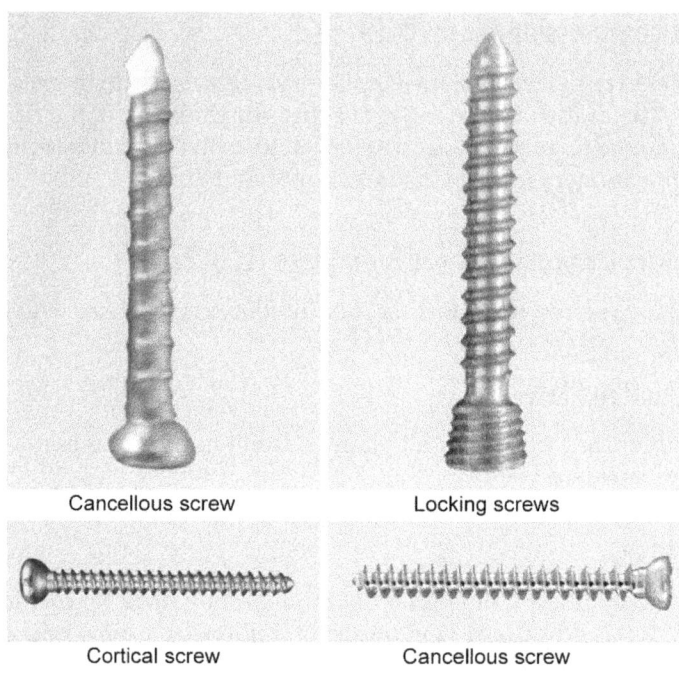

Fig. 2: Screws.

They are available in various sizes, according to the diameter of the head and the sizes being imprinted on the stem.

■ AUSTIN MOORE'S PROSTHESIS (AMP)

- ❖ This is a self-locking type of variety
- ❖ It has head, neck, collar, shoulder and stem
- ❖ Head is spherical in shape, which fits into the acetabulum like the head of the femur
- ❖ Neck is constriction just below the head
- ❖ Collar sits on the calcar femorale of femoral neck after its proper insertion. It has a small hole placed laterally, which is used for extraction of prosthesis when required, and also for assessing and controlling anteversion of the prosthesis, done by inserting a Steinman pin or straight artery forceps through the hole, when the prosthesis is inserted into the proximal femoral medullary cavity
- ❖ The shoulder is sharp edged, which snugly fits into the medullary part of the greater trochanter and prevents rotation of the prosthesis within the medullary canal
- ❖ The stem is inserted into the medullary canal of the femur. It is quadrangular in cross section which prevents rotation. The tip is smooth, blunt and tapering, which prevents accidental fracture of the lateral femoral cortex if not inserted. It has two fenestrations, which makes the prosthesis lighter

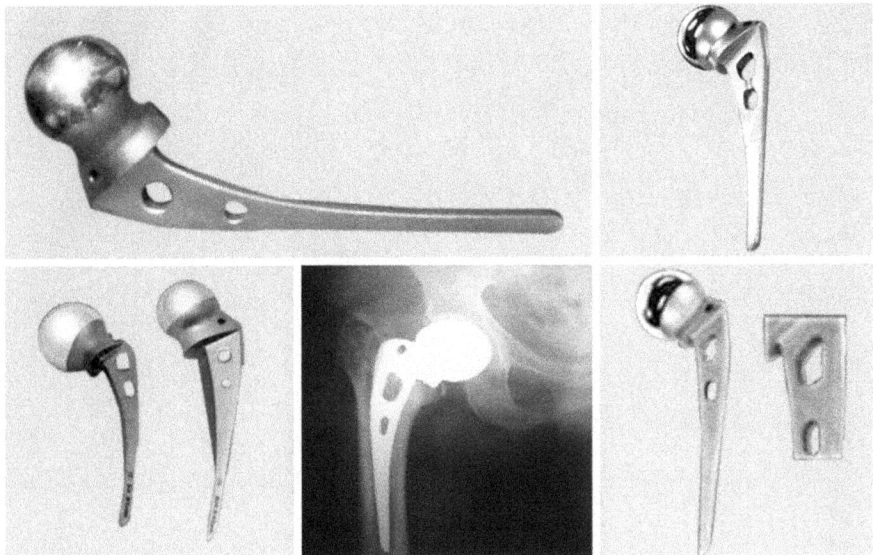

Fig. 3: Austin Moore's prosthesis.

and also make it self-locking, because it allows bone growth through the fenestrations, which locks the prosthesis and fixes it rigidly
- About 1.25 cm of calcar femorale must be present for AMP prosthesis, if not then, Thompson's prosthesis should be used
- Disadvantage of hip hemiarthroplasty operation is that after 10–12 years, joint-congruency will loss and there will be limitation of mobility, along with pain at the hip, which may require total hip replacement later on
- Sterilization by autoclaving (Fig. 3).

Indications/Uses

For hemiarthroplasty, in hip operation for fracture neck of the femur. Primarily indicated in case of old fracture of neck of femur of more than 3 weeks duration in elderly persons (more than 65 years of age), where the chances of union of the fracture segments is very little, as 3 weeks have already passed and the patient mostly has poor general health.

THOMPSON'S PROSTHESIS

- Similar to AMP, with minor differences like, it has no fenestrations in the stem and no hole in the collar, and also not having the shoulder. So it is not a self-locking variety of prosthesis like AMP
- It is always used with bone cement for its firm fixation, so it is very difficult to extract or remove, when required. But the advantage of using bone cement is that, very early mobilization and weight bearing can be started, as early as on 2nd or 3rd postoperative day
- Sterilization by autoclaving (Fig. 4).

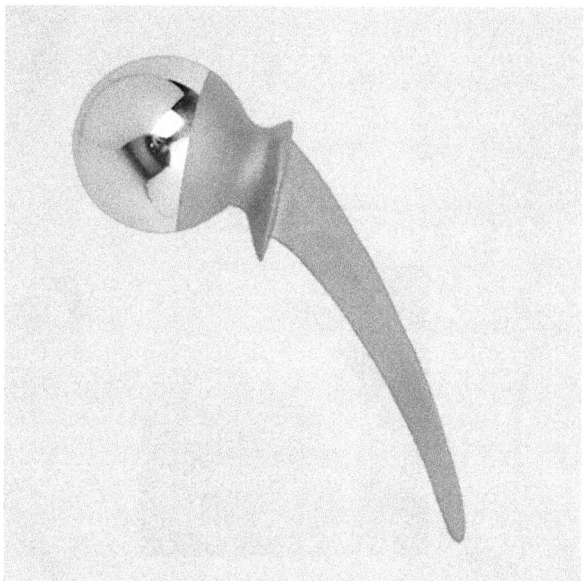

Fig. 4: Thompson's prosthesis.

Indications/Uses

Used for hemiarthroplasty, in hip operation for fracture neck of the femur. Primarily indicated in case of old fracture of neck of femur of more than 3 weeks duration in elderly persons (more than 65 years of age), where the chances of union of the fracture segments is very little, as 3 weeks have already passed and the patient mostly has poor general health, when the length of calcar femorale is less than 1 cm.

■ BIPOLAR PROSTHESIS

- ❖ These prosthesis has polyethylene cuff over the head of the femur, so acetabulum does not get destroyed like in case of AMP and Thompson's prosthesis
- ❖ It may be modular or nonmodular
- ❖ Modular prosthesis can be dismantled into components
- ❖ Modular bipolar prosthesis can be converted to total hip arthoplasty, simply by changing the acetabulum (Fig. 5).

■ INTRAMEDULLARY NAILS (IM NAILS)

Nowadays, these nails are routinely used in clinical practice for fracture of shaft of long bones.

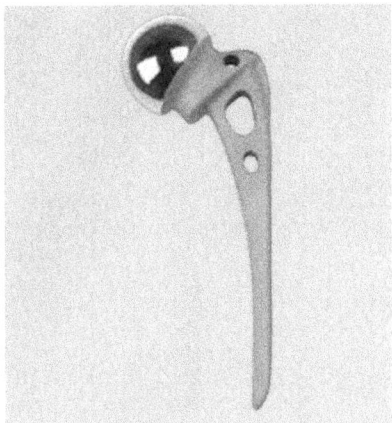

Fig. 5: Bipolar prosthesis.

The principles for fracture fixation by an intramedullary nail are:
1. 3 point fixation: A straight nail is introduced in a curved canal.
2. It is a load shearing implant.
3. It allows for dynamization and compression at the fracture site, which hastens healing.

The interlocking nails of femur, tibia and humerus have two eyes or fenestrations at both the ends (total 4 on a nail), which are used for fixing the nail.

- IM interlocking nails for femur, are cylindrical in cross section, curved anterolaterally and having both ends blunt
- IM interlocking nails for tibia, are cylindrical in cross section, slightly angulated (13°) or bend at proximal 1/3rd, i.e. at the junction of upper 1/3rd and lower 2/3rd of the nail and having both the ends blunt
- IM interlocking nails for humerus, are cylindrical in cross section, slightly angulated at proximal 1/3rd, and having both ends blunt
- IM nails for ulna are squared in cross section, straight and its one end is blunt, while the other end is sharp pointed
- IM nails for radius, are square in cross section, straight and its one end is blunt, while the other end is beveled and smooth (Fig. 6).

RUSH NAIL

- Available in different diameters and lengths
- Its one end is beveled and the other end is bent like a hockey stick, and having cylindrical shaft in between them
- Hockey stick like end prevents migration of the nail intraosseously. It also provides grip for its easy extraction, when required
- The beveled end easily and smoothly goes into the medullary canal, when hammered
- It does not prevent rotational movements at the fracture site, as there is no interlocking mechanism as in the IM interlocking nails (Fig. 7).

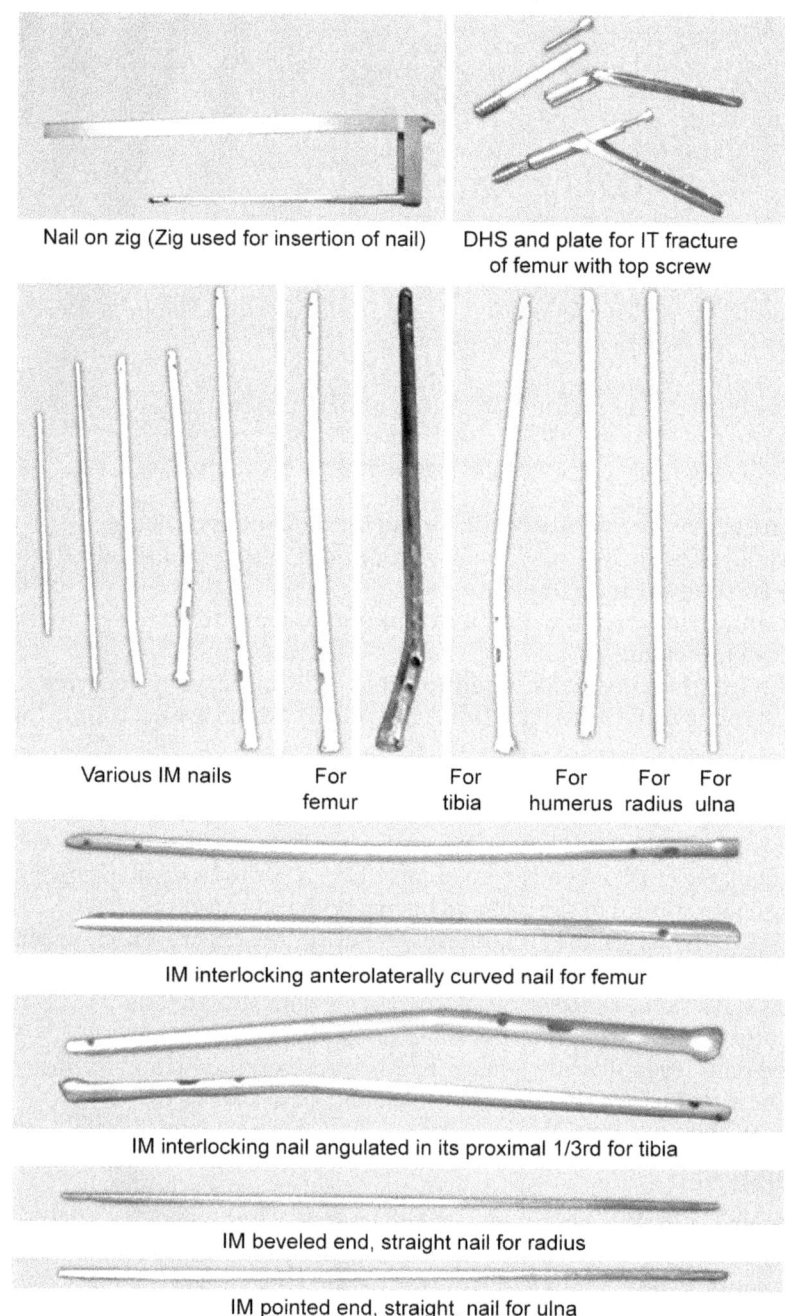

Fig. 6: Intramedullary nails.

Chapter 22: Orthopedics Implants

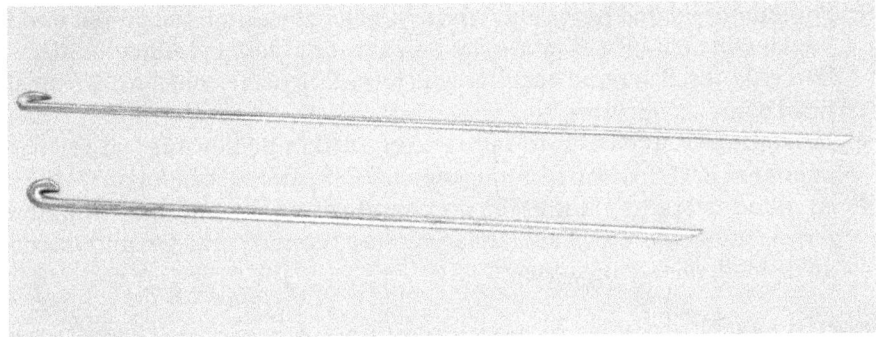

Fig. 7: Rush nail.

Uses

- In definitive fixation of fractures like fracture both-bones forearm
- Fracture fibula in distal 1/3rd
- Rarely used for distal humeral fracture dislocation.

K-WIRE

- Most commonly used implant in orthopedic surgery
- Available in various diameters from 1 mm to 3 mm
- It has sharp trocar pointed ends and cylindrical shaft in between the two sharp ends
- Some nails may have diamond-shaped pointed ends
- It has to be drilled (inserted) using high speed power drill, as hand drills may bend the wire (Fig. 8).

Uses

- For definitive fixation of the fractures, after their reduction like supracondylar and lateral condyle fracture of the humerus in a child, fracture metatarsals and metacarpals, fractures radial neck, percutaneous fixation of Colles' fracture, fracture of surgical neck humerus, etc.

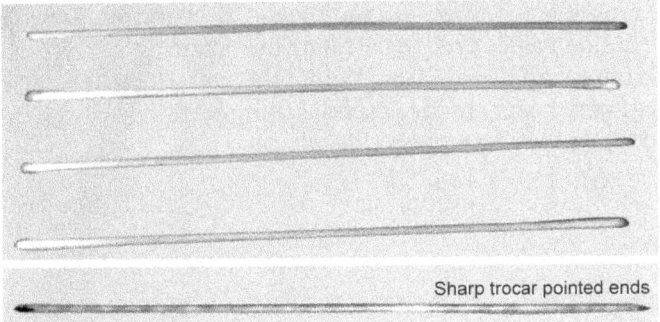

Fig. 8: K-wire.

- ❖ For temporary and provisional fixation before selecting the proper sized implant for definitive fixation of fractures around knee and elbow like distal humerus, distal femoral fractures with intra-articular extensions, proximal tibial complex fractures, etc.
- ❖ In fixation of navicular to tallus after Turco's posteromedial release operation in CTEV, also in application of JESS external fixation in CTEV
- ❖ As an adjuvant implant in tension band wiring operations of fracture patella, olecranon, supracondylar fracture humerus, medial and lateral ankle malleoli fractures, etc.

KUNTSCHER'S INTRAMEDULLARY NAIL (K-NAIL)

- ❖ German surgeon Kuntscher made this nail for fixing fracture of shaft femur
- ❖ It is hollow incomplete tube and there is a slot or gap in the circumference of the whole of the nail which allows it to bend slightly on the tensile surface of the femur (anterolateral)
- ❖ As it is hollow, it maintains bone marrow continuity and preserves bone nutrition, and also allows guidewire to pass, when it is used
- ❖ It has clover-leaf cross section, which prevents its rotation within the medullary cavity
- ❖ It has two blunt ends, which reduces the chances of cortical break while insertion
- ❖ It has one eye or fenestration at each end (total two eyes on the nail) which are used for extraction of the nail, by inserting the hook of the nail extractor into the eye
- ❖ Medullary cavity is reamed over a guidewire, sometimes from one end after aligning the ends until cavity is uniform
- ❖ Nail of correct size, correct diameter should be used
- ❖ A guidewire is driven along medullary canal through the end of bone and approached through the skin incision. Nail is passed over this and driven down the medullary canal through the fractured site after it has been reduced into the distal fragment
- ❖ Clinically, the length of the nail is calculated by measuring length from the tip of the greater trochanter to the lateral knee joint minus 2 cm taken on the non-affected thigh and radiologically by digital X-rays, with exact magnification values used to calculate the length
- ❖ Splintering of the cortex, migration of the nail, stuck nail, fat embolism, breakage of the nail, are the potential complications
- ❖ Nowadays, not used routinely (Fig. 9).

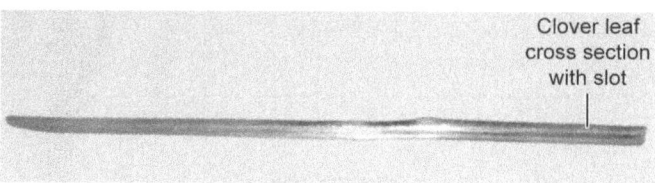

Fig. 9: K-nail.

Uses

For fixation of diaphyseal fractures of the femoral shaft.

S-P NAIL

- It was designed by Smith Peterson, so its name
- On cross section, it is three flanged
- Various modifications are there now
- It is available in different sizes: 4½ inches – 5¼ inches
- It is triflanged, each flange is 0.3 cm thick (1/8 inches). Flanges are thin to minimize destruction of spongy bone during insertion
- The flanges are meant for taking a hold in the surrounding bone and prevent rotational strain at the fracture site
- It has a central canal to pass guidewire and nail can be 'threaded' on a guidewire
- Cannulated nail can stand more stress than solid nail
- Sharp conical tip
- Circular flat base has grooves for screw or nailing and plating. Made up of an inert alloy
- Triflanged nail permits maximum surface of nail in contact with the bone fragments and fixed properly, also it causes less bone destruction. Originally designed nail was cylindrical
- Its position should be confirmed by plain X-ray by AP and lateral views or with C-arm during operation, if available
- Not used nowadays (Fig. 10).

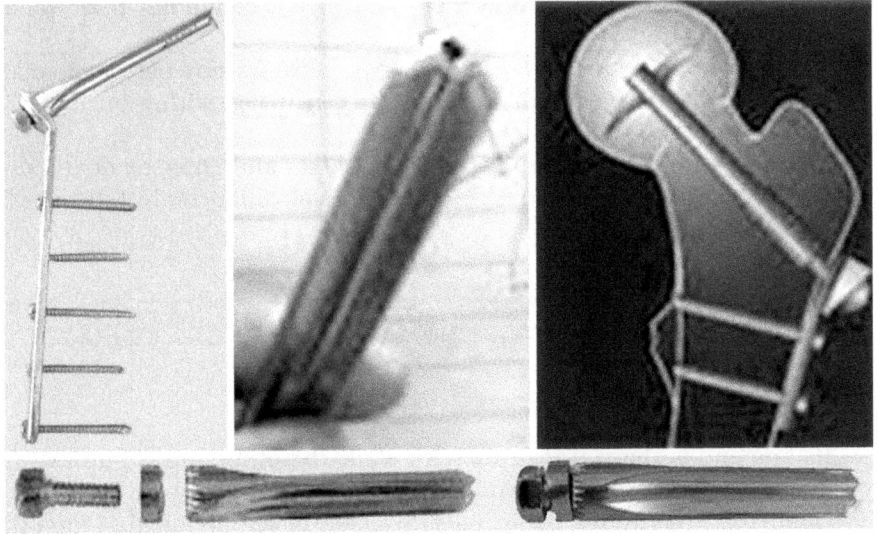

Fig. 10: S-P nail.

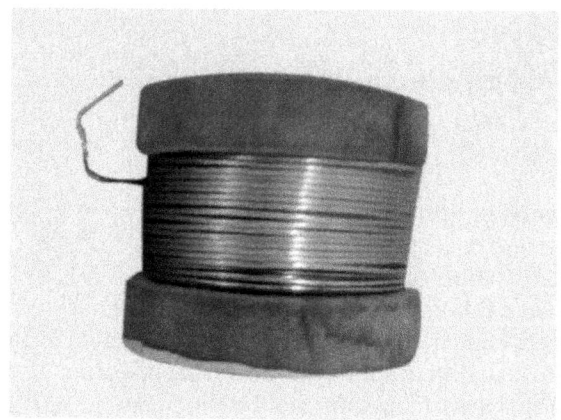

Fig. 11: Stainless steel wire.

Uses

For internal fixation of the fracture neck of the femur.

STAINLESS STEEL WIRE

- It is extremely inert
- Available in different sizes from 6 to 5-0 (Fig. 11).

Uses

- Closure of midline sternotomy incision, which is commonly performed in CVTS surgeries
- In orthopedic operations, for suturing bones like fracture patella, medial malleolus of tibia, olecranon fracture, bone encirclage wiring, etc.
- Interdental wiring or fracture mandible
- Earlier used in herniorrhaphy for hernia repair and Thiersch operation done for anal encirclement in case of rectal prolapse, but not used nowadays.

BOHLER'S PIN (STEINMANN) WITH ROTATING STIRRUP

STEINMANN PIN

- Its one end is sharp trocar pointed, while the other end is blunt with quadrangular cross section and having rounded smooth shaft
- Diameter varies from 4-6 mm and is available in various lengths (Fig. 12).

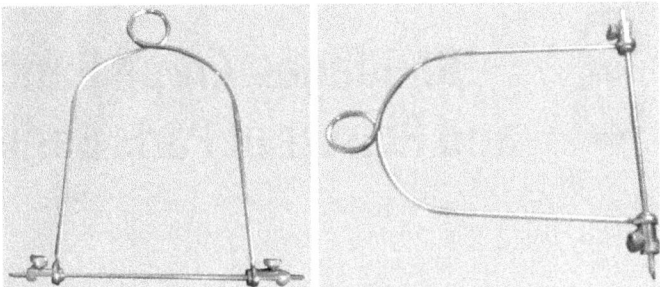

Fig. 12: Steinmann pin with rotating stirrup.

BOHLER'S STIRRUP

- It is 'U' shaped and has a rounded crossing loop for inserting and tying the nylon traction cord and the 2 ends of the limbs of the 'U' are used to fix the Steinman pin through the stirrup
- Steinman pin is drilled through the bone under local anesthesia and traction is applied through the stirrup, which can rotate freely on the pin. This enables to alter the line or direction of traction, according to the need of the patient, without rotating or moving the pin within the bone
- The pin exercises direct pull on the lower fragment, and displacement like backward angulation and rotation can easily be corrected
- The point at which the pin enters the bone should lie away from the joint, so that joint does not suffer
- The sites where skeletal traction can be given are proximal tibial, distal femoral, distal tibial and calcaneal
- Pin tract infection, physical injury, damage to the adjacent nerve, ligamentous damage are the potential complications of inserting Steinman pin.

Uses of Steinmann Pin

Mainly used for giving skeletal traction to the limbs, mostly lower limbs.

May be Used

- For fracture reduction and internal fixation of the fracture segments
- For external fixation.

CHAPTER 23

Bandages, Crepe Bandages and Plaster of Paris Bandages

■ COTTON BANDAGES

- ❖ Bandage is defined as 'a piece of material used to cover, support, immobilize or exert pressure to a part of the body'
- ❖ A roller bandage is defined as 'a length of material wound into a compact firm roll'
- ❖ Various lengths and sizes are in use, according to the part to which the bandage is to be applied and the need (Fig. 1).

Uses

- ❖ As a first aid measure in the treatment of the injured, particularly to control bleeding by compression
- ❖ To protect a surgical wound, against infection
- ❖ To hold surgical dressings or other local applications in place
- ❖ To hold the splint securely
- ❖ To prevent or reduce swelling by compression.

■ COTTON CREPE BANDAGE (ELASTOCREPE)

- ❖ This is smooth surface cotton crepe bandage, which provides greater compression and support then the ordinary crepe bandage

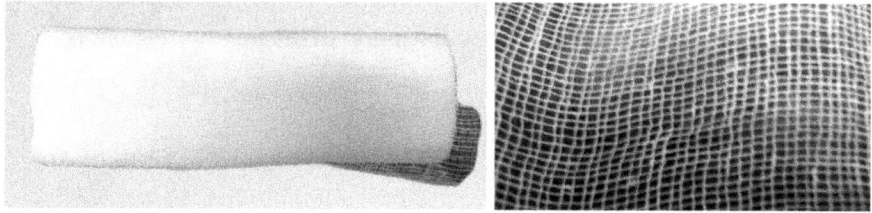

Fig. 1: Open-weave cotton bandage.

Chapter 23: Bandages, Crepe Bandages and Plaster of Paris Bandages

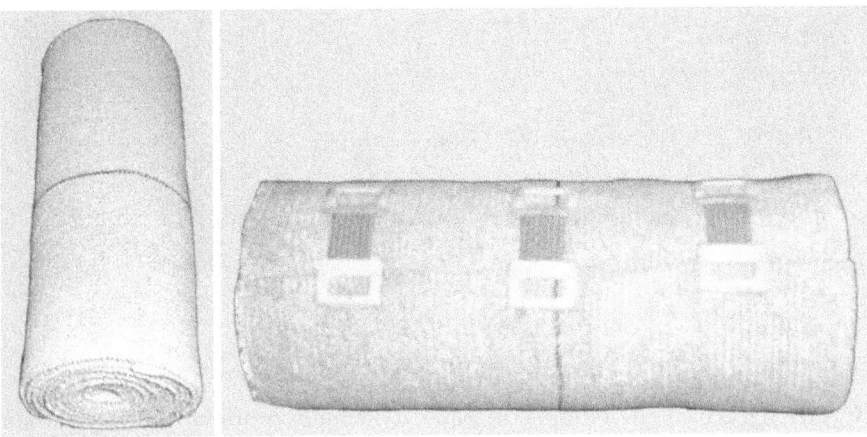

Fig. 2: Crepe bandage.

- It is light and woven
- Various sizes as per its width like 3/4/6 inches
- It has considerable elasticity, and it stretches to nearly twice of its length, but regains its original length readily
- This elasticity gives firm, but controlled compression
- It can be incorporated with strong rubber threads which provide even greater compression and support than the cotton crepe bandage
- 'Blue line' woven into the center of the bandage and running throughout, provides a visual guide to the amount of overlap, that should be allowed in the application of the bandage (Fig. 2).

Uses

- For compression bandaging, in case of sprain
- For compression dressing, to control bleeding
- In case of varicose veins of the leg. It is applied from the great toe towards the knee, after emptying the lower limb veins by elevating the leg
- To prevent or reduce the swelling by compression in soft tissue inflammation or contusion
- To assist in the correction of the deformity
- To immobilize a part or restrict its movement
- To afford support to the part of the body.

■ PLASTER OF PARIS BANDAGE

- It is machine made, plaster of Paris impregnated bandage of 3/4/6 inches width
- Chemical name is 'hemihydrated salt of calcium sulfate' ($CaSO_4 \cdot 1/2H_2O_2$)

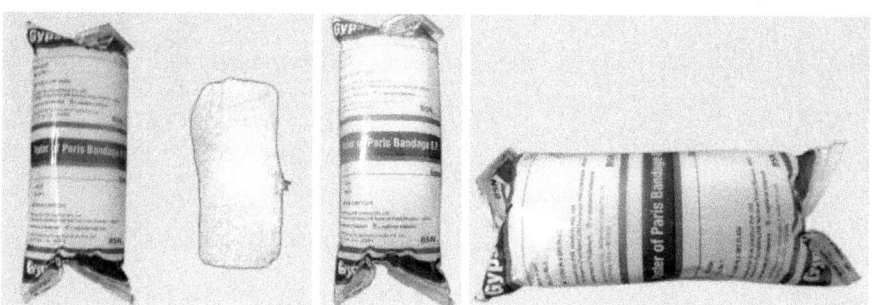

Fig. 3: Plaster of Paris bandage.

- When it is soaked or dipped in water, it becomes mouldable first and then becomes hard due to exothermic reaction. The anhydrous hemihydrated salt of calcium sulfate converted to hydrated calcium sulfate (Gypsum) (Fig. 3).

$$CaSO_4 \cdot 1/2H_2O + 1/2H_2O \longrightarrow CaSO_4 \cdot H_2O$$

Uses

- As a cast or slab for definitive or temporary treatment, after correction of any fracture or dislocation, correction of deformities, etc.
- To immobilize a skin grafted part of the body near a joint, to prevent the accidental graft removal by joint movements.

Section 6

Suture Materials Used in Surgical Practice

Section Outline

24. Classification and Description of Suture Materials
25. Needles
26. Different Types of Suture Materials

CHAPTER 24
Classification and Description of Suture Materials

■ INTRODUCTION

Sutures are used in the surgical practice, to hold the approximated tissue, till the normal process of healing is complete.

■ CLASSIFICATION OR TYPES

Depending on the Source or Origin

Natural
- They are obtained from the natural resources and protein in nature
- Their absorption is by cellular response
- They are having less tensile strength, than synthetic suture material.

Example: Catgut, silk, linen, cotton.

Synthetic
- They are made artificially and carbohydrate in nature
- They get absorbed in tissue by hydrolytic action
- They are having higher strength than natural suture material.

Example: Vicryl (Polyglactin 910 or polyglycolic acid), vicryl rapide, monocryl, PDS, dexon, prolene (Polypropylene), nylon, monofilament polyamide (Ethilon), polyester (Ethibond), metallic wires.

Depending on the of the Suture Material in the Tissues

Absorbable Sutures
These sutures get absorbed in the tissues either by enzymatic digestion or by phagocytosis.
1. **Natural absorbable sutures:** Plain and chromic catgut.
2. **Synthetic absorbable sutures:** Polyglycolic acid (Dexon), polyglactin 910 (Vicryl), polyglactin 910 rapide (Vicryl rapide), poliglecaprone 25 (Monocryl), polydioxanone (PDS).

Non-Absorbable Sutures

These sutures remain in the tissues for indefinite period without getting absorbed.
1. **Natural non-absorbable sutures:** Silk, linen thread, cotton.
2. **Synthetic non-absorbable sutures:** Polypropylene (Prolene), monofilament polyamide (Ethilon), polyester (Ethibond), nylon.

Depending on the Number of Strands in the Suture Materials

Monofilament

- It consists of single strand of fiber
- It is smooth and strong, and chances of bacterial contamination are less
- It is stiff like wire, so knotting property is not good. The knot tide looses easily and slips, so at least 6–8 throws needed while suturing and knotting this type of suture to secure the knot from slipping.

Example: Polypropylene, catgut, polyamide (Ethilon), polydioxanone (PDS), monocryl, etc.

Polyfilament

- It consists of multiple strands of fibers braided together
- It is easier to handle, and the knot tied does not slip, so 2–3 knots are sufficient to secure a knot
- Disadvantage of this suture is that, bacteria may lodge in the crevices of the sutures, so chances of infection of the wound are more, if this suture is used as compared to the monofilament, and so these sutures are not suitable in presence of infection.

Example: Silk, linen, polyglycolic acid (Dexon), polyglactin 910 (Vicryl), polyester (Ethibond), etc.

Characteristic of an Ideal Suture Material

It should have:
- Adequate tensile strength, to maintain the tissue approximation till healing of the tissue takes place
- Incite minimal tissue reaction
- Easy handling property
- Smooth for passage of suture through the tissue causing less trauma to the tissue
- Good knotting quality or security
- Nonallergenic and noncarcinogenic

Chapter 24: Classification and Description of Suture Materials

- It should not have memory (inherent capability of suture to return or maintain its original shape as it has been kept in the foil pack)
- Easily available and cost effective or cheap.

Descriptions of Different Labeling in a Foil Pack

Suture materials are provided in a sterile pack.

Number of Suture Material

- Number of suture material, indicates thickness of the suture
- Depending on the thickness of the suture, the No. may be 2, 1, 0, 1-0, 2-0, 3-0, 4-0, etc.
- Higher the number, thicker the suture, like No. 2 is thicker than 1
- But, if '0' is prefixed by the higher numbers, then the sutures become finer or less thick, like 3-0 is finer and thinner than 2-0 suture.

Type of Suture in the Pack

Absorbable or nonabsorbable, chemical name of the suture and brand name of the suture (which may vary according to manufacturer).

Length of the Suture Material in the Pack

Variable length like 45 cm, 76 cm, 90 cm, 152 cm, etc.

Description of the Needle

- Most of the needles are curved and atraumatic (eyeless), as the suture is inserted or imbricated at the end of the needle by special technique
- May be of different sizes according to their length like 16 mm, 22 mm, 30 mm, 40 mm, 45 mm, etc.
- May have different curvatures like half circle (1/2), 3/8th circle, 1/4th circle, 5/8th circle
- Depending on the type of sharp end it may be: Round body, cutting, reverse cutting, blunt tip, taper cut.

Other Descriptions which are not Necessary to Mention in the Examinations

- Name of the manufacturer
- Manufacturer license No., manufacture date, expiry date
- Price of the pack
- Company code for a particular suture
- Lot No. or batch No. of the suture.

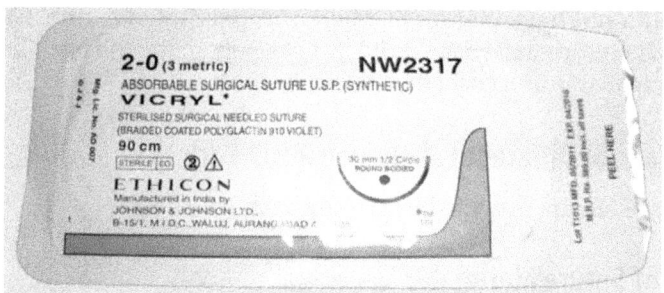

Fig. 1: Sterilized suture pack containing polyglactin (VICRYL) No. 2-0.

How to Describe the Suture Material in the Foil Pack?

This is a sterile suture pack containing synthetic absorbable suture, no. 2-0, polyglactin 910, on a atraumatic, 1/2 circle, round bodied needle, with needle length of 30 mm and suture length of 90 cm, made by company ethicon, by trade name 'VICRYL' (Fig. 1).

CHAPTER 25

Needles

INTRODUCTION

Made up of stainless steel.
It has three parts: Point, shaft and eye.

Classification

- **According to the shape:** Straight or curved
  - *If curved:* Half (1/2) circle, 5/8th circle, 3/8th circle, 1/4 th circle
- **According to the edge:** Cutting or noncutting (round body)
- **According to the tip:** Triangular or rounded, blunt tip, taper cut
- **According to the eye:** Traumatic (needle with eye for threading a suture) or atraumatic (eyeless).

Depending on the type of sharp end, it may be: Round body, cutting, reverse cutting.

Sterilized by dipping them in lysol in case of traumatic needle, whereas atraumatic needles are provided in a sterilized pack with the suture (Fig. 1).

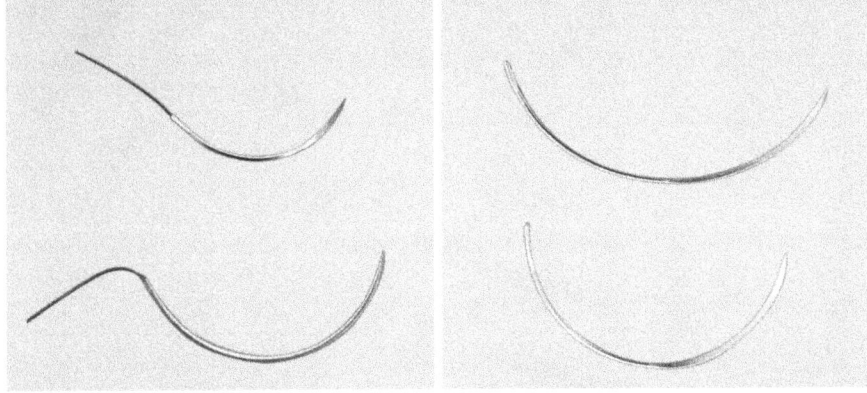

3/8th circle curved atraumatic (eyeless) needle

3/8th circle (upper) and ½ circle curved (lower) traumatic (with eye) needles

Fig. 1: Different types of needles used in surgical practice.

Uses

- Curved, round body atraumatic needles, are used for suturing peritoneum, muscles, and for doing intestinal and vascular anastomosis
- Curved cutting needles, are used for suturing skin, fascia
- Blunt pointed needles, are used for suturing friable vascular tissue like liver, spleen, etc.

CHAPTER 26

Different Types of Suture Materials

ABSORBABLE SUTURE MATERIALS

1. NATURAL ABSORBABLE SUTURE MATERIAL

Catgut (Plain and Chromic Catgut)

- It is a natural, absorbable, monofilament suture material. It is 99% collagen
- Packed in yellow (plain catgut) or khaki color (chromic catgut) foil
- Derived from the submucosa of sheep's intestine, after stripping the mucosa and muscular layers and leaving behind the tubes of submucosa, which are preserved by salting and freezing
- It is also derived from the serosa of the cattle's or beef's intestine
- It is absorbed by the process of enzymatic digestion by proteolytic enzymes and absorption rate depends upon size of suture, and whether it is plain or chromic catgut
- Plain catgut, if treated with 20% chromic acid, it becomes chromic catgut
- Chromic acid alters its property, so durability and tensile strength of the suture is increased, i.e. it stays for a longer duration in the tissues maintaining its tensile strength for a longer time than plain catgut
- Plain catgut loses 50% tensile strength in tissues in 2 or 3 days (unreliable after 48 hours), and loses all its tensile strength in 15 days, and gets completely absorbed in the tissue and disappears from the body within 60 days
- Chromic catgut loses 50% tensile strength in tissues in 7 days, and loses all its tensile strength in 28–30 days, and gets completely absorbed in the tissue and disappears from the body within 90–100 days
- It is sterilized by gamma irradiation and is supplied in a presterilized pack containing isopropyl alcohol
- In infected tissue, catgut gets absorbed earlier than non-infected tissue
- Thickness of catgut ranges from 7/0 to 7 (Fig. 1).

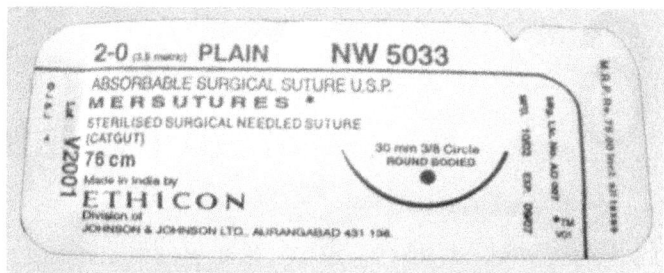

No. 2-0, plain catgut, on 3/8th circle round bodied needle.

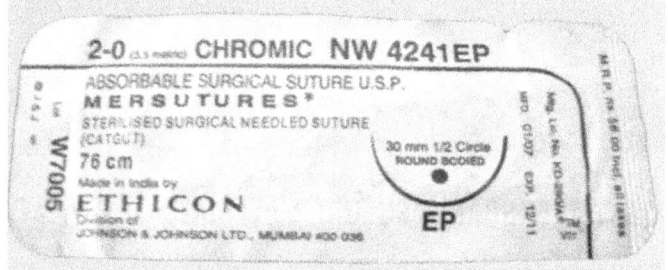

No. 2-0, chromic catgut, on 1/2 circle round bodied needle.

Fig. 1: Different types of catgut—plain and chromic in presterilized packs.

Uses

Uses of Plain Catgut

- To tie or ligating the small subcutaneous bleeding vessels to achieve hemostasis, during every surgical procedure
- To approximate the subcutaneous tissue, during closure of the incision
- To suture the cut margins of prepuce, during circumcision
- Suturing of the wounds of the lip and oral cavity
- Suturing mucosa of the genitourinary tract in case of pyelolithotomy, ureterolithotomy, cystolithotomy, so that it dissolves fast and does not act as a nidus for future stone formation.

Uses of Chromic Catgut

- Suturing cut muscles, during closure of the incisions, where the muscles are cut like cholecystectomy by right subcostal incision, nephrectomy or nephrolithotomy via lumbar incision, appendicectomy by Rutherford Morrison incision, etc.
- Suturing anterior or posterior rectus sheath, in laparotomy through paramedian incisions
- For bowel anastomosis, after small or large gut resection

- While doing gastrojejunostomy
- For biliary-enteric anastomosis
- Suturing peritoneum while closing abdominal incisions
- During appendectomy, to ligate the mesoappendix till base, ligating and invaginating the base of the appendix into the cecum, during burying of its stump by purse string suture.
- Synthetic absorbable sutures like polyglactin 910 (Vicryl) and polyglycolic acid (Dexon) are replacing the catgut suture for most of its uses, as catgut being an animal protein, evokes sterile inflammatory tissue reaction, which leads to rapid loss of its tensile strength and makes its use unreliable.

2. SYNTHETIC ABSORBABLE SUTURE MATERIAL

- Prepared artificially
- Strong as compared to the natural absorbable sutures, and maintains tensile strength in tissue for longer time than natural suture material
- It gets absorbed by hydrolysis and elicits minimal tissue reaction
- They have excellent handling properties, once tied, knots get secured and does not slip easily
- Sterilized by ethylene oxide and supplied in a presterilized pack
- Available in different sizes, different lengths, with different types of needles.

POLYGLACTIN 910 SUTURES
(Vicryl: Trade Name by Ethicon)

- Synthetic, absorbable polyfilament suture material, packed in violet foil and suture is also violet in color
- Sterilized by gamma irradiation
- It loses its tensile strength in 28–30 days, and gets completely absorbed in the tissue and disappears from the body in 80–90 days
- It gets absorbed by hydrolysis and not by enzymatic digestion, hence incites less tissue reaction as compared to the catgut, so preferred over catgut in every surgery nowadays
- Available in different sizes like 1, 1-0, till 9-0 and length like 90 cm, 70 cm or 45 cm, etc.
- Needle may be of different sizes of 40 mm, 30 mm, etc., and may be round bodied, cutting or taper cut (Fig. 2).

Uses

Vicryl used in all situations where chromic catgut is used, like:
- Suturing cut muscles during closure of the incisions where muscles are cut, like cholecystectomy by right subcostal incision, nephrectomy or nephrolithotomy via lumbar incision, appendicectomy by Rutherford

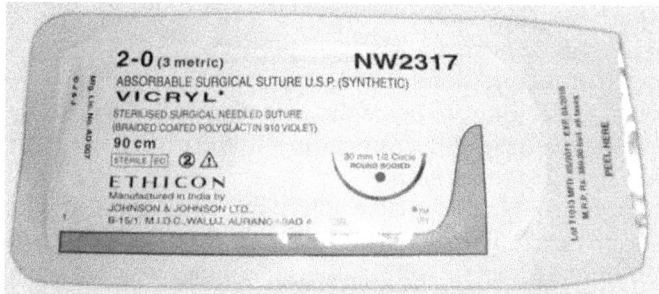

No. 2-0, polyglactin, on 1/2 circle, round bodied needle.

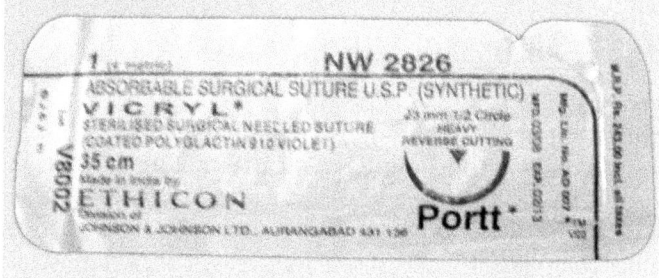

No. 1, polyglactin, on 1/2 circle, reverse cutting needle.

Fig. 2: Polyglactin 910 (Vicryl) in presterilized packs.

- Morrison incision, closure of thoracotomy, etc.
- Suturing anterior or posterior rectus sheath in laparotomy, through paramedian incisions
- For intestinal anastomosis, after small or large gut resection
- While doing gastrojejunostomy
- For biliary-enteric anastomosis like choledochoduodenostomy, choledochojejunostomy, hepaticojejunostomy
- Suturing peritoneum, while closing the laparotomy incisions
- During appendicectomy, to ligate the mesoappendix till base, ligating and invaginating the base of the appendix into the cecum, during burying of its stump by purse string suture
- During urological procedures like pyeloplasty, ureter or pelvis repair, closure of the bladder after cystolithotomy, etc.

Vicryl Rapide Suture

- Variety of polyglactin 910 suture
- Vicryl rapide is rapidly absorbed and loses its tensile strength early as compared to vicryl, which is achieved by exposure of coated vicryl to gamma irradiation
- Vicryl rapide loses its tensile strength in 10–12 days, and gets completely absorbed in the tissues and disappear from the body in 42 days.

Uses

- Vicryl rapide used in all situations where plain catgut is used, like:
- For continuous subcuticular sutures like closing neck incision in thyroid surgery, as its gives better cosmetic effect than interrupted silk skin sutures
- To approximate the subcutaneous tissue, during closure of the incision in every surgery
- To suture the cut margins of prepuce, during circumcision
- Suturing of the oral mucosa.

NONABSORBABLE SUTURES

1. NONABSORBABLE NATURAL SUTURES

Silk, Mersilk

- It is a natural, non-absorbable, polyfilament suture material
- Silk is derived from the cocoon of silkworm larvae
- Supplied in a sterile pack without needle (Sutupak), and also on eyeless needle
- May also be supplied in silk reels, which is nonsterile and have to be sterilized by autoclaving
- Handling property is best than any other suture, and it knots securely
- Sterilized by gamma irradiation and dyed black, so black in color
- Provided in sky blue or light green color foil
- Silk maintains tensile strength for a longer time, and loses it over a period of 2 years
- Mersilk is available in different sizes from 1 to 7-0, in different lengths 45 cm, 76 cm, 90 cm, with different types of needles 16 mm, 22 mm, 30 mm, etc. with 1/2 circle, 3/8th circle curvatures (Fig. 3).

Uses

Uses of Silk (Sutupak)

No. 1 or 1-0 sutures are used as a ligature:
- To ligate the cystic duct and cystic artery, during cholecystectomy
- During small and large gut resection anastomosis, to ligate the mesenteric vessels
- To ligate the pedicles, during splenectomy and nephrectomy
- For ligating major blood vessels
- During vasectomy and tubectomy.

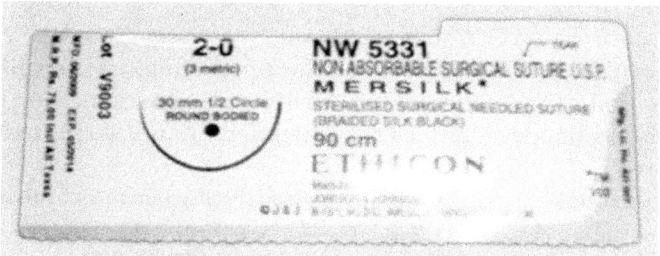

No. 2-0 braided silk, on ½ circle round bodied needle.

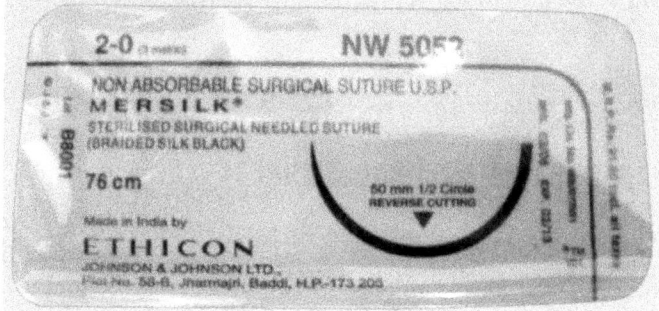

No. 2-0 braided silk, on ½ circle reverse cutting needle.

Fig. 3: Silk in presterilized packs.

Uses of Mersilk

- For skin closure with interrupted sutures, for approximation of the skin edges
- For suturing the contused lacerated wound, incised wounds, etc.
- For fixing the edges of the skin graft, to the recipient area
- For taking outer seromuscular sutures, in small gut resection anastomosis
- For repair of tendon, nerve, etc.

Linen And Cotton Thread

- It is prepared from cotton and is cheap and easily available
- It is natural, non absorbable, polyfilament suture material
- It has an excellent knotting property, but has low tensile strength
- Sterilization by autoclaving or keeping it in the formalin chamber (Fig. 4).

Uses

Tying pedicles and as ligatures.

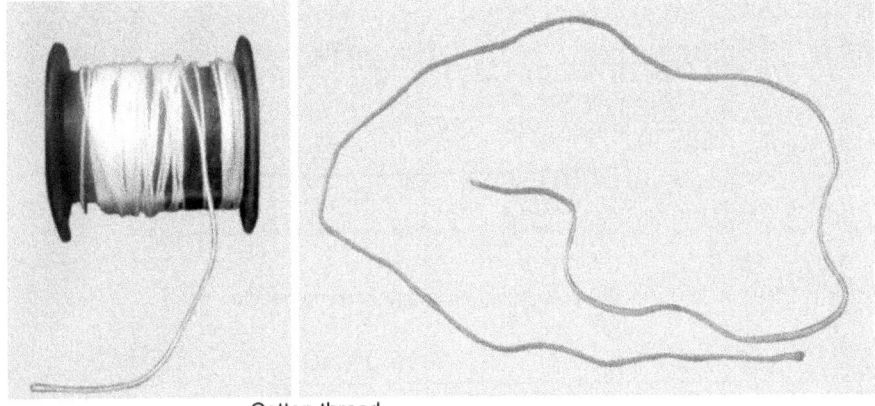

Cotton thread

Fig. 4: Cotton thread bundle.

2. NONABSORBABLE SYNTHETIC SUTURES

Monofilament Polyamide
(ETHILON: Trade Name of Monofilament Polyamide by Ethicon)

- It is a synthetic, nonabsorbable, monofilament suture and is a variety of nylon
- It maintains tensile strength for a longer time, and starts losing it after 1 year
- It is an inert suture and incites minimal tissue reaction and easily passes through the tissues
- It has a memory and has poor knot security, so require at least 4–5 throws for proper secured knotting, to prevent it from slipping
- Provided in a presterilized pack (Fig. 5).

Uses
- For closure of skin incisions, to approximate the skin edges
- For suturing the contused lacerated wounds, incised wounds, etc.
- For closing midline laparotomy incision, by mass closure technique, mainly linea alba
- For repair of posterior wall of inguinal canal, during herniorrhaphy and darning
- Finer sutures can be used in vascular and cardiovascular surgeries, also in plastic surgeries.

Nylon
- It is a synthetic, nonabsorbable, monofilament suture, white in color

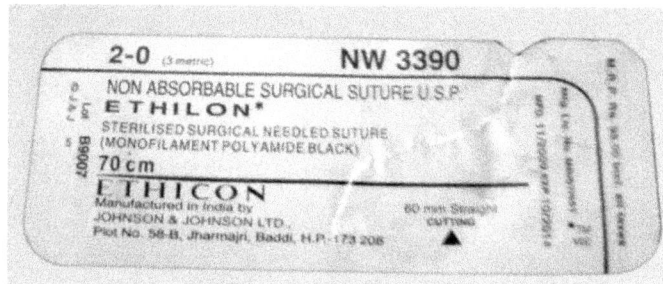

No. 2-0 polyamide, on straight cutting needle.

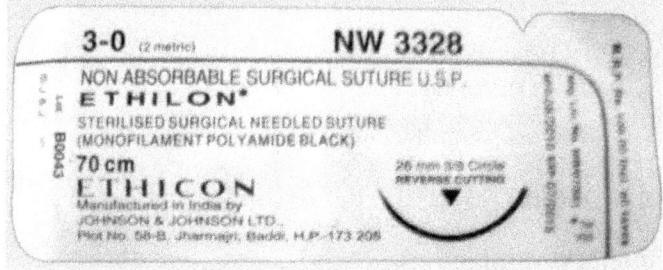

No. 3-0 polyamide, on 3/8th circle reverse cutting needle.

Fig. 5: Polyamide (ETHICON) in presterilized packs.

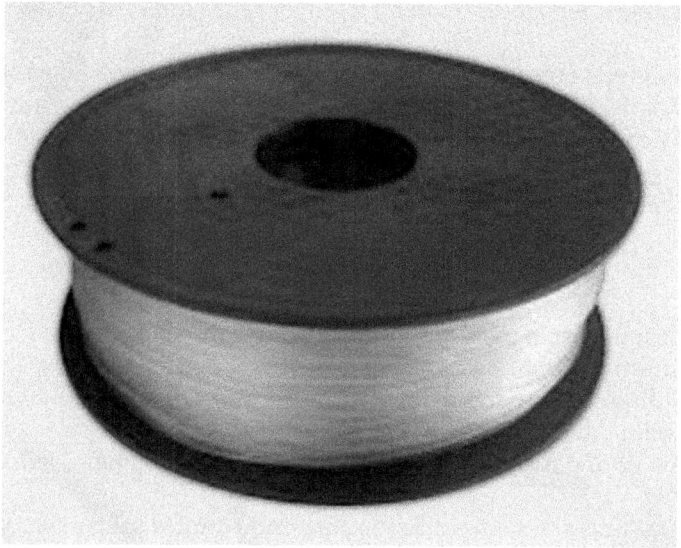

Fig. 6: Nylon bundle.

- It has high tensile strength, and maintains its tensile strength for indefinite period
- Sterilization by autoclaving or by keeping it in the formalin chamber (Fig. 6).

Uses

Same as monofilament polyamide suture.

Polypropylene
(Prolene: Trade Name of Polypropylene by Ethicon)

* It is a synthetic, monofilament, nonabsorbable suture material
* It maintains tensile strength for indefinite period
* It is a inert suture, and incites minimal tissue reaction and is non-biodegradable
* It slides through the tissues easily
* It is available in a variety of eyeless needles (atraumatic) in various sizes from 8-0 to 1
* Mesh used in repair of hernias, are also made up of polypropylene
* Provided in a presterilized pack (Fig. 7).

Uses

* For closure of midline laparotomy incision, by mass closure technique, mainly linea alba
* No. 1-0 or No.1 is used for herniorrhaphy, for repair of the posterior wall of the inguinal canal
* For repair of incisional, umbilical, epigastric hernias
* For tension sutures, during closure of the laparotomy incision, where there are chances of postoperative burst abdomen
* Finer sutures 4-0, 5-0, 6-0 are used in vascular surgery like vascular anastomosis like repair of an aneurysm, major arterial injuries, coronary artery bypass grafting, etc.

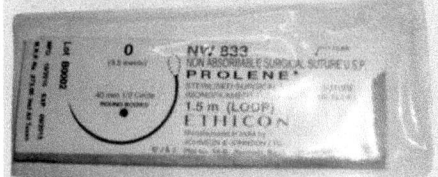
No. 0 polypropylene, on 1/2 circle round bodied needle.

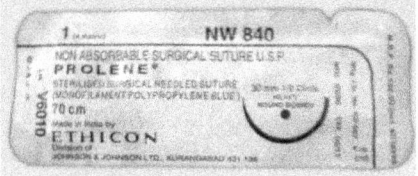
No. 1 polypropylene, on 1/2 circle round bodied needle.

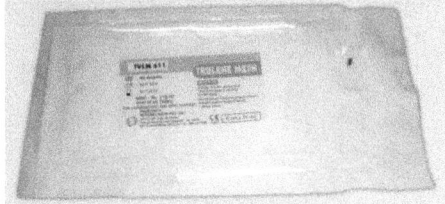
Polypropylene mesh in a presterilized pack

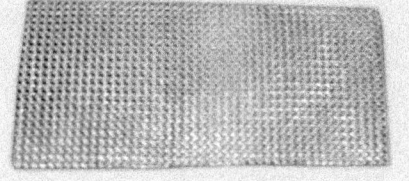
Polypropylene mesh

Fig. 7: Different types of polypropylene sutures and mesh.

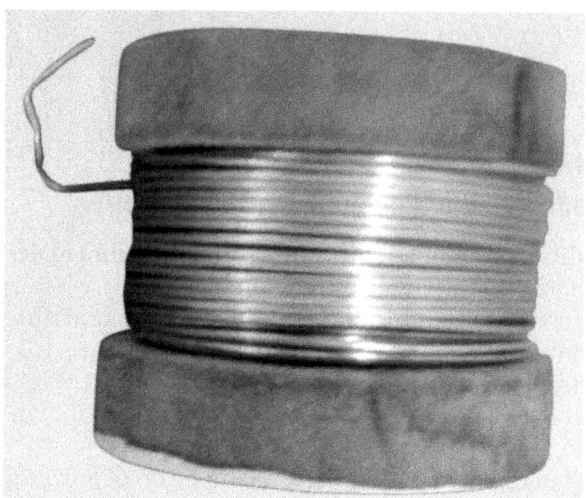

Fig. 8: Stainless steel wire.

- For repair of nerve, tendon injuries
- In plastic surgeries.

Stainless Steel Wire

- It is having very high tensile strength
- It is extremely inert
- Suturing with stainless steel require perfect technique, as too tight suturing may cause tissue necrosis and may pull and tear the tissue
- Barbs on the ends of the steel can traumatize the surrounding tissues
- Available in different sizes from 6 to 5-0 (Fig. 8).

Uses

- Closure of the midline sternotomy incision, which is commonly performed in CVTS surgeries
- In orthopedic operations, for suturing bones like fracture patella
- Interdental wiring for fracture mandible
- Earlier used in herniorrhaphy for hernia repair and Thiersch' operation done for anal encirclement in case of rectal prolapse.

Section 7

Anesthesia Equipments

Section Outline

27. Airways
28. Equipments for Tracheal Intubation
29. Equipments for Ventilation
30. Equipments for Regional Anesthesia
31. Commonly Used Drugs in Anesthesia

CHAPTER 27

Airways

GUEDEL'S OR OROPHARYNGEAL AIRWAY

- It is anatomically-shaped airway, to be inserted through the mouth above the tongue into the oropharynx, to maintain the patency of the upper airway
- It is made up of hard plastic, to prevent occlusion of the air channel, if the patient bites the oropharyngeal airway
- It may be made up of metal or silicone
- Metallic is made up of stainless steel, but not used routinely nowadays
- Designed in different sizes from No. 1 to 5, to fit the majority of patients from children to adults
- Both the ends are open, one end has to be kept in the patient's mouth, while the other end with its bite block, is placed outside the mouth
- The curved body of the airway contains the air channel
- It is flattened anteroposteriorly and curved laterally
- The bite portion is straight and fits between the teeth
- Sterilized it by autoclaving for 15 minutes or by boiling for 3 minutes (Fig. 1).

Uses

Patient's airway is kept patent by preventing the tongue and epiglottis from falling backwards in unconscious patient, to prevent obstruction of the airway
- To prevent tongue bite, in semiconscious or irritable patient
- During ventilating a patient with mask, to prevent tongue from falling backwards and obstructing the airway

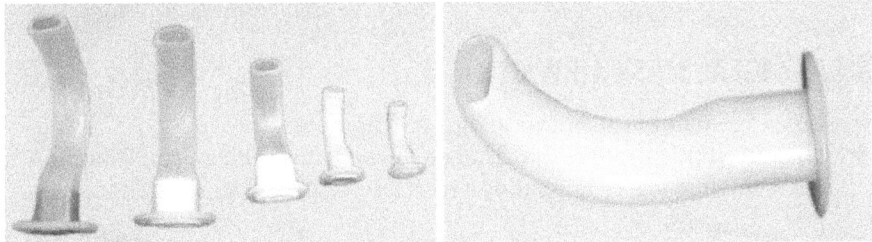

Fig. 1: Oropharyngeal (Guedel's) airways.

- During postanesthetic recovery when patient is not fully conscious, to prevent tongue from obstructing the airway
- Suction catheter can be passed through the airway, to aspirate the oropharyngeal secretions
- Airway can be used along with the endotracheal tube, to prevent kinking of the tube due to its biting in a conscious patients.

Complications of Putting the Oropharyngeal Airway

- Can cause trauma and injury to different structures in the oropharynx
- Trauma can occur to the teeth if the patient bites on the airway
- If inserted in a patient, whose pharyngeal reflexes are insufficiently depressed, there is a risk of gag reflex stimulation and vomiting.

NASOPHARYNGEAL AIRWAY

- It is inserted through the nose into the nasopharynx, bypassing the mouth and the oropharynx
- The distal end is beveled, which is left facing and lies just above the epiglottis and below the base of the tongue when inserted
- The body is rounded and curved
- The proximal end has a flange
- It is not recommended in coagulopathy, nasal sepsis and deformities (Fig. 2).

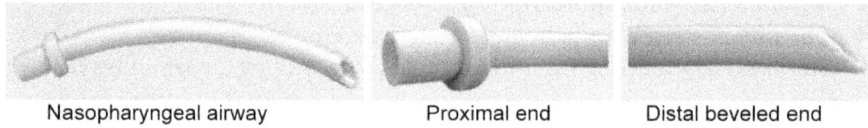

Nasopharyngeal airway   Proximal end   Distal beveled end

Fig. 2: Nasopharyngeal airway.

Uses

- It is an alternative to the oropharyngeal airway if the mouth cannot be opened, or if an oral airway does not relieve the obstruction
- It is better tolerated by semi-awake patient, than the oral airway.

LARYNGEAL MASK AIRWAY (LMA)

- It is a transparent tube of wide internal diameter
- It has an elliptical cuff at the distal end, which resembles a small face mask and is inflated via a pilot balloon with a self-limiting valve

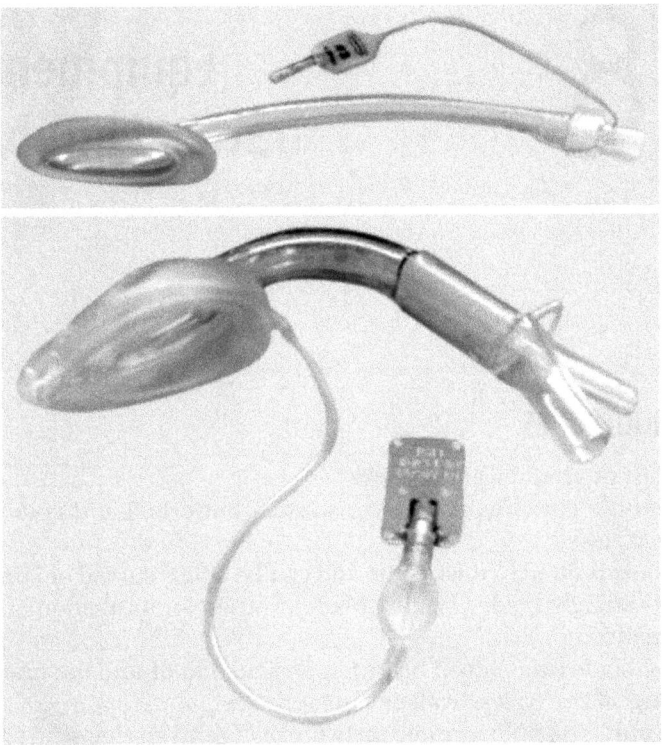

Fig. 3: Laryngeal mask airway.

- Cuff has to be deflated and lubricated before use, and it is inserted through the mouth, which lies over the larynx after insertion
- Once the cuff is in position, it has to be inflated (Fig. 3).

Uses

- It is a very useful device, used as an alternative to either the face mask or ETT during anesthesia, for spontaneous and controlled ventilation
- It has a role as an aid in difficult intubation, as a narrow lumen ETT can be inserted into the trachea through it (intubating LMA). Intubating LMA allows blind tracheal intubation
- The reinforced version, can be used for head and neck surgery.

Complications in Using LMA

- LMA does not protect against the aspiration of gastric contents
- Rotation of LMA may result in ineffective ventilation or airway obstruction.

CHAPTER 28

Equipments for Tracheal Intubation

■ LARYNGOSCOPES

- ❖ It consist of a handle and a blade
- ❖ The handle contains the power source (batteries) and is designed in different sizes
- ❖ The blade is fitted to the handle and can be either curved or straight
- ❖ Usually straight blade (Magill's blade), is used for intubation of neonates and infants
- ❖ Curved blade (Macintosh blade), is designed to fit into the oral and oropharyngeal cavity. It is available in four sizes
- ❖ Light source is a bulb screwed on to the blade and an electrical connection is made, when the blade is opened for use
- ❖ Different designs and shapes exist (Fig. 1).

How to Perform Laryngoscopy

- ❖ Blade is inserted through the right angle (corner) of the mouth and advanced gradually pushing the tongue to the left and away from the view, until the tip of the blade reaches the vallecula

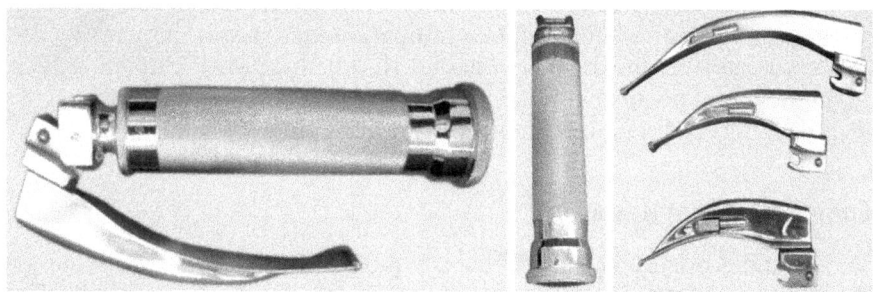

Handle attached with blade   Handle   Curved (Macintosh) blade

Fig. 1: Laryngoscope.

- ❖ Blade has a small bulbous tip to lift the larynx
- ❖ The laryngoscope is lifted upwards elevating the larynx and allowing the vocal cords to come into the view.

Uses

- ❖ To perform direct laryngoscopy
- ❖ To aid in the endotracheal tube intubation.

Complications During Laryngoscopy

Risk of trauma and bruising to the different structures in the oropharynx like epiglottis, and is more when the blade is straight.

ENDOTRACHEAL TUBES (ETT)

- ❖ It is made up of Indian red rubber or plastic. Nowadays, mostly plastic tubes are in use
- ❖ The plastic tubes are made up of polyvinyl chloride (PVC), and have a radiopaque line running along their length, that enables their position to be determined on chest X-rays
- ❖ May be cuffed or non-cuffed. Cuff is attached near the distal or beveled end (patient's end)
- ❖ The cuff when inflated with air provides an airtight seal between the tube and the tracheal wall. This airtight seal protects the patient's airway from aspiration of the oropharyngeal secretions into the trachea and subsequently into the lungs. It also allows efficient ventilation during intermittent positive pressure ventilation (IPPV), by preventing the inhaled air from returning back by the side of the tube
- ❖ Balloon should be inflated with air and never with normal saline or distilled water, as if it ruptures or leaks catastrophic complication like aspiration pneumonitis can occur
- ❖ Cuff is connected to its pilot balloon, which has a self-retaining valve for injecting air. The pilot balloon also indicates whether the balloon is inflated or not. After intubation, the cuff is inflated until no gas leak can be heard during IPPV
- ❖ Cuffed tubes are used in adults only
- ❖ It has different numbers, according to the internal diameter of the tube from number 1.5 to 11, which is marked on the outside of the tube in millimeters (mm)
- ❖ No. 1.5 to 4 ETT are non-cuffed, whereas ETT from No. 4.5 onwards are cuffed (non-cuffed tubes are also available)
- ❖ As the number of tube increases, its diameter increases. Number indicates internal diameter of the tube in millimeters (mm)

- Length taken from the tip of the tube is marked in centimeters (cm) on the outside of the tube
- Usually tubes No. 1.5 to No. 6, are used in pediatric patients and their size depends on the basis of the age and height of the patient. No. 6.5 to 7.5 used in average size adult female and No. 8 to 9 used in average size adult male
- Connectors connect the ETT to the breathing system, made up of plastic or metal. Standard connector has universal 15 mm diameter at the proximal end, irrespective of the number of the tube
- An introducer (stylet) is used to adjust the curvature of the ETT to help, to direct the tube through the vocal cords
- Plastic tubes are provided in presterilized pack, while rubber tubes are reusable after cleaning and sterilizing it, by autoclaving or boiling it for 3 minutes.
- Can be inserted orally or nasally
- Indications of nasal intubation are: Surgery where access via mouth is necessary (e.g. oral or dental operations) and patients requiring long-term ventilation in intensive care units, where patient tolerates a nasal tube better and cannot bite the tube. Nasal intubations are usually avoided in children up to the age of 8–11 years, due to hypertrophy of the adenoids in this age group which may cause profuse bleeding if nasal intubation is performed
- Confirmatory test for successful endotracheal intubation is $EtCO_2$ monitoring and fiberoptic bronchoscopy (Fig. 2).

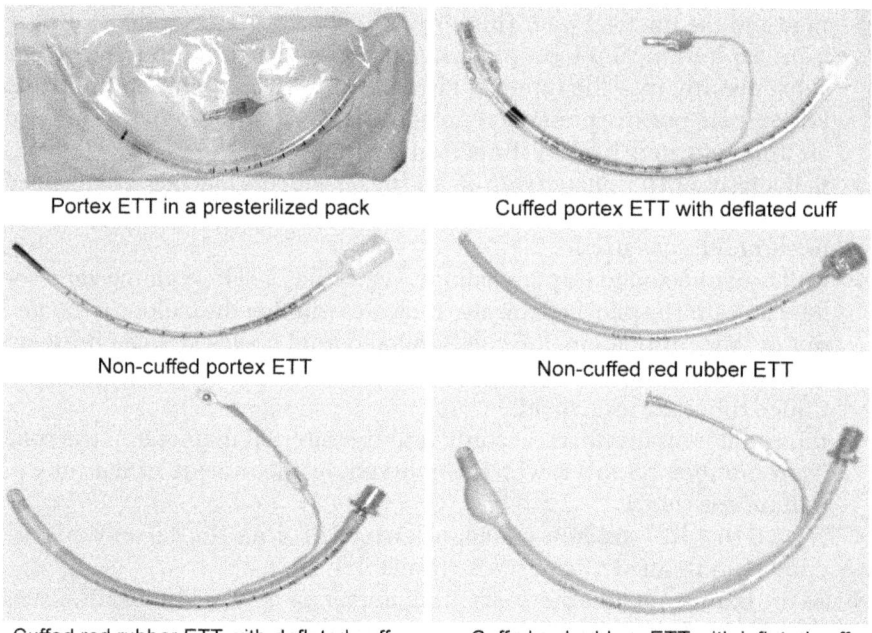

Fig. 2: Endotracheal tubes.

Uses

- For securing patient's airway, to give positive pressure ventilation to the patient of respiratory distress (gasping) or respiratory arrest, by inserting an appropriate number endotracheal tube (ETT), and connecting it to the artificial manual breathing unit (Ambu) bag and oxygen
- To give oxygen and inhalational anesthetic agents, during any surgery done under general anesthesia.

Problems in Practice with ETT Intubation

- Obstruction of the ETT by kinking, herniation of the cuff, occlusion by oropharyngeal secretions, foreign body or the bevel lying against the wall of the trachea
- Esophageal intubation or intubation in one of the bronchus (endobronchial intubation)
- Trauma and injury to the various tissues and structures during and after intubation.

CONNECTOR

- It is made up of metal or plastic
- Its one end is connected to the outer end of the endotracheal tube, which can vary as per the size of tube, whereas the outer (proximal) end has universal diameter of 15 mm (Fig. 3).

Uses

Connectors connect the ETT to the breathing system.

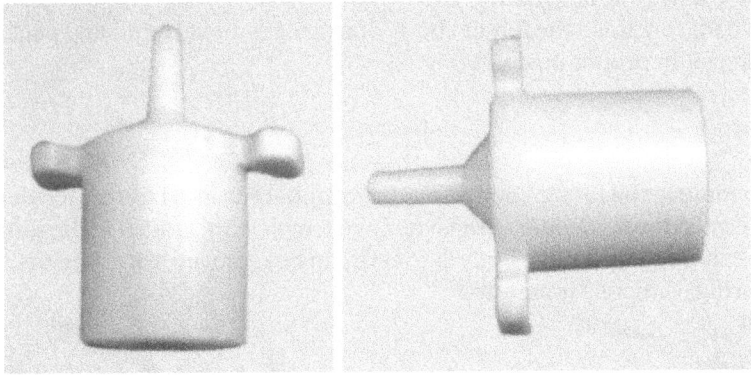

Fig. 3: Plastic connectors.

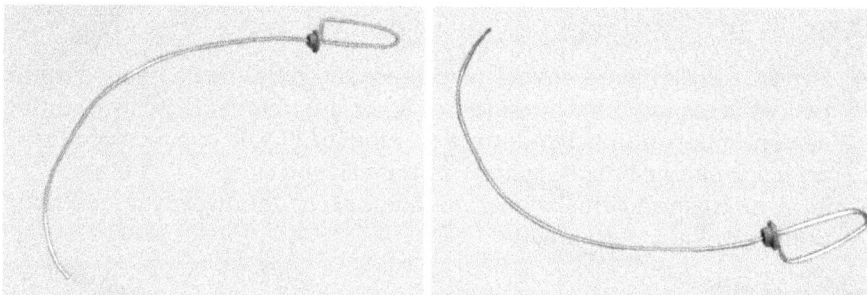

Fig. 4: Stylet.

STYLET

- It is made up of stainless steel or aluminum
- It is curved and mouldable, to mould as per the curve of the endotracheal tubes (Fig. 4).

Uses

It is inserted inside the endotracheal tube, while intubating the patient.

MAGILL'S FORCEPS

- Designed in such a manner, for its easy use within the mouth and oropharynx
- It has finger bows, and pair of shafts and blades
- This instrument is curved at blades, in such a way that the holding hand will not obstruct the vision of the person working with it
- The tip of the instrument is rounded, fenestrated and having transverse serrations like swab holding forceps, for firm holding of the things in its tip without slipping them
- The tip can grasp the foreign body during its removal or during packing to direct it in proper position (Fig. 5).

Uses

- To remove the foreign body from the oropharynx and larynx. Accidentally ingested foreign bodies can be removed, which are lodged in the pharynx. Also iatrogenic foreign body like teeth can be removed, if avulsed or broken during (difficult) intubation

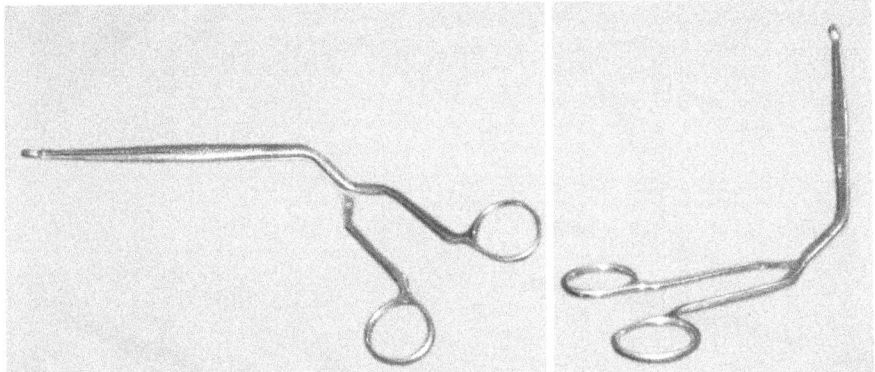

Fig. 5: Magill's forceps.

- To clear the oropharynx from thick secretions, solid vomitus, blood clots, etc. in unconscious patients or in immediate postoperative period
- For packing of nasal cavity to stop bleeding from the nostrils in case of spontaneous epistaxis or due to nasal trauma
- For packing oropharynx, to prevent aspiration of blood and oral secretions, while doing tonsillectomy or during oral surgeries
- For inserting and removing of throat packs
- During ETT intubation, they can be used for guiding the ETT towards the larynx and vocal cords into the trachea, in nasal as well as oral intubation
- For guiding nasogastric tube into the pharynx, if having difficulty in inserting it.

SUCTION CATHETER

- It is made up of PVC (Polyvinyl chloride)
- It is a having a blunt tip along with side hole, to prevent blockage of the catheter and allow free drainage
- The tip is blunt and smooth, to prevent trauma to the oropharynx
- The other end is dilated, and it is attached to the suction tubing while suction (Fig. 6).

Uses

- To suck the secretions of the oropharynx, for preventing its aspiration, in an unconscious patient

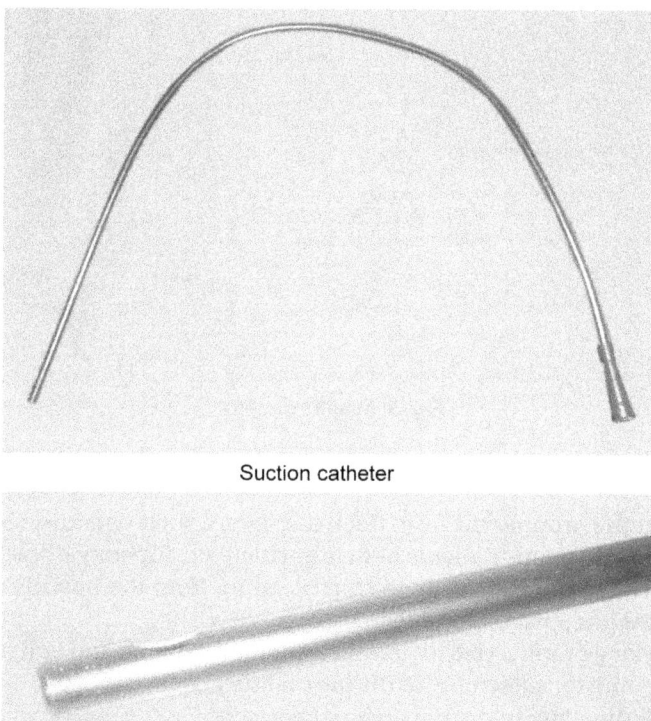

Suction catheter

Tip of suction catheter

Fig. 6: Suction catheter.

- ❖ To suck the secretions of the oropharynx, before inserting an endotracheal tube, to clear the oropharynx for better vision, while intubating a patient
- ❖ It can be inserted through the lumen of the endotracheal tube, laryngeal mask airway, oropharyngeal airway, to suck the secretions and clear the oropharynx to prevent aspiration.

CHAPTER 29

Equipments for Ventilation

AMBU BAG (AMBULATORY MANUAL BREATHING UNIT)

- This is a means of providing manual intermittent positive pressure ventilation (IPPV)
- It is a compact, portable, self-inflating bag with a one way valve and a connection for adding oxygen at one end
- Shape of the self-inflating bag is automatically restored after compression, which allows fresh gas to be drawn from the reservoir
- Oxygen reservoir can be added to increase FiO_2 (Forced inspiratory oxygen volume) delivered to the patient
- Non-rebreathing one way valve (Ambu valve) has three ports:
    a. Inspiratory inlet allowing the entry of fresh gas during inspiration
    b. Expiratory outlet allowing the exit of exhaled gases
    c. Connection to the face mask or tracheal tube (Fig. 1).

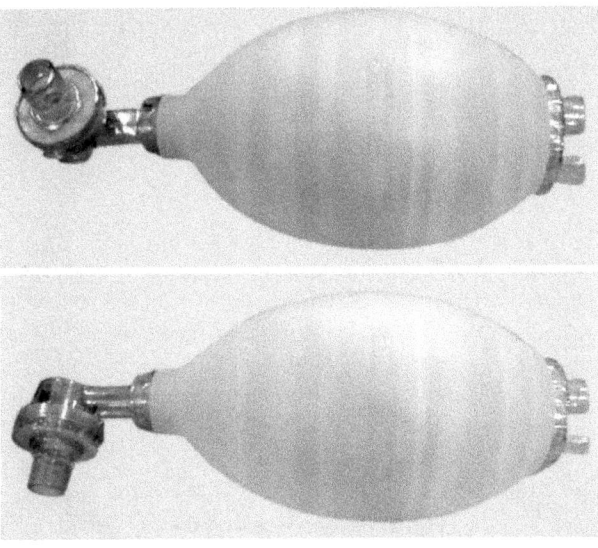

Fig. 1: Ambu bag with non-rebreathing valve.

Uses

- Used during resuscitation, transport and short-term ventilation
- Ambu valve is suitable for both IPPV and spontaneous ventilation.

OXYGEN RESERVOIR

This has to be attached to one pole of the Ambu bag adjacent to the port, where oxygen tubing is attached (Fig. 2).

Uses

It is attached to the Ambu bag to increase FiO_2, whenever required in emergency when ventilator is not available, as the oxygen is delivered from the reservoir bag.

NON-REBREATHING VALVE
(Fish Mouth Valve)

- It has two limbs with open ends, which are connected to each other at right angle
- The limb having adjustable pressure releasing valve, has to be attached to the Ambu, through which excess of pressure will be released while giving IPPV. The other limb is attached to the connector of the ETT of the patient
- When Ambu is compressed and ventilation (manual IPPV) is given, air (oxygen) in the Ambu enters in the ETT through the unidirectional valve,

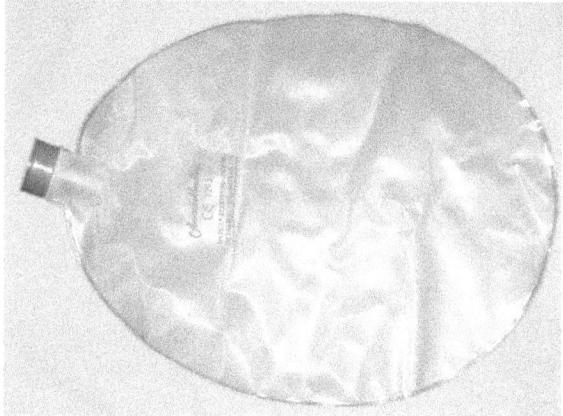

Fig. 2: Oxygen reservoir bag.

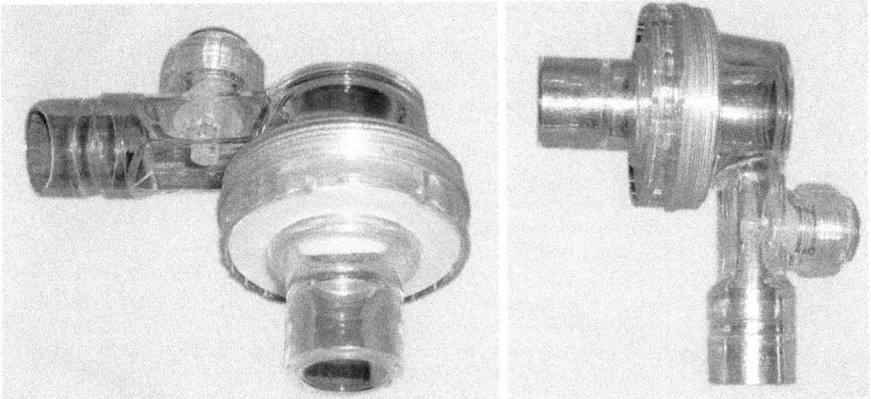

Fig. 3: Non-rebreathing valve.

whereas it will not allow the patients exhaled air (carbon dioxide) to return back into the Ambu (Fig. 3).

Uses

- Its one limb has to be connected to the pediatric Ambu bag, and the other limb to the patients ETT. The valve allows unidirectional flow of air (oxygen) from Ambu to the patient, and prevents patients exhaled carbon dioxide to return back into the Ambu which can be subsequently given to the patient, if return back.

ANGLE (UNIVERSAL) CONNECTOR

- It is a plastic tube, having 2 limbs with open ends, which are connected to each other at right angle
- Its one end is attached to the connector of the ETT, while the other end to the corrugated antistatic rubber tubing which is attached to the ventilator (Fig. 4).

Uses

It act as a connector, to connect the ETT to the tubings of the ventilator.

RESERVOIR BAG

- It is made up of antistatic rubber or plastic, and ellipsoidal in shape
- Available in volumes from 0.5 to 6 liters. Standard adult size is 2 liters which is commonly in use

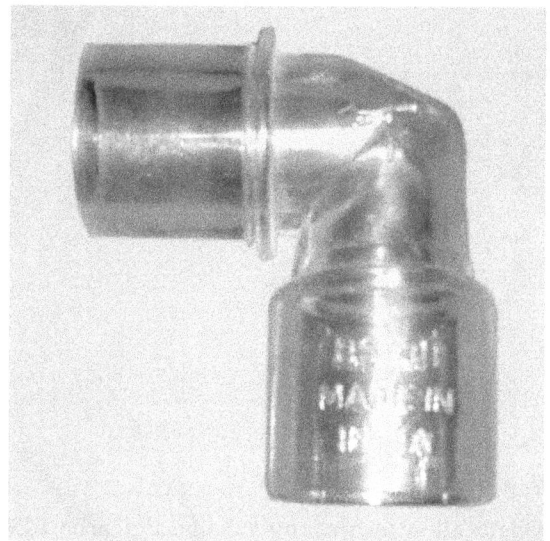

Fig. 4: Angle connector.

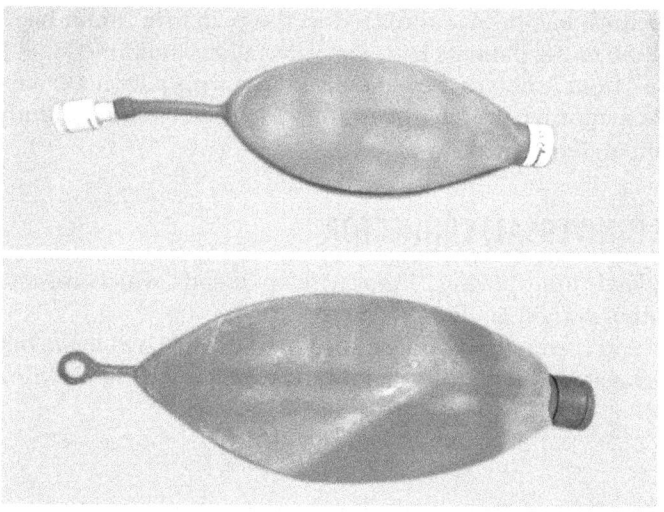

Adult reservoir bag (below) of 1.5 lit without valve and pediatric reservoir bag (above) of 0.5 lit with valve

Fig. 5: Reservoir bag.

- ❖ Smallest size for pediatric use is 0.5 liter. Pediatric reservoir bag has a valve at its other pole, which can be adjusted as per patients required tidal volume (Fig. 5).

Uses

- It accommodates the fresh gas flow during expiration, acting as a reservoir available for the following inspiration
- Acts as a monitor of the patient's ventilatory pattern, during spontaneous breathing
- Can be used to assist or control ventilation
- Limits pressure builds up in the breathing system
- Bigger sized bag can be used, for inhalational induction in adults like sevoflurane.

CORRUGATED ANTISTATIC RUBBER TUBE

It is made up of antistatic rubber material, so does not transfer heat and electricity (Fig. 6).

Uses

Commonly used in closed circuit, Mapleson type A open circuit.

FACE MASKS

- They are designed to fit the face anatomically
- Available in different sizes from No. 1 to 5, to fit patients of different age groups from neonates to adults

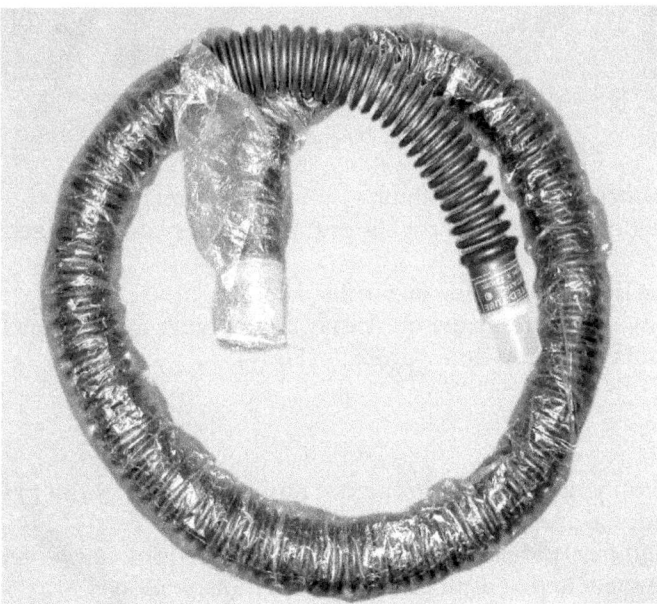

Fig. 6: Corrugated antistatic rubber tube.

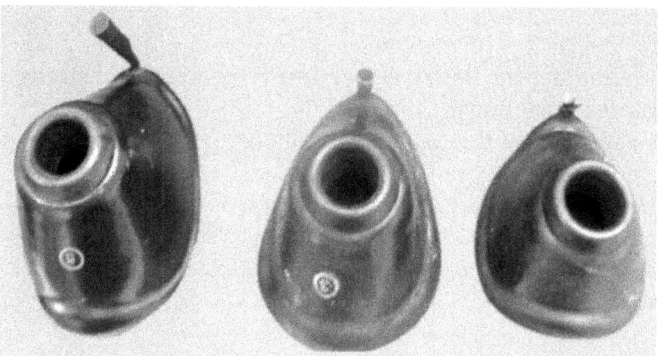
Different sizes of rubber face masks

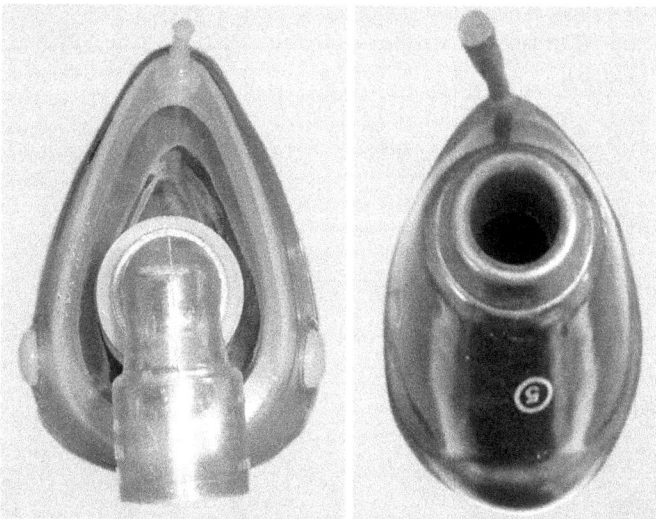
Plastic face mask with connector   No. 5 face mask

Fig. 7: Face masks.

- ❖ It is connected to the breathing system, via the angle piece
- ❖ It is made up of silicone rubber or transparent plastic or black antistatic rubber
- ❖ Body of the mask rests on an air-filled cuff
- ❖ Excessive pressure by the mask may cause injury to the branches of the trigeminal or facial nerves, eyeballs (Fig. 7).

Uses

- ❖ Commonly used during induction and ventilation of the patient with inhalational anesthetic drugs
- ❖ Through transparent masks vomitus and secretions can be seen, which can be suctioned or aspirated to prevent its aspiration

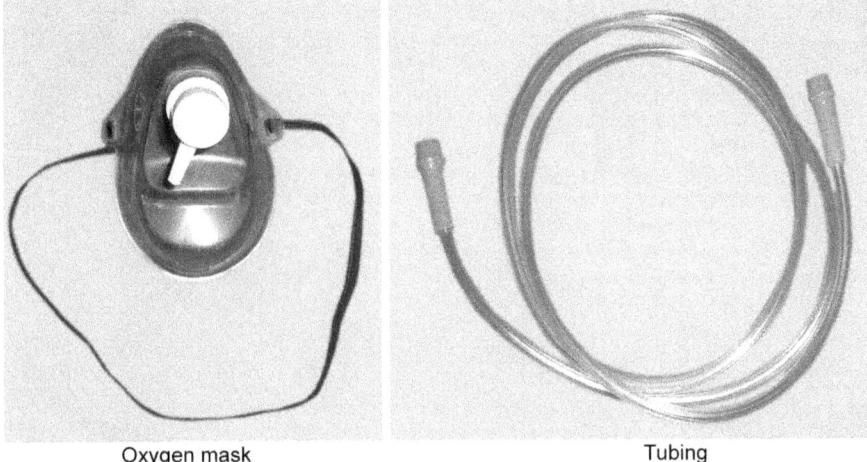

Oxygen mask Tubing

Fig. 8: Face mask and tubing.

- Air-filled cuff helps to ensure a snug fit over the face and minimizes the mask's pressure on the face
- Causes an increase in dead space up to 200 mL in adults.

OXYGEN MASK AND TUBING

- Available in different sizes for pediatric and adults
- It loosely fits covering the nose and the mouth
- Lower end is oval and corresponds to the chin and fits over the chin, while its upper end corresponds to the root of the nose
- Tubing attached to its connector, delivers oxygen from the oxygen cylinder, Boyle's machine to the patient, through the mask (Fig. 8).

Uses

To deliver oxygen to the patient.

'T' PIECE

- It is designed like 'T'
- The end of the 'T' is attached to the endotracheal or tracheostomy tube, one limb of the 'T' is attached to the oxygen cylinder and the other limb of 'T' is open to the atmosphere, which is wrapped with gauze piece, to avoid the sucking of foreign bodies like insects through it during inspiration
- Made up of plastic and provided in a presterilized pack (Fig. 9).

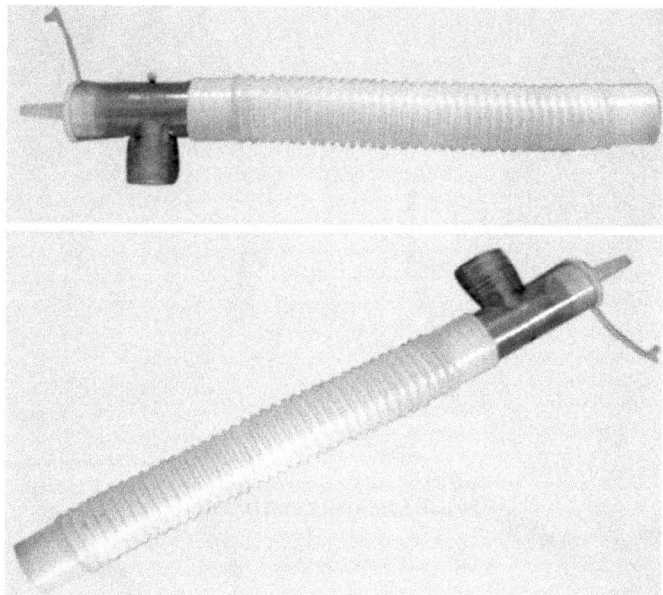

Fig. 9: 'T' tube.

Uses

- It is attached to the ETT or tracheostomy tube, while weaning the patient from the ventilator to know, whether the patient is able to take spontaneous respiration or not
- Oxygen can be given intermittently through the limb of the 'T' piece, if patient is not maintaining its oxygen saturation by other limb of the 'T' tube with atmospheric oxygen only.

CHAPTER 30

Equipments for Regional Anesthesia

■ SPINAL NEEDLE

- It is a long needle with two ends, one end is beveled, sharp and pointed to prick the skin and subcutaneous tissue to reach the subarachnoid space, while other end is dilated, which is universal irrespective of the size of the spinal needle, to snugly fit to the syringe used for giving the drug for spinal anesthesia
- It has a transparent hub, to identify the flow of cerebrospinal fluid (CSF) quickly
- It has a stylet, which is used to prevent core of tissue occluding the lumen of the needle during its insertion. It also strengthens the shaft. It has to be withdrawn once the tip of the needle is positioned and confirmed in the subarachnoid space
- The bevel can be cutting or pencil like
- Its length varies from 5–15 cm, but the 10 cm version is most commonly used
- It is available in sizes from no. 18 G–32 G (gauze) in diameter. But more than 29 G are rarely used in clinical practice. As the number increases, the diameter of the needle decreases
- Nowadays, small diameter spinal needles (mostly 25 or 26 G) are used for lumbar puncture as well as for giving spinal anesthesia, to prevent post-spinal headache, which is more common with large diameter needles
- 28 G nylon, open-ended spinal microcatheters can be inserted through the needle, which allows top-ups to be administered
- It is provided with needle protector (plastic cap or covering), to prevent accidental pricking by its sharp end, while it is not in use and during its transport
- Lumbar puncture is done below L_1 or L_2 space, generally at L_3 or L_4 space
- Provided in presterilized pack (Fig. 1).

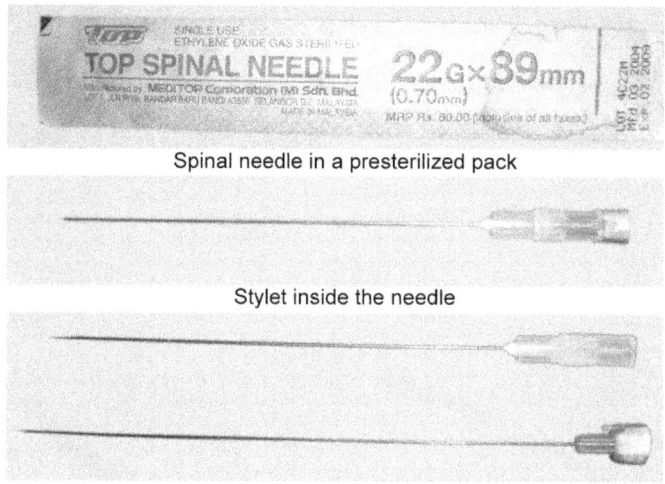

Fig. 1: Spinal needle.

Uses

- For lumbar puncture, to obtain or drain the cerebrospinal fluid (CSF) for diagnostic as well as therapeutic purposes
- To inject spinal anesthesia, by giving drugs like sensorcaine (heavy) or lignocaine (heavy), before the surgeries which has to be done under spinal anesthesia
- Can be used to give intrathecal injections of antibiotics and cytotoxics.

Contraindications for Lumbar Puncture

- Raised intracranial tension (ICT)
- Spine deformities like scoliosis, kyphosis, etc.
- Local sepsis.

Complications of Lumbar Puncture

- Incidence of postspinal dural headache is directly proportional to the gauge of the needle used and number of the punctures made through the dura mater which can be prevented by using small gauge spinal needles and giving head low position after lumbar puncture
- Postspinal paraparesis
- Iatrogenic infections
- Sudden death due to tonsillar herniation.

EPIDURAL CATHETER

- It consists of a soft catheter, filter, large bore epidural needle, catheter introducer and a syringe to confirm the epidural space (loss of resistance device)
- The catheter is transparent, malleable tube made up of either nylon or Teflon, and is 90 cm long. Its distal end has 2 or more side ports with a closed and rounded tip with markings at 5 centimeters intervals (with additional 1 cm markings between 5 to 15 cm), and the proximal end is connected to a Luer Lock and a filter. It should not be advanced more than 5 cm inside the epidural space (Usually 3–5 cm)
- The epidural needle is 10 cm in length and is provided with a stylet introducer. Commonly 10 cm Tuohy needle with the oblique bevel (Huber point) is commonly used. Usually 16 G or 18 G needle are used.
- It has 1 cm markings, to enable the anesthetist to determine the distance between the skin and the epidural space
- The filter acts as a filter for bacterial, viral and foreign bodies
- The syringe has a special low resistance plunger, which is used to identify the epidural space by loss of resistance to either air or saline.
- After infiltrating local anesthetic drug (2% lignocaine) in the skin and subcutaneous tissue around the space through which the epidural catheter has to be inserted, large bore needle is introduced through the skin and the subcutaneous tissue in the epidural space, which is confirmed by loss of resistance to the syringe
- After confirming the epidural space, introducer is attached to the syringe and epidural catheter is introduced through it into the epidural space
- Catheter is fixed to the skin with adhesive tape and anesthetic drug is given through it
- Provided in a presterilized pack
- A combined spinal-epidural technique is becoming more popular nowadays, and is possible by using 26 G spinal needle of about 12 cm length with a standard 16 G Tuohy needle. The advantage of this combined technique is that, surgical procedure can be started early, as the effect of spinal anesthesia starts early and the surgeon does not have to wait for the effect of epidural anesthesia to be achieved, as it takes longer time for the anesthetic effect of epidural anesthesia, if used alone (about 20–30 minute) (Fig. 2).

Uses

- In case of prolonged surgeries, epidural catheter is introduced and anesthetic drug top-up is given through it till the surgery is completed, which is not possible in case of spinal anesthesia, as in that the effect of the anesthetic drug starts weaning off after 2–3 hours

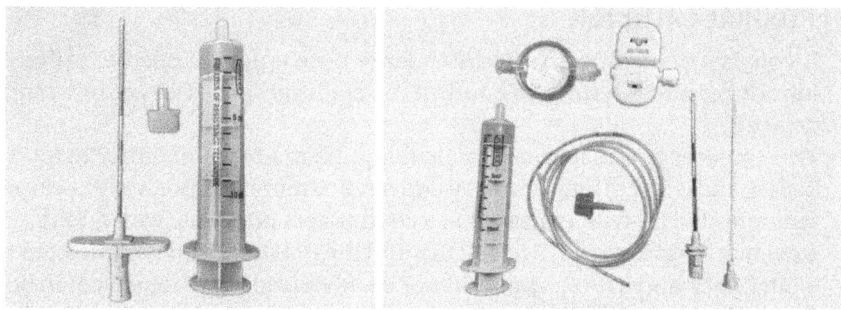

Loss of resistance syringe and epidural needle   Complete epidural set with epidural catheter

Fig. 2: Epidural catheter set.

- Postoperative analgesia by opiates can be given till the catheter is in situ, so need for other analgesic drugs by intravenous or intramuscular route is not needed in such cases
- Nowadays, catheter is introduced before the delivery to provide analgesia during the labor, known as 'labor analgesia'.

CHAPTER 31

Commonly Used Drugs in Anesthesia

■ BUPIVACAINE HYDROCHLORIDE IN DEXTROSE INJECTION (ANAWIN SENSORCAINE Heavy, 5%)

- ❖ It is provided in 4 mL ampoule
- ❖ It contains bupivacaine hydrochloride (5 mg) in dextrose (80 mg) injection
- ❖ As it contains dextrose, it is called as 'heavy' (i.e. hyperbaric)
- ❖ Depending upon the time of surgery and level of anesthesia required 1/2/2.5/3/3.5 or whole 4 mL can be given
- ❖ 4 mL drug has maximum effect for about 4 hours
- ❖ Maximum recommended dose is 2–3 mg/kg. It is not recommended for intravenous use (Fig. 1).

Uses

For giving spinal anesthesia in the surgeries, which has to be done under spinal anesthesia.

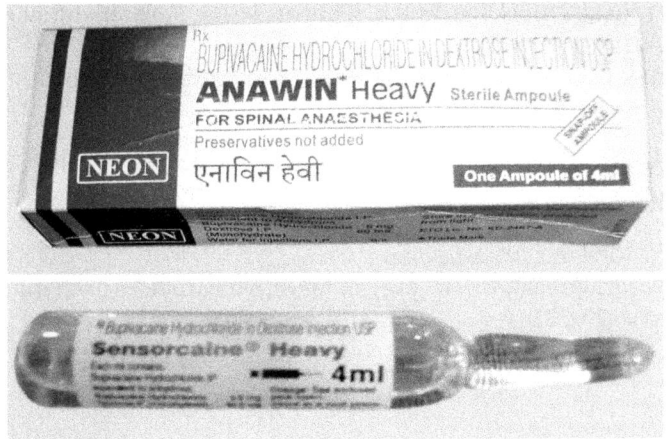

Fig. 1: Bupivacaine hydrochloride in dextrose injection USP.

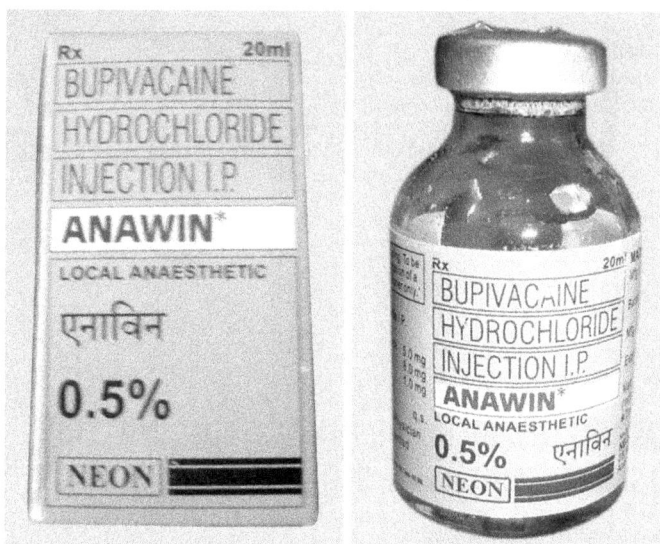

Fig. 2: Bupivacaine hydrochloride injection IP.

■ BUPIVACAINE HYDROCHLORIDE INJECTION (ANAWIN 0.5%)

- It is an amino type of local anesthetic drug, provided in 20 mL vial
- It contains bupivacaine hydrochloride 5 mg in each mL (0.5%)
- Maximum recommended dose is 2 or 3 mg/kg. It is not recommended for intravenous use (Fig. 2).

Uses

- For giving caudal anesthesia and analgesia in children up to 5 years of age
- Nerve (plexus) block like brachial plexus block, isolated upper and lower limb blocks
- It can also be used for local infiltration, for surgeries under local anesthesia.

■ LIGNOCAINE HYDROCHLORIDE AND DEXTROSE INJECTION (LOX Heavy 5%)

- It is provided in 2 mL ampoule
- It is having lignocaine (53.3 mg) along with dextrose, in each mL, so called as 'heavy' (Fig. 3).

Uses

For spinal anesthesia, but the duration of its action is very short as compared to sensorcaine, i.e. hardly half an hour to one hour.

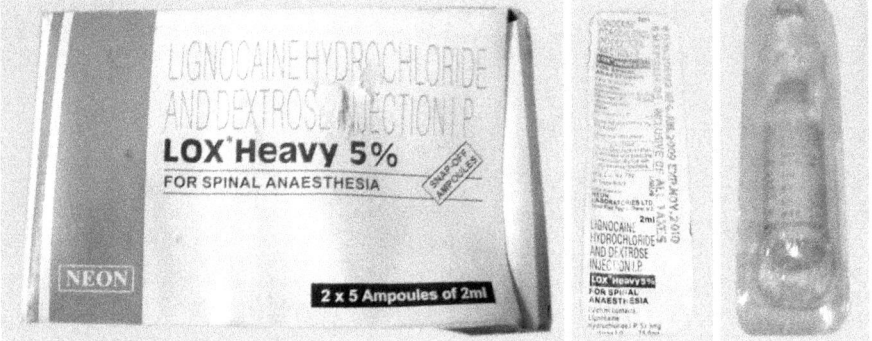

Fig. 3: Lignocaine hydrochloride and dextrose injection IP.

■ LIGNOCAINE HYDROCHLORIDE (XYLOCAINE 1% or 2%)

- It is an amide type (aminoamides) of local anesthetic drug
- It is provided in concentration of 1% and 2% in 30 mL vial (1% means each mL contains 10 mg of the drug, 2% means 20 mg/mL)
- Each mL contains lignocaine hydrochloride IP: 21.3 mg, sodium chloride: 6.0 mg, and preservative methylparaben IP 1 mg
- It has to be administered after a test dose, by infiltrating lignocaine 0.1 mL subcutaneously in the forearm of the patient by raising a subcutaneous bleb. The infiltrated area is with a marker. Observe the marked area, for hypersensitivity reactions like itching, redness, increase in its size, etc. If such reactions occurs, it means patient is sensitive to lignocaine and patient should not be operated under local anesthesia using lignocaine
- During infiltration of lignocaine, the syringe should be aspirated first before infiltrating the drug locally through small bore needle, to confirm that the needle is in the subcutaneous plain and not in any of the adjacent blood vessel. This has to be done, to prevent accidental injection of lignocaine directly into the blood vessel
- As it contains preservative (methylparaben), so should never be given intravenously
- Safe dose is 4 mg/kg body weight, and it will be toxic to the patient if it exceeds more than 5 mg/kg (Fig. 4).

Uses

- As a local anesthetic drug, for surgeries to be done under local anesthesia.
- It has to be infiltrated all around the swelling to be excised like cyst, lipoma, lymph node, etc.
- Suturing of any wound over the body under local anesthesia
- Infiltrating skin with lignocaine along the line of incision, while doing venesection

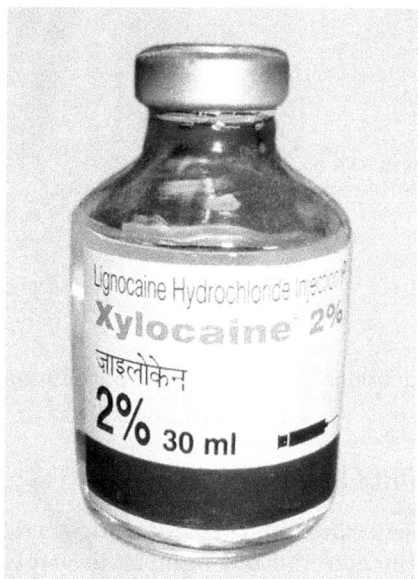

Fig. 4: Lignocaine hydrochloride injection IP (Xylocaine 2%).

- Preferably used for giving ring block at the base of the fingers and toes for drainage of pulp abscess, excision of nail in case of paronychia, etc.
- For giving penile block during circumscision for phimosis and dorsal slit for reduction of paraphimosis in adults.

LIGNOCAINE WITH ADRENALINE (LOX 2%)

- It is provided in concentration of 2% in 30 mL vial (1% = 10 mg/mL, 10% = 100 mg/mL)
- Each mL contains lignocaine hydrochloride IP: 21.3 mg, adrenaline I.P.: 0.005 mg, sodium chloride IP: 6.0 mg, sodium metabisulfite IP: 0.5 mg and preservative methylparaben 1 mg
- As in this, adrenaline is combined with lignocaine, adrenaline causes vasoconstriction of the blood vessels, so bleeding will be less while dissection of the tissue is done during the operation, duration of the effect of lignocaine is more prolonged and also less amount of lignocaine is required than using plain lignocaine
- To be used cautiously in patient having hypertension
- Safe dose is 7 mg/kg body weight, and it will be toxic to the patient if it exceeds more than 7 mg/kg, so more amount of drug can be infiltrated than plain lignocaine (Fig. 5)

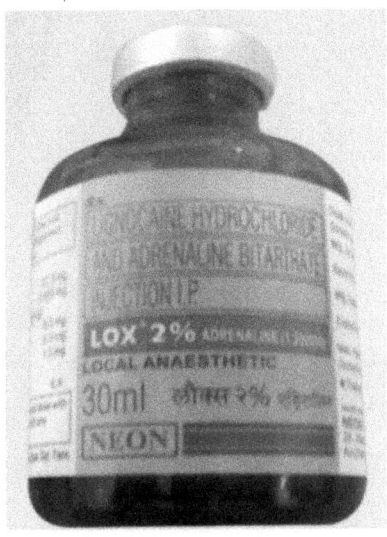

Fig. 5: Lignocaine hydrochloride 2% with adrenaline injection IP.

Uses

Same as plain lignocaine, except strictly contraindicated and not used for ring block of fingers, toes and for penile block, due to catastrophic complication of ischemia and gangrene of the part, where it has been used, as most of them are having end arterial blood supply.

LIGNOCAINE HYDROCHLORIDE INJECTION (XYLOCARD 2%)

- It contains 2% lignocaine without preservative (methylparaben), which is present in all other preparations of lignocaine, which are used as a local anesthetic agent
- It is provided in 50 mL vial. Each mL contains lignocaine hydrochloride IP: 21.3 mg, sodium chloride: 6.0 mg
- It is given intravenously, as it free of preservative.

Dose: As an antiarrhythmic agent 1–2 mg/kg intravenously (Fig. 6).

Uses

In ventricular arrhythmias like ventricular tachycardia, ventricular ectopics, etc.

LIGNOCAINE SPRAY

- It is provided in a 50 mL glass bottle with spray mounted at its neck

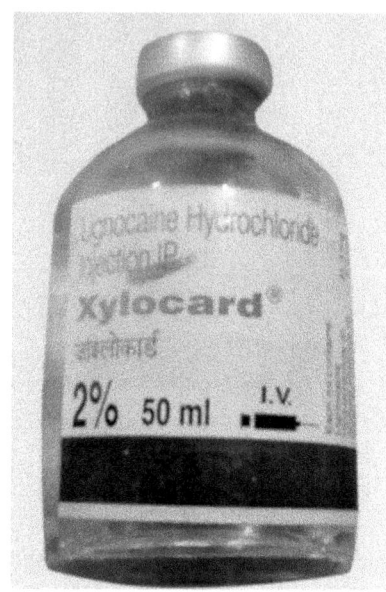

Fig. 6: Lignocaine hydrochloride injection IP (Xylocard 2%).

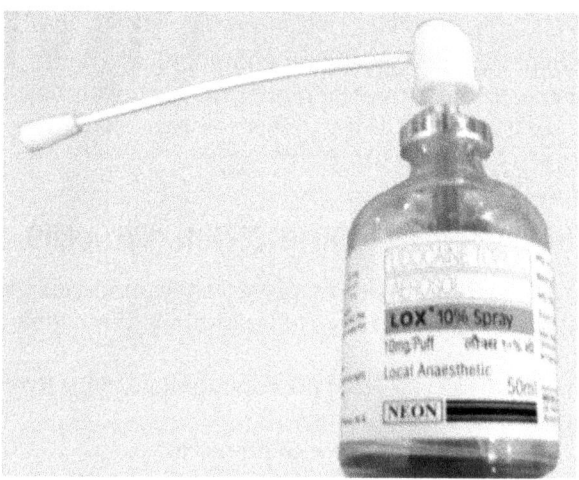

Fig. 7: Lignocaine topical aerosol (LOX 10% spray).

- It contains lidocaine USP, at a concentration of 10%, i.e. 10 mg/puff
- Each mL contains lidocaine USP 100 mg, with ethanol IP 30.4% V/V (Fig. 7).

Uses

- To anesthetize the oropharynx, before endotracheal tube intubation
- To anesthetize the oropharynx, during upper gastrointestinal (GI) endoscopy, for easy passage of the endoscope.

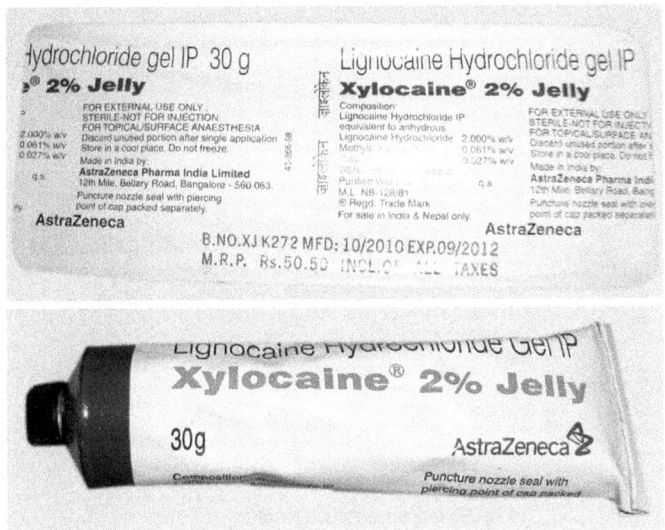

Fig. 8: Lignocaine hydrochloride gel IP (Xylocaine 2% jelly).

LIGNOCAINE HYDROCHLORIDE GEL (Xylocaine 2% Jelly)

- It contains lignocaine hydrochloride gel IP
- Provided in concentration of 2% gel, in a sterile tube (Fig. 8).

Uses

- For topical and surface anesthesia
- It provides lubrication as well as anesthetizes the surface on which it is applied
- Used before inserting a nasogastric tube. Lidocaine gel is applied at the tip and body of the tube and also in the nostril through which it has to be passed
- Before periurethral catheterization, lignocaine jelly is pushed into the urethra through the external urethral meatus with a syringe, to anesthetize as well as lubricate the entire urethra for easy passage of the catheter. 10 minutes have to wait after inserting the gel in the urethra, to get its maximum anesthetic effect for easy catheterization
- Lignocaine ointment is also available which contains lidocaine hydrochloride in a concentration of 5%, in a sterile tube, which is mostly applied per anally before defecation in case of fissure-in-ano, to anesthetize the anal canal to prevent excessive pain during defecation.

ADRENALINE TARTRATE INJECTION

- It is an endogenous catecholamine, with alpha and beta action. Positive inotropic action (Fig. 9)

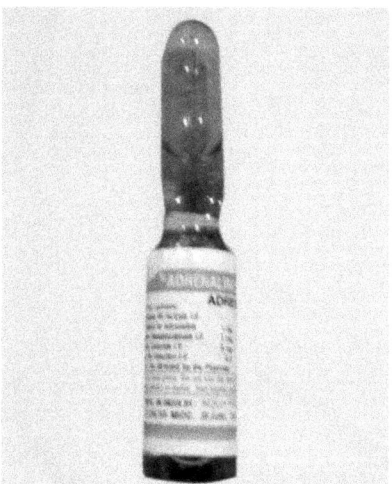

Fig. 9: Adrenaline tartrate injection.

- It causes tachycardia, hypertension, vasoconstriction, b-2 mediated bronchodilation and hyperglycemia. Provided in 1 mL vial.
- Each mL contains adrenaline bi-tartrate IP 1 mg, sodium metabisulfate
- IP: 1 mg, Sodium chloride IP: 8 mg, for IV/IM use
- 1:1000 contains 1 mg/mL
- 1:10000 contains 100 mg/mL
- 1:200000 contains 5 mg/mL.

Dose

- 0.1 mL/kg of 1 : 10000 (10 mg/kg) for intravenous purpose
- 0.1 mL/kg of 1 : 1000 (100 mg/kg) [ETT]
- 0.05–1 mg/kg/min iv infusion
- Maximum dose for infiltration 2 mg/kg.

Uses

- As an emergency drug to stimulate the heart in cardiopulmonary resuscitation (CPR), to increase blood pressure (BP), heart rate, myocardial contractility (stimulates heart)
- In hypotension, resistant to dopamine, it is used as a continuous infusion to increase BP
- In treatment of atropine resistant bradycardia
- In anaphylactic shock
- As a local infiltration with local anesthetic drug, to prolong its duration of action and to reduce blood loss by vasoconstriction
- As a bronchodilator.

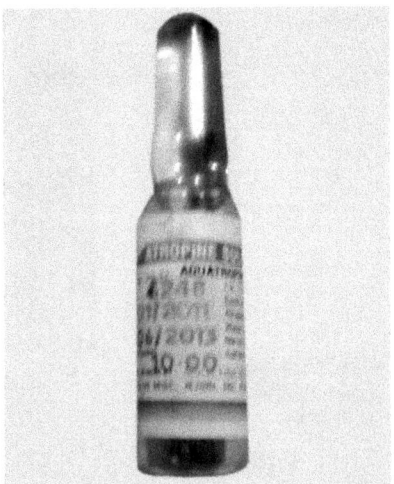

Fig. 10: Atropine sulfate injection.

ATROPINE SULFATE INJECTION

- It is an anticholinergic drug
- It causes predominantly tachycardia, due to vagal blockade at AV and sinus node, crosses blood brain barrier
- It decreases secretions, relaxes bronchial smooth muscle
- Provided in 1 ml vial. Each mL contains atropine sulfate IP: 0.60 mg, for IV/IM use (Fig. 10).

Dose: 10–20 mg/kg (Pediatric), 300–600 mg/kg in adults maximum 3 mg in cardiac arrest.

Uses

- In treatment of bradycardia, vagal syncopal attack due to vagal stimulation during intraoperative period
- In organophosphate poisioning
- To reduce secretions, it is used as a premedication drug before any operative procedure under anesthesia
- Prevention of muscarinic effects of neostigmine, postoperatively at the time of reversal of anesthesia, from neuromuscular blocking drugs.

GLYCOPYRROLATE (PYROLATE) INJECTION

- It is provided in 10 mL vial and also in 1 mL ampoule, for intravenous/intramuscular use
- Each mL contains glycopyrrolate USP 0.2 mg and benzyl alcohol 0.9% V/V as a preservative (Fig. 11).

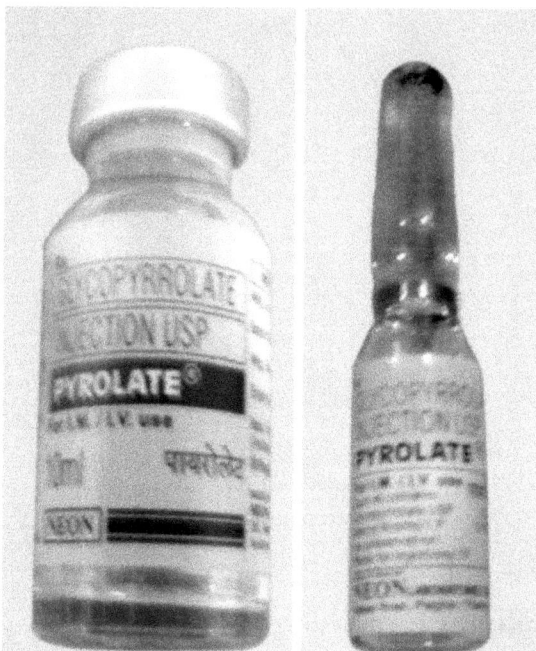

Fig. 11: Glycopyrrolate injection USP.

Uses

- To reduce the secretions, it is used as a premedication drug before any operative procedure under anesthesia
- It causes less tachycardia as compared to atropine.

ONDANSETRON

- 5-HT3 receptor antagonist
- It is an anti-emetic drug.

Dose: 8 mg given 1 hour before anesthesia, and 2 more doses of 8 mg postoperatively at 8 hours intervals (Fig. 12).

Uses

- As a premedication drug, to prevent postoperative nausea and vomiting, before any operative procedure under anesthesia
- To prevent nausea and vomiting, associated with highly emetogenic chemotherapy or radiotherapy.

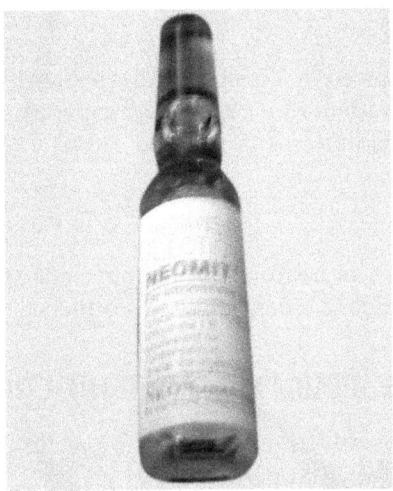

Fig. 12: Ondansetron injection.

■ HYDROCORTISONE SODIUM SUCCINATE INJECTION

- ❖ It is a short acting endogenous steroid, with anti-inflammatory and potent mineralocorticoid action
- ❖ It causes hyperglycemia, hypertension, psychic disturbance, muscle weakness, fluid retention
- ❖ It is provided in 100 mg vial in powdered form, which has to be reconstituted with one ampoule of 5 mL sterile water provided with it for IV/IM use
- ❖ Each vial contains hydrocortisone sodium succinate equivalent to 100 mg hydrocortisone IP, sodium phosphate IP and sodium acid phosphatase IP as a buffering agent (Fig. 13).

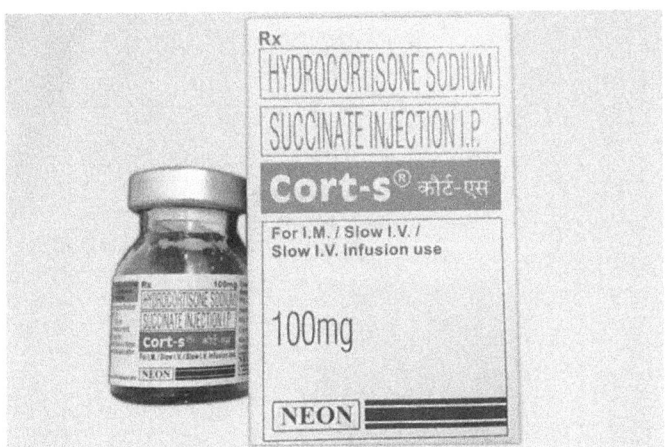

Fig. 13: Hydrocortisone sodium succinate injection IP.

Dose

- 4 mg/kg bolus followed by 2–4 mg/kg qds (pediatric)
- 25 mg at induction, then 25 mg qds in intraoperative period
- For adrenal suppression 50–200 mg qds.

Uses

As an emergency drug, in treatment of anaphylactic shock, bronchospasm, laryngeal edema, allergic reactions, thyroid storm, etc.

DEXAMETHASONE SODIUM PHOSPHATE INJECTION (DEXONA)

- It is a long acting steroid, provided in 2 mL vial, for IV/IM injection
- Prednisolone derivative corticosteroid
- It cause less sodium retention than hydrocortisone
- Each mL contains dexamethasone sodium phosphate IP equivalent to dexamethasone phosphate 4 mg, methylparaben IP 0.15% W/V, propylparaben IP 0.02% W/V (Fig. 14).

Dose

- 4–8 mg (adult)
- 200–400 mg/kg (pediatric)
- Dexamethasone 0.75 mg = prednisolone 5 mg.

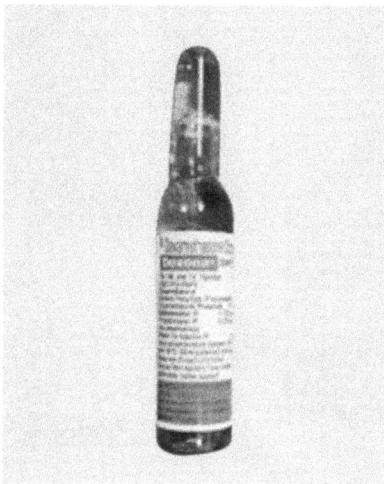

Fig. 14: Dexamethasone sodium phosphate injection IP.

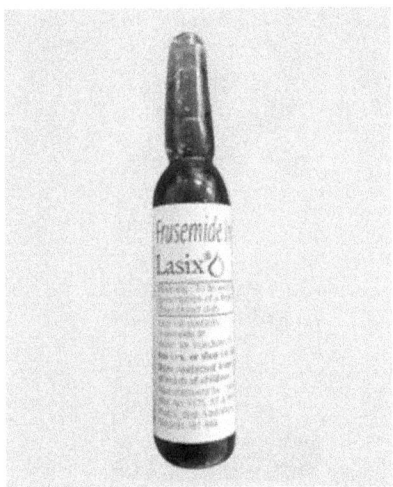

Fig. 15: Furosemide injection IP.

Uses
- As an emergency drug, in the treatment of anaphylactic shock, bronchospasm, laryngeal edema, allergic reactions, etc.
- To decrease cerebral edema as a adjuvant drug to mannitol, in head injury patients, also to decrease cerebral edema postoperatively in craniotomy patients
- As an antiemetic.

FUROSEMIDE (LASIX)

It is a loop diuretic, provided in 2 mL vial. Each mL contains furosemide IP 10 mg (Fig. 15).

Uses
For diuresis in the treatment of congestive cardiac failure (CCF), pulmonary edema, cerebral edema, early stages of renal failure due to renal causes.

MIDAZOLAM (MEZOLAM)
- It is a short acting benzodiazepine, provided in 5 or 10 mL vial for IV/IM use
- Each mL contains midazolam BP 1 mg with benzyl alcohol IP 1% V/V (Fig. 16).

Uses
- As a anxiolytic drug, as a premedication in preoperative period for sedation
- To provide sedation for short cases
- As a anticonvulsion drug.

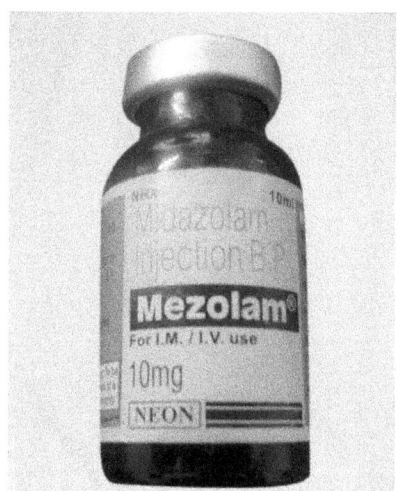

Fig. 16: Midazolam injection BP.

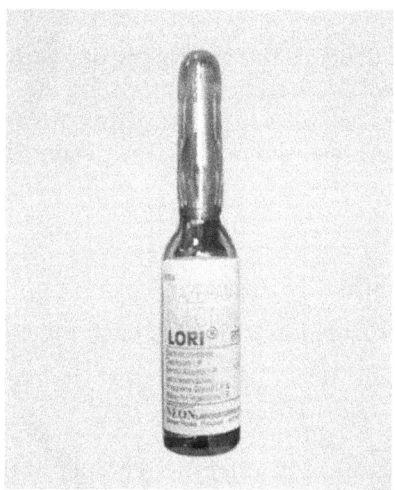

Fig. 17: Diazepam injection IP.

DIAZEPAM (CALMPOSE)

- It is a short acting benzodiazepine, provided in 2 mL vial, for IV/IM use
- Each 2 mL contains, diazepam IP 10 mg, and benzyl alcohol 1.5% V/V (Fig. 17).

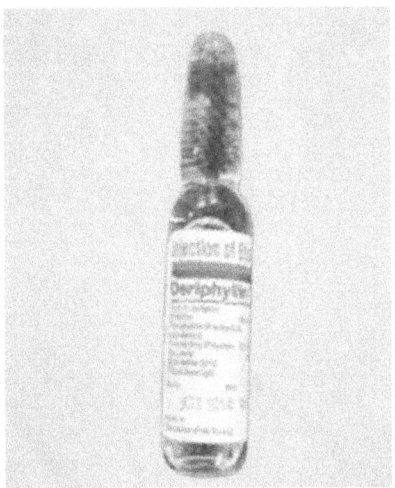

Fig. 18: Etofylline and theophylline injection IP.

■ INJECTION OF ETOFYLLINE AND THEOPHYLLINE (DERIPHYLLIN)

- ❖ It is a bronchodilator drug, provided in 2 mL for IV/IM use
- ❖ Each mL contains etofylline IP 85: 84.7 mg, theophylline IP anhydrous equivalent to theophylline IP hydrate 25.3 mg (Fig. 18).

Uses

In treatment of bronchospasm, bronchial asthma, chronic obstructive pulmonary disease.

■ THIOPENTONE SODIUM (THIOSOL SODIUM)

- ❖ It is an ultrashort acting barbiturate, available in yellowish powdered form
- ❖ It is used as 2.5% solution (25 mg/mL)
- ❖ It is a potent anticonvulsant
- ❖ It produces myocardial and respiratory depression, peripheral vasodilatation and hypotension
- ❖ Dose: 4–5 mg/kg body weight intravenously (Fig. 19).

Uses

For induction and maintenance of general anesthesia, while performing procedures under anesthesia.

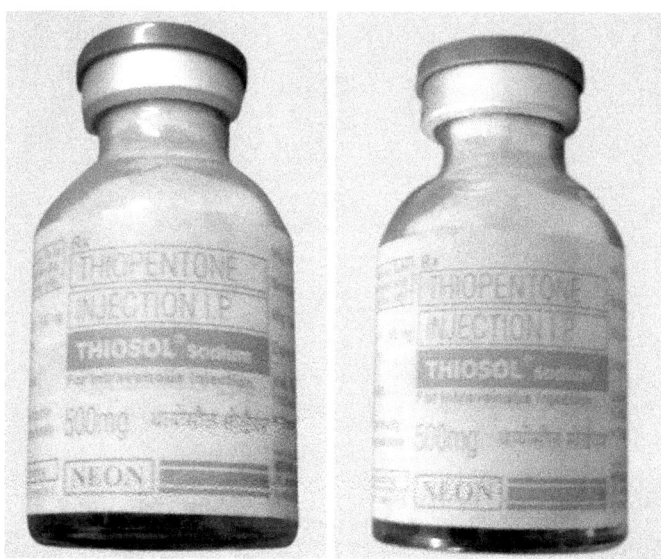

Fig. 19: Thiopentone sodium IP.

■ KETAMINE HYDROCHLORIDE INJECTION (ANEKET)

- ❖ It contains ketamine hydrochloride 50 mg in each mL, for IV/IM use
- ❖ It is a phencyclidine derivative, NMDA receptor antagonist
- ❖ It produces dissociative anesthesia and intense analgesia
- ❖ It causes tachycardia, hypertension, bronchodilation and respiratory depression in high doses, when given rapidly
- ❖ It also causes vivid and unpleasant hallucinations, delirium
- ❖ It is provided in 2 mL ampoule and also in 10 mL vial (Fig. 20).

Dose: 1–2 mg/kg for IV use, 5–10 mg/kg for IM use. For IV Infusion: 1–3 mg/kg/h.

Uses

For induction and maintenance of general anesthesia, while performing procedures under general anesthesia.

■ PROPOFOL INJECTION (NEOROF)

- ❖ It is highly lipid soluble and formulated in a white, aqueous emulsion (milky white) containing soybean oil and egg phosphate
- ❖ It contains 10 mg/mL and provided in 10, 20, 50 mL vial, for intravenous use
- ❖ Recovery is rapid
- ❖ It causes cardiovascular and respiratory depression (Fig. 21).

Dose: 2–2.5 mg/kg for IV use.

Chapter 31: Commonly Used Drugs in Anesthesia

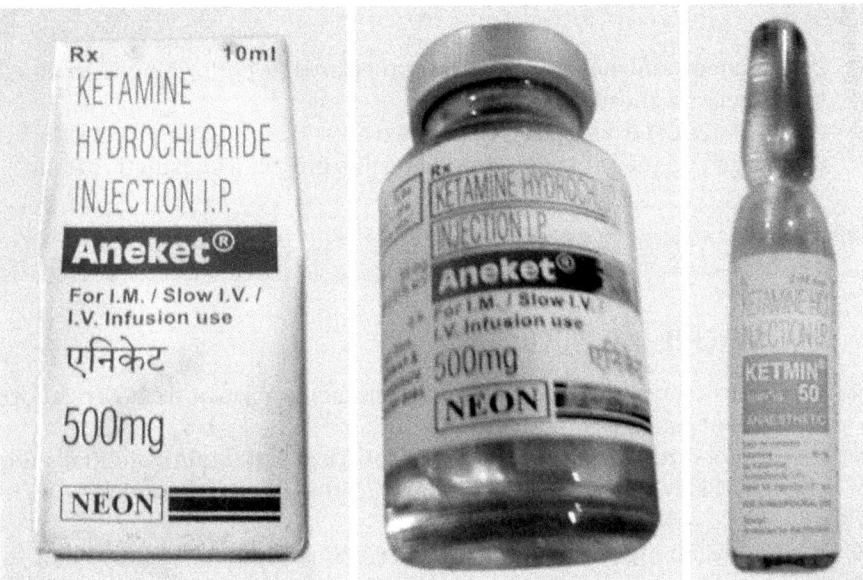

Fig. 20: Ketamine hydrochloride IP in 10 mL vial and 2 mL ampoule.

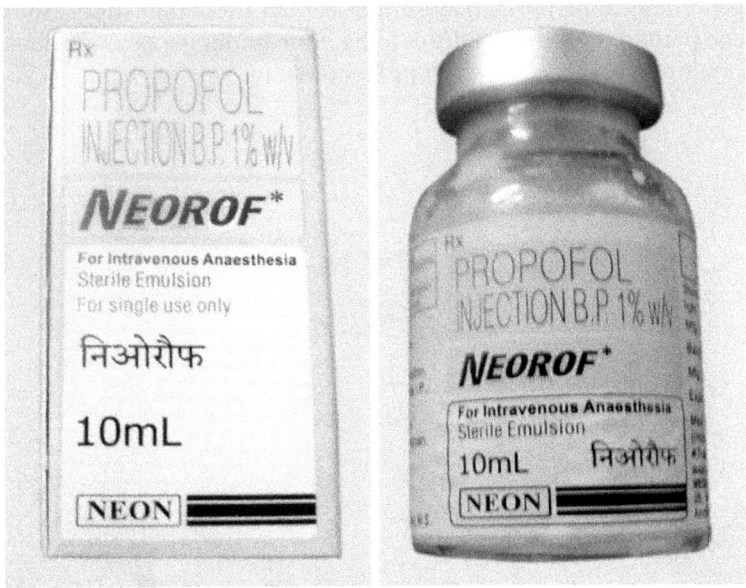

Fig. 21: Propofol injection BP 1% W/V.

Uses

- For induction and maintenance of anesthesia, while performing procedures under general anesthesia
- It is mostly used as a 'day care anesthetic' agent, as patient can be discharged on the same day after using this drug as a anesthetic agent.

MUSCLE RELAXANTS

SUCCINYLCHOLINE (SUCOL)

- It is a ultrashort acting depolarizing muscle relaxant with very short duration of action (2 minutes)
- It gives good relaxation to facilitate intubation, but if intubation fails the patient is likely to resume spontaneous breathing early preventing hypoxic injury
- It contains 50 mg/mL and provided in 1 mL ampoule, 10 mL vial or in powdered form also which has to be reconstituted.

Dose: 1–1.5 mg/kg body weight for intravenous use (Fig. 22).

Uses

- Given intravenously to facilitate endotracheal intubation, during induction of the patient for the procedures to be done under general anesthesia
- To maintain paralysis for short procedures.

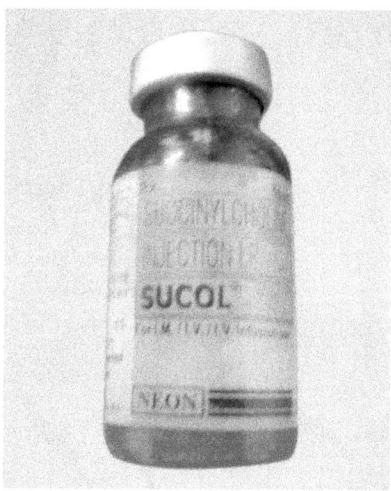

Fig. 22: Succinylcholine injection IP.

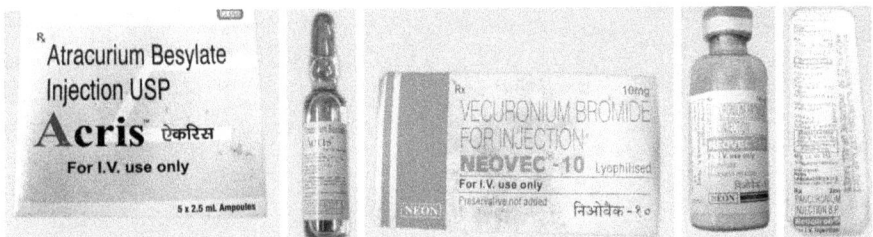

Atracurium besylate injection   Vecuronium bromide injection   Pancuronium injection

Fig. 23: Muscle relaxants.

ATRACURIUM/PANCURONIUM/VECURONIUM/ROCURONIUM

These are long acting non depolarizing muscle relaxants causing muscle paralysis (Fig. 23).

ATRACURIUM BESYLATE

It contains atracurium besylate 10 mg/mL and provided in 2.5 mL ampoule for intravenous use.

Uses

- For muscle paralysis, while performing procedures under general anesthesia with intermittent positive pressure ventilation (IPPV) or controlled ventilation
- To maintain paralysis in a patient in intensive care unit on a ventilator.

NEOSTIGMINE METHYLSULFATE

- It contains neostigmine methylsulfate IP 0.5 mg in each mL
- It is provided in 5 mL vial for intramuscular, slow intravenous and subcutaneous use
- It is a cholinesterase inhibitor; parasympathomimetic drug
- It blocks the action of cholinesterase, thus increasing the amount of acetylcholine in the neuromuscular junction
- It can cause the muscarinic effects of acetylcholine such as bradycardia, bronchoconstriction, etc. Hence, it is always combined with atropine or glycopyrrolate, to counteract these effects (Fig. 24).

Dose: 0.05–0.08 mg/kg body weight intravenously.

Uses

- For reversal of non-depolarizing neuromuscular blockade given during general anesthesia

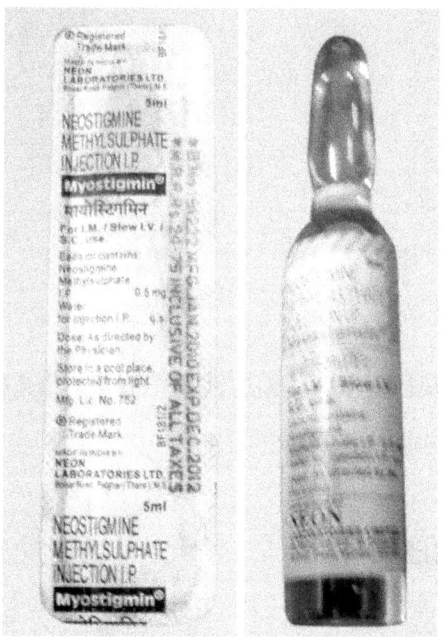

Fig. 24: Neostigmine methylsulfate injection IP.

- Also used in treatment of myasthenia gravis, paralytic ileus and postoperative urinary retention.

INHALATIONAL ANESTHETIC AGENTS

■ HALOTHANE/SEVOFLURANE/ISOFLURANE/DESFLURANE

They are given through the endotracheal tube, from the container of the inhalational anesthetic drug attached to the Boyle's machine, via the antistatic rubber tubings.

■ HALOTHANE

- It is a volatile inhalational anesthetic agent
- It is a colorless liquid with pleasant smell
- It depresses myocardial contractility and cardiac output. Also causes arrhythmias (Fig. 25).

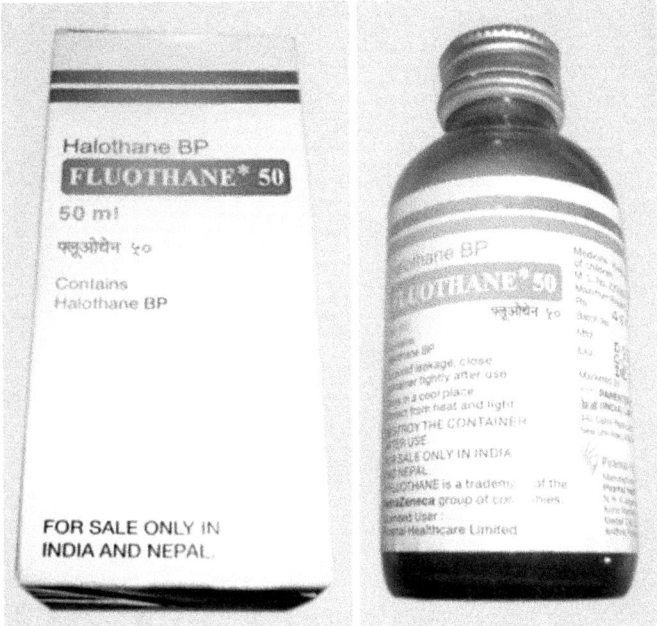

Fig. 25: Halothane BP.

ISOFLURANE

- It is a halogenated ether, with pungent smell
- It is preferred over halothane, in patients with cardiac disease and patients with raised intracranial pressure, as it causes less cardiac depression and less cerebral vasodilatation than halothane.

SEVOFLURANE AND DESFLURANE

- They are newer general inhalational anesthetic agents
- Induction and recovery is faster than halothane, and they also produces minimal cardiac depression
- Sevoflurane is popular in children, for induction of general anesthesia.

Uses

For induction and maintenance of general anesthesia.

Section 8

Surgical (Operative) Procedures

Various surgical (operative) procedures are there in the general surgical practice. But in this book, only those procedures are described, which are usually asked in the table viva of operative procedures and instruments in general surgery, in undergraduate and postgraduate examinations

Students should follow the systematic approach, to explain the surgical procedures as described in this book.

The procedures described in this section, are broadly divided into major and minor surgical procedures.

Most of the major surgical procedures are usually done under general or regional anesthesia (spinal or epidural anesthesia), whereas, minor surgical procedures are done under local anesthesia.

Section Outline

32. Preoperative Preparation of the Patient Prior to Surgical Procedures
33. Preparation of the Patient on the Operation Table Prior to the Procedures
34. Major Operative Procedures
35. Minor Operative Procedures

CHAPTER 32

Preoperative Preparation of the Patient Prior to Surgical Procedures

■ PREPARATION OF THE OPERATIVE AND SURROUNDING AREA

- ❖ Remove hair from the skin of the operative and adjacent area preoperatively, by shaving, threading or by application of epilating cream
- ❖ Shaving is not a good procedure, as it may cause microscopic cuts in the skin, where bacterial proliferation can occur overnight, if shaving has been done prior to a day before the surgery. If shaving has to be done, it should be done in the morning hours of the day of surgery or just preoperatively on the operation table. Removal of the hair by applying epilating cream is a better option than shaving, as the risk of skin cuts and their subsequent contamination will not occur unlike with shaving.

Prophylaxis against Tetanus by Injecting Tetanus Toxoid

Injection tetanus toxoid 0.5 mL intramuscularly should be given preoperatively in every young and adult patients, but not routinely in children till 15 years of age, as most of them are immunized as per the National Immunization Schedule.

Injection Lignocaine Hydrochloride (Xylocaine) Sensitivity Test

- ❖ This test has to be done, if the surgical procedure is planned under local or spinal anesthesia.
- ❖ It is done by infiltrating 1% or 2% xylocaine subcutaneously in the forearm of the patient by raising a subcutaneous bleb. The infiltrated area marked with a skin marker.
- ❖ Observe the marked area, for hypersensitivity reactions like itching, redness, increase in the size of the bleb, etc. If such reactions occurs, it indicates patient is sensitive to lignocaine and that patient should not be operated, under local or spinal anesthesia, in which lignocaine is used.

Fasting or Nil by Mouth (NBM)

Patient should be kept fasting or nil by mouth for at least 6–8 hours prior to the proposed time of surgery, if the procedure has to be done under regional or general anesthesia.

Written and Informed Consent

- ❖ Detailed information about the planned surgical procedure, other alternative procedures, advantages and disadvantages of the planned as well as its alternative options, risk of anesthesia to be given for the opted procedure, intraoperative and postoperative complications also should be explained to the patient and his/her relatives in their own language
- ❖ Consent has to be taken prior to the procedure by taking signature or left thumb impression of the patient in case of adults and that of parents or guardian, if the patient is minor (less than 18 years of age), after explaining them everything as described above in their own language.

CHAPTER 33

Preparation of the Patient on the Operation Table Prior to the Procedures

Following step-by-step approach, should be followed on the operation table before starting any procedure.

Anesthesia

Anesthesia has to be given as per the surgeon's and anesthetist's preference according to requirement of the patients operative procedure, which are described in subsequent chapters along with the procedures.

Position of the Patient for the Surgery

Patient has to be positioned on the operation table in such a way that, it should give easy accessibility of the operative area to the operating surgeon.

Antiseptic Cleaning of the Operative Area

Operative and surrounding adjacent area should be thoroughly cleaned (scrubbed) with swab soaked in antiseptic solution, before starting any procedure, to make the operative, as well as the adjacent area sterile and free of microorganisms.

Various Antiseptic Solutions in Use

- **Povidine iodine:** Application of 2–3 layers of povidine iodine. It releases iodine slowly and provides longer duration of antiseptic effect.
- **Tincture iodine and spirit (Isopropyl alcohol):** Cleansing with tincture iodine and spirit.
- **Cetrimide (Savlon) and spirit:** Cleansing with cetrimide and with spirit.

For abdominal operations (laparotomy), skin from the mid chest to mid thigh level should be cleaned.

Draping the Operative Area

❖ Draping means placement of sterile sheets or towels surrounding the operative area and fixing it with towel clips, to isolate the operative area from the rest of the unsterile area of the body
❖ It prevents contamination of the sterile operative area during surgery from the adjacent unsterile area.

After strictly following the above step-by-step approach, the procedure can be started.

CHAPTER 34

Major Operative Procedures

■ APPENDICECTOMY

Definition

Removal of the appendix from the body (abdominal cavity).

Indications

- ❖ Acute appendicitis
- ❖ Recurrent or chronic appendicitis
- ❖ Mucocele of the appendix
- ❖ Carcinoma or carcinoid tumor of the appendix confined to the mucosa and tip or body of the appendix, and not involving the base of the appendix.

Contraindications

Appendicular mass.

Techniques

Open and laparoscopic appendicectomy.

■ OPEN APPENDICECTOMY

Definition

Removal of the appendix from the peritoneal cavity, by dissecting appendix from its tip to base by open surgical approach.

Anesthesia

Mostly done under regional anesthesia like spinal anesthesia, and rarely under general anesthesia if required as in case of children.

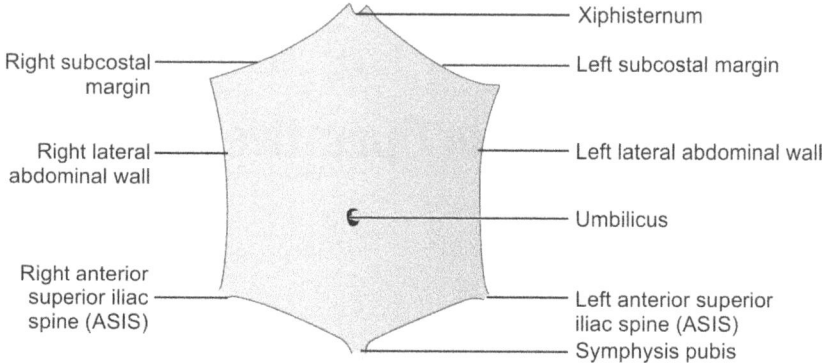

Fig. 1: Prototype diagram for different incisions over anterior abdominal wall.

Position of the Patient on the Operation Table

Supine position.

Prototype diagram of abdomen showing different quadrants of the abdomen for easy understanding of the incisions of different procedures shown in Fig. 1

Incisions

Different incisions can be employed for appendicectomy like (Fig. 2):
A. McBurney's gridiron incision (Most commonly used and preferred incision)
B. Rutherford Morrison incision
C. Lanz's incision
D. Right lower paramedian incision
E. Lower midline incision.

Steps of the Procedure

Parts are painted with antiseptic solution and draped with sterile sheets.

McBurney's Gridiron Incision

- ❖ It is a muscle splitting, 5–6 cm oblique skin incision in right iliac fossa, perpendicular to the right spinoumbilical line (line joining the anterior superior iliac spine to the umbilicus on right side of the abdomen), centring over the McBurney' point (Point situated on medial 2/3rd and lateral 1/3rd of the right spinoumbilical line) described by McArthur (McBurney's incision)
- ❖ Subcutaneous tissue incised in the same line as that of the skin incision
- ❖ Superficial circumflex iliac artery is identified in the subcutaneous fat and ligated
- ❖ External oblique aponeurosis is identified by direction of its fibers (fibers running downwards, forwards and medially)
- ❖ A nick (small incision) is given with the surgical blade, parallel to the fibers of external oblique aponeurosis. It is then extended laterally as well as medially along the direction of its fibers to expose the internal oblique muscle

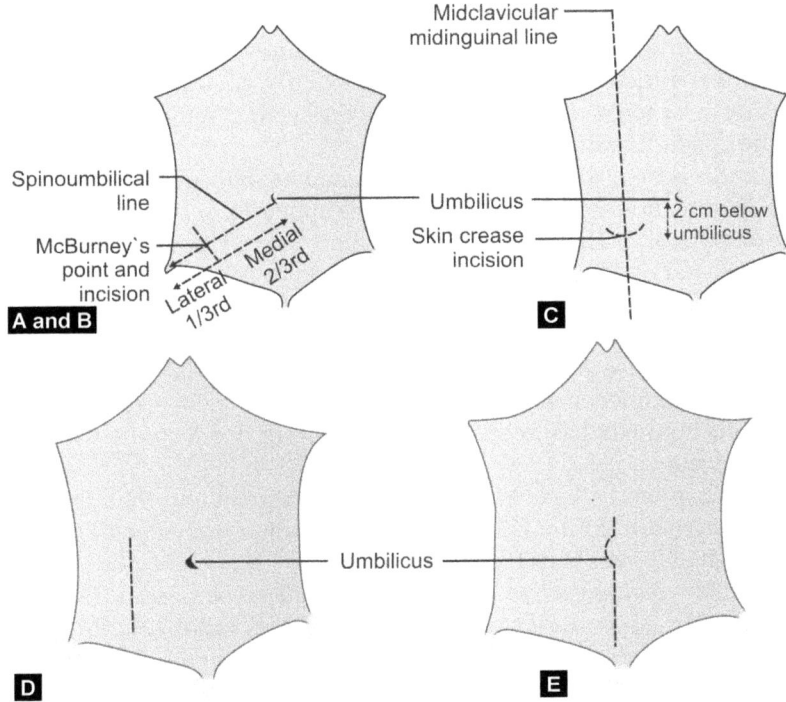

Figs. 2A to E: Different incisions for appendicectomy; (A and B) McBurney's grid iron incision, Rutherford Morison incision; (C) Lanz's incision; (D) Right lower paramedian incision; (E) Lower midline incision.

- A Mayo's scissor or medium sized curved hemostatic forceps is thrushed with closed blades through the fibers of the internal oblique and transversus abdominus muscle and then the blades are opened up to split both these muscles along the direction of their fibers
- Two Langenbach's right angled retractors are inserted through the split fibers of these muscles, which are then retracted to reach and expose the peritoneum
- Moist packs are kept around the incision before opening the peritoneum, to avoid contamination of the skin and adjacent tissue with the peritoneal contents like pus, after opening the peritoneum
- Peritoneum is lifted up by two curved hemostatic forceps and a nick (small incision) is given over the peritoneum with the surgical blade, which is then incised cautiously with fine scissor along the line of skin incision, to open the peritoneal cavity, talking care not to injure the underlying bowel (small and large intestine)
- If serous exudates or pus is present in the peritoneal cavity, it has to be sucked with the sucker (suction cannula) before it escapes through the incision
- Cecum is identified by its pale color, presence of three tenia coli and absence of the mesentery

- Cecum is grasped with moist sponge or plain dissecting forceps and delivered into the wound till the appendix comes into the view
- If there is difficulty in localizing the appendix, then it can be found by tracing three tenia coli along the wall of the cecum. At their junction, base of the appendix will be found
- Appendix is held with the help of nontraumatic Babcock's forceps one at the tip and another one at the base of the appendix
- Mesoappendix is clamped with one or more curved mosquito hemostatic forceps, and divided and ligated with thread or silk, from apex up to the base of the appendix
- Mobilized appendix is held upward with the Babcock's forceps applied at its tip and its base is crushed with straight hemostatic forceps close to the cecal wall for few seconds and then removed
- Another hemostatic forceps is applied 0.5 cm distal to the previously crushed site
- Crushed appendix base is first ligated with thread and then transfixed with absorbable suture (Vicryl No. 2-0, on round body needle) through the crushed lumen of its base
- Appendix is divided with a knife close to the distal hemostatic forceps
- Stump of the appendix is swabbed with povidone-iodine solution or spirit
- Appendix is removed from the operative area along with the swab, knife and hemostatic forceps holding the body of the appendix to prevent contamination of the surrounding area
- Burying the base of the appendix is surgeon's preference, which is not done nowadays by most of the surgeons
- If the base (stump) of the appendix has to be buried or invaginated, a purse string suture of absorbable suture material (Vicryl No. 2-0, on round body needle) is taken circumferentially all around the ligated stump (1 cm from the stump), through the seromuscular coat of the cecal wall. Alternatively a 'Z' suture can be taken through the cecal wall to bury the stump
- Stump of the appendix is held by plain dissecting forceps and then the purse string suture is tightened
- The stump is invaginated (buried) in the cecal wall while tightening the purse string or 'Z' suture
- If there is edema of the cecal wall, or if the appendix is gangrenous or if the appendix is perforated at its base, then invagination of the stump should never be tried and it is absolutely contraindicated in such circumstances. In such cases, appendix should only be doubly ligated at its base with thread even without crushing and then removed
- Check for hemostasis from the appendix stump, adjacent bowel, mesentery and raw peritoneal area
- The terminal ileum is brought outside the wound up to 2 feet proximal to the ileocecal junction to check for associated Meckel's diverticulum, which has to be managed accordingly if found pathological

- Drainage of the peritoneal cavity is usually not needed in case of appendicitis without complications. It can be done by inserting abdominal drain in right iliac fossa or in the pelvis, in cases of complicated appendicitis like appendicular abscess or perforation with significant peritoneal contamination
- Peritoneum is closed with continuous absorbable suture (Vicryl No. 2-0, on round body needle)
- Retractors are removed and transverses abdominis and internal oblique muscles approximated with absorbable suture (Vicryl No. 2-0, on round body needle) if required
- External oblique aponeurosis is sutured with continuous absorbable suture (Vicryl No. 2-0, on round body needle)
- Subcutaneous tissue is approximated with absorbable suture (Vicryl No. 2-0, on round body needle)
- Skin is sutured with interrupted nonabsorbable suture (Nylon or silk No. 2-0/3-0, on cutting needle) or by subcuticular sutures for better postoperative scar
- Sterile adhesive dressing is applied.

The above described removal of appendix is anterograde appendicectomy, which is commonly employed.

Other Recommended Incisions for Appendicectomy

Rutherford Morrison Incision

Gridiron incision can be converted to Rutherford Morrison incision by cutting the internal oblique and transversus abdominus muscles along the line of the skin incision. It is useful and necessary in cases of paracecal or retrocecal appendix and also in cases of appendicular abscess or perforation, when gridiron incision is inadequate for giving proper access to the inflamed appendix and adjacent area.

Right Lower Paramedian Incision

Preferred in case of appendicular abscess or perforation, for proper exposure of the peritoneal cavity, drainage of pus and for giving thorough peritoneal lavage to remove the pus and pus flakes.

Lower Midline Incision

Employed in patients in whom diagnosis of appendicitis is in doubt and in case of female patients where gynecological or obstetric causes for acute right lower quadrant abdominal pain are suspected.

Lanz's Incision

Transverse skin crease cosmetic incision, preferred in female patients, located 2 cm below the umbilicus, centring on mid clavicular-mid inguinal line.

Retrograde Appendicectomy (Dissection of the Appendix from Base to its Tip)

- ❖ When the appendix is retrocecal or retrocolic, the tip of the appendix may not be easily visualized and accessible and difficult to find, or in cases where it is firmly adherent to the surrounding structures (terminal ileum, cecum, omentum, etc.), then it cannot be easily delivered into the wound
- ❖ In such cases, the base of the appendix is freed and divided first between the hemostatic forceps, the base ligated, transfixed and then the remainder of the body of the appendix is freed from base to tip and delivered out of the wound.

Postoperative Complications

Early Complications

- ❖ Wound infection and wound gape
- ❖ Intra-abdominal abscess (pelvic abscess): If pus is not drained and peritoneal lavage is not given properly
- ❖ Postoperative paralytic ileus
- ❖ Faeces fistula due to leakage of faeces from the appendicular stump, because of slipping of ligature of the stump or due to iatrogenic trauma causing rupture of the cecal wall during dissection.
- ❖ Hemorrhage due to slipping of the ligature of the appendicular artery, from the raw peritoneal area, from mesenteric tear of the surrounding bowel.

Late Complications

- ❖ Postoperative adhesive intestinal obstruction
- ❖ Incisional hernia is a late rare complication.

LAPAROSCOPIC APPENDICECTOMY

Diagnostic as well therauptic in case of child-bearing age women.

Anesthesia

Mostly done under general anesthesia and rarely done under regional anesthesia like spinal or epidural anesthesia.

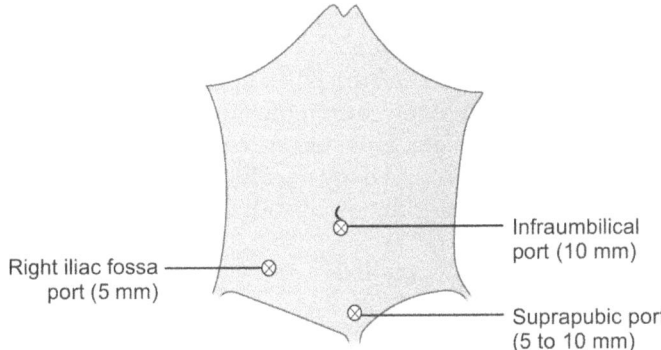

Fig. 3: Port sites for laparoscopic appendicectomy.

Position of the Patient on the Operation Table

Head down (Trendelenburg) position supplemented by left lateral tilt, which encourages gravitation of the small bowel towards the upper and left side of the abdomen, i.e. away from the cecum to expose the cecum and the appendix.

Incision

Three 1 cm incisions are required for port insertion. Infraumbilical 10 mm port for telescope, one 5 mm port in right iliac fossa and another 5 or 10 mm port in left iliac fossa or in suprapubic region (Fig. 3).

Steps of the Procedure

- Parts are painted with antiseptic solution and draped with sterile sheets
- Pneumoperitoneum is created by insufflating carbon dioxide through the Hasson's cannula or Veress needle, through the umbilicus or through the infraumbilical incision
- Telescope is inserted into the peritoneal cavity through the infraumbilical port
- One 5 mm port is inserted in the peritoneal cavity through right iliac fossa and another 5 or 10 mm port is inserted through left iliac fossa or suprapubic region under direct vision of the laparoscopic port
- Appendix is exposed by displacing terminal ileum and cecum using atraumatic grasping forceps like Babcock's forceps
- Mesoappendix is ligated to secure appendicular artery by ligatures or clips or cauterized by using bipolar coagulation
- Base of the appendix is encircled and ligated by two absorbable sutures (Catgut or vicryl ligatures by intracorporal knotting or by loop) with Roeder knot or by external knot snugged down with a knot pusher (extracorporal knotting)

- Appendix is removed from the body from the 10 mm port, after cutting its base in between the two ligatures
- Base of the appendix not to be buried like open appendicectomy
- After complete removal of the carbon dioxide from the peritoneal cavity through the ports or incisions, port sites are closed with absorbable sutures (Vicryl or catgut no. 2-0, round body needle)
- Skin incisions are sutured with non-absorbable sutures (Nylon or silk no. 2-0/3-0, on cutting needle)
- Sterile adhesive dressing is applied.

Advantages of Laparoscopic Appendicectomy Over Open Appendicectomy

- More rapid recovery
- Shorter stay in hospital and earlier discharge from the hospital
- Less postoperative pain
- Quicker return to normal activities
- Shortened time off from work
- Decrease wound complications and less wound infection
- Acceptable and better cosmetic scar
- Postoperative complications like postoperative adhesions, incisional hernia are rare.

Disadvantages of Laparoscopic Appendicectomy

- Requires general anesthesia
- Port site hernia.

Postoperative Complications of Laparoscopic Appendicectomy

Same as open appendicectomy, but much less as compared to it due to less tissue handling.

TREATMENT OF APPENDICULAR MASS

- Initial treatment is conservative known as 'Ochsner Sherren regimen' by keeping patient nil by mouth with intravenous fluid supplementation along with broad spectrum intravenous antibiotics
- Conservative management should be given, even if the patient has been taken on the operation table for appendicectomy, and anesthesia has also been given, if the appendicular lump is palpable
- Regime consists of observing and examining the patient regularly on hourly basis, to know whether the patient is responding to the conservative regime or not
- Majority of appendix masses (90%) resolves by this regime

- If patient responds to the conservative regime, 'interval appendicectomy' should be done after 6–8 weeks in such cases. This much time is sufficient, for the inflammation of the adjacent viscera (bowel) to subside and appendicectomy can be carried out easily without much risk of intra- and postoperative complications
- If appendicectomy is tried in such cases in acute phase, it inadvertently leads to formation of fecal fistula, due to injury to the adjacent bowel like terminal ileum, ascending colon and cecum while dissecting the appendix from the dense adhesions present between the inflamed appendix and the adjacent bowel.

Vitals to be Monitored and Criteria to Stop the Conservative Regimen are

1. **Extent of the mass:** Increase in the size of the mass (Extent of the mass is marked on the anterior abdomen wall and its size monitored regularly)
2. **Pulse rate:** Increase in the pulse rate (tachycardia)
3. **Body temperature:** Fever (Increasing pyrexia)
4. **Abdominal pain:** Increased abdominal pain (Suggestive of local or generalized peritonitis).

TREATMENT OF APPENDICULAR ABSCESS

- Failure of resolution of an appendix mass or continuous spiking (high-grade fever) suggests pus within phlegmonous mass (appendicular abscess)
- USG/CT abdomen and pelvis is diagnostic of such condition
- Emergency percutaneous drainage or laparotomy by midline or right paramedian incision is indicated in such cases, for drainage of pus and peritoneal lavage
- If the appendix is found easily and does not have dense adhesions with the adjacent viscera, appendicectomy can be done safely, otherwise should not be tried in such cases
- More often appendicectomy is impossible and the abscess cavity should only be washed with normal saline to remove pus and postoperatively to be drained by the abdominal drain in right iliac fossa or in the pelvis.

CHOLECYSTECTOMY

Definition
Removing gallbladder from the abdominal cavity.

Indications
Most common indication is recurrent biliary colic due to gallbladder stones.

Other Indications are

- ❖ Symptomatic gallstone disease
- ❖ Acute or chronic cholecystitis
- ❖ Empyema of the gallbladder
- ❖ Emphysematous cholecystitis
- ❖ Ascending cholangitis
- ❖ Gallbladder perforation
- ❖ Gallbladder neoplasm
- ❖ Cholecystoenteric fistula.

Indications in Asymptomatic Gallstones

- ❖ Large stone >3 cm due to risk of malignancy
- ❖ Multiple small stones due to chances of stones passing into the common bile duct, causing obstruction to bile flow leading to obstructive jaundice
- ❖ Stones associated with polyp
- ❖ Calcified gallbladder (Porcelain) due to risk of malignancy
- ❖ Gallstones in a patient with diabetes mellitus
- ❖ Congenital anomalies of gallbladder
- ❖ Patient with congenital hemolytic anemia.

Techniques

Done by open as well as laparoscopic technique.

Anesthesia

Both procedures are mostly done under general anesthesia, and rarely under regional anaesthesia like spinal or epidural anesthesia.

OPEN CHOLECYSTECTOMY

Position of the patient on the operation table: Supine.

Incisions (Figs. 4A to D)

A. Right subcoastal incision (Kocher's incision): Most commonly preferred incision
B. Right paramedian incision: Rectus splitting or rectus displacing
C. Right upper quadrant transverse incision
D. Upper midline incision (When simultaneous common bile duct exploration has to be done).

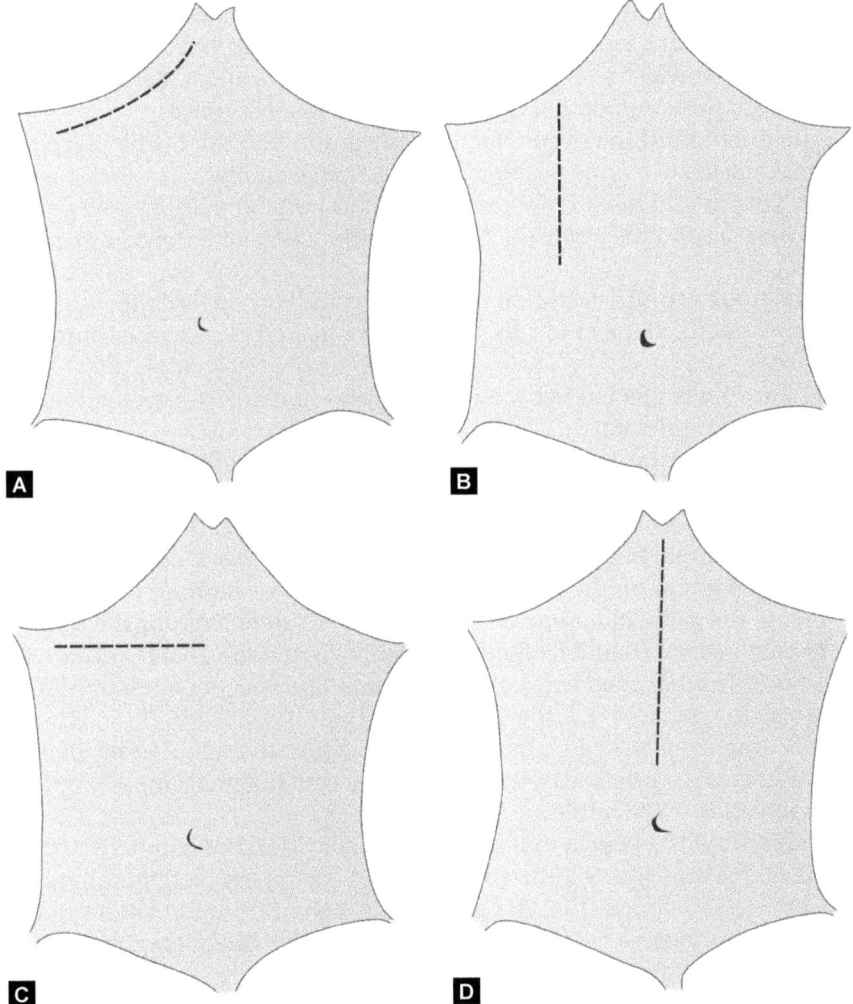

Figs. 4A to D: Different incisions for open cholecystectomy: (A) Right subcostal incision; (B) Right paramedian incision; (C) Right upper quadrant transverse incision; (D) Upper middle incision.

Steps of the Procedure

- 'Fundus first cholecystectomy' is most commonly employed technique for open as well as laparoscopic cholecystectomy in which gallbladder is dissected from its fundus down to the cystic duct.
- Separation of the gallbladder is commenced first at the fundus, after dividing its peritoneal reflections on each side with scissors, where it is reflected on to the liver.
- Any adhesions or peritoneal folds connecting the gallbladder to the duodenum or colon are divided and bleeding points are ligatured.

- Gentle traction is applied to the fundus of the gallbladder with sponge holding forceps and dissection carried out towards the cystic duct and cystic artery which should be clearly identified before their division to avoid injury to the common bile duct or to the right hepatic artery.
- The junction of the cystic duct and common bile duct is displayed by snipping the overlying peritoneum by gauze stripping.
- An absorbable ligature (Vicryl 2-0, round body needle) is now placed loosely around the cystic duct close to its junction with the common bile duct.
- Any stones in the cystic duct should be milked towards towards the gallbladder and the cystic duct clamped or ligated close to the Hartman's pouch.
- Cystic duct is opened between the ligatures and any stone remaining in the duct is removed.
- Cannula can be introduced into the cystic duct for intraoperative cholangiography to identify common bile duct stones at the time of surgery.
- After operative cholangiography, cannula is removed and the ligature close to the common bile duct is fully tightened and the cystic duct is divided.
- Gentle traction on the cystic duct and gauze dissection up to the upper part of the gallbladder neck reveals the cystic artery crossing the triangle of Calot, which should be doubly ligated with nonabsorbable suture (Silk or linen) and divided between the ligatures and specimen removed from the abdomen.
- Bleeding from the raw area of the liver (from the gallbladder bed), if present can be arrested by simple pressure with hot moist mop or by light coagulation with diathermy electrode.
- Drain should be kept in the subhepatic space (Morrison's pouch) as there may be postoperative biliary leakage from the cystic duct stump due to slipping of ligature, from the gallbladder bed or from the common bile duct if has been accidently punctured during cholangiography and also for oozing of blood from gallbladder bed.
- Wound is closed in layers by mass suture technique or layer by layer by suturing cut muscles with absorbable sutures (Vicryl 2-0, round body needle).
- Skin closed with interrupted nonabsorbable sutures (Silk or nylon 2-0, cutting needle).

In retrograde cholecystectomy, dissection and ligation of the cystic duct and cystic artery are done first and then fundus approached and gallbladder removed from its bed.

LAPAROSCOPIC CHOLECYSTECTOMY

Most popular method nowadays due to avoidance of large muscle cutting incision.

Position of the Patient on the Operation Table

Supine with 15° reverse Trendelenberg position (Head up position).

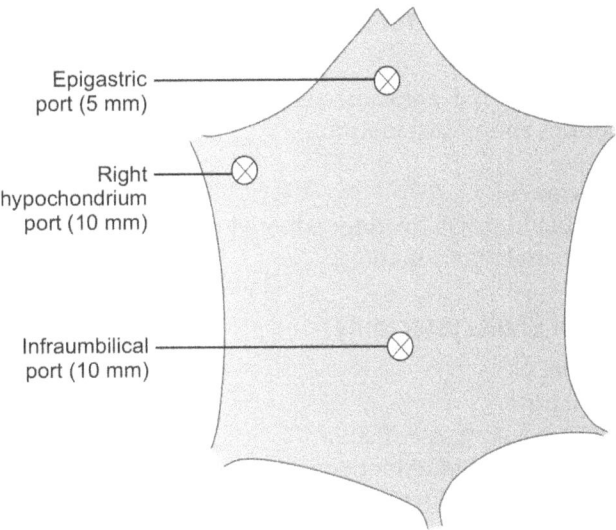

Fig. 5: Port sites for laparoscopic cholecystectomy.

Incision

Three 1 cm incisions are required for port insertion. Infraumbilical 10 mm port for telescope, one 5 mm port in epigastrium for holding the gallbladder at its fundus and another 10 mm port in the right hypochondrium for dissection, suction, GB removal, etc (Fig. 5).

Steps of the Procedure

- Pneumoperitoneum created with carbon dioxide with Veress needle or by open method by Hassan's cannula by subumbilical incision
- Rest of the procedure is same that of open cholecystectomy as described earlier.

Advantages of Laparoscopic Cholecystectomy Over Open Cholecystectomy

- Shorter stay in the hospital
- Less postoperative pain
- Fast recovery
- Quicker return to normal activities
- Shortened time off from work
- Less wound infection
- Acceptable and better cosmetic scar
- Postoperative complications like postoperative adhesive obstruction, incisional hernias are rare.

Absolute Contraindications for Laparoscopic Cholecystectomy
- Pregnancy
- Patient's infirmity for general anesthesia
- Previous upper abdominal incison
- Obesity
- Lung emphysema
- Difficult gallbladder (Gallbladder adhered to the surrounding structures or with congenital malformation).

Complications of Cholecystectomy
- Bile duct injury
- Bile duct stricture
- Postoperative biliary leak or fistula
- Hemorrhage from gallbladder bed
- Complications like bile duct injury, are more common in laparoscopic than open cholecystectomy.

CIRCUMCISION

Definition
Excision of the preputial foreskin to expose the glans penis and external urethral meatus.

Indications
- Most commonly performed for ritual reasons in Muslims and Jews (most common indication)
- In true phimosis with balanoposthitis and obstruction to the urinary flow
- In adults, mostly done for inability to retract the foreskin for intercourse
- For an abnormally tight frenulum
- Recurrent balanitis and chronic infection like balanitis xerotica obliterans (BOX)
- Paraphimosis
- Prior to radiotherapy (RT) for carcinoma of penis.

Anesthesia
- In pediatric age group patients, it is done under general anesthesia (GA) or caudal block
- In adults, it is done under penile ring block by infiltrating 1 or 2% plain lignocaine (without adrenaline) all around the base of the penis.

Position of the Patient on the Operation Table
Supine position.

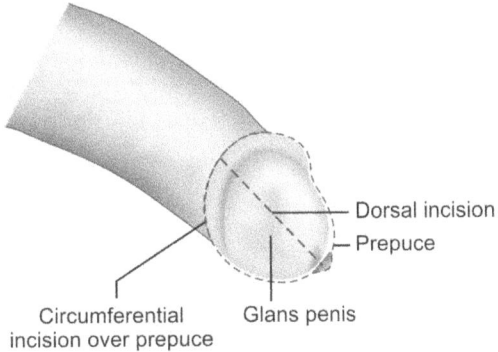

Fig. 6: Incision for circumcision.

Incision

Dorsal midline incision (12'O clock position) up to 1 cm of the corona glandis and from midline dorsal incision at the corona glandis, circumferential incision in the penile skin is taken around the penis at the level of corona glandis using knife towards the frenulum (Fig. 6).

Steps of the Procedure

- Parts are painted with antiseptic solution and draped with sterile sheets.
- Adhesions between the prepuce and the glans penis are separated up to the corona glandis by curved hemostatic mosquito forceps.
- Opening of the prepuce is held by three mosquito hemostatic forceps, one on either side of the preputial orifice (3 and 9'O clock position) and one in the midline inferiorly at the midline raphe, where frenulum is attached (6'O clock position) and all of them are pull on gentle stretch.
- Prepuce is then split or divided in midline dorsally (12'o clock position) up to 1 cm of the corona glandis.
- From midline dorsal incision at the corona glandis, circumferential incision in the penile skin taken around the penis at the level of corona glandis, using knife towards the frenulum.
- Inner layer of each flap is incised with a second circumferential incision, 5 mm distal to the outer layer of prepuce.
- The cut margins of prepuce (inner and outer layers) are sutured together circumferentially with interrupted absorbable sutures (Plain catgut or vicryl rapide 3-0, on atraumatic round body needle) to stop bleeding from the cut edges of the prepuce.
- Four in one or box suture taken at the frenulum to secure the frenular artery, before dividing the preputial skin at the frenulum and the redundant prepucial skin excised.
- Bipolar diathermy can also be used to coagulate the cut edges of the prepuce to achieve hemostasis.
- Sterile adhesive dressing applied.

Precautions to be Taken While Doing Circumcision

- Monopolar diathermy should be avoided due to fear of coagulation of the body of the penis
- Preparation of lignocaine with adrenaline is strictly contraindicated and not used, as it causes vasoconstriction and gangrene of the penis.

Postoperative Complications

- Bleeding from the cut edges of the prepuce, if not properly secured with the interrupted sutures or from the frenular artery due to slippage of the ligature at the frenulum
- Wound infection
- Removal of too much of preputial skin can lead to bending or bowing of the penis in future after erection
- If less preputial skin is removed, it can lead to paraphimosis or recurrent phimosis
- Injury to the glans penis, while excising the prepuce
- Injury to the external urethral meatus can lead to urethral stricture.

Guillotine method and plastibell ring techniques are used in infants and children for circumcision.

OPERATIONS FOR REPAIR OF INGUINAL HERNIA

Italian surgeon, Eduardo Bassini had done the first hernia repair in 1884, and reported it in 1887, and so called as **'Father of Modern Herniorrhaphy'**.

Repair of Inguinal Hernia Consists of

- Excision of the hernial sac (herniotomy) along with
- Repair of the stretched internal (deep) inguinal ring (in case of indirect inguinal hernia)
- Repair or reconstruction of the fascia transversalis (in case of direct inguinal hernia)
- Further reinforcement of the posterior wall of the inguinal canal (in case of direct as well as indirect hernia also) which must be achieved without tension.

In infants and children up to 15 years of age, herniotomy alone is sufficient to treat the congenital hernia, as in them patent processes vaginalis is the sole cause of inguinal hernia and hernia is not due to the weakened posterior wall of the inguinal canal (fascia transversalis) as in adults, so repair of posterior wall is not necessary in them which has to be done in adults.

Repair of the deep inguinal ring is an important step in repairing the indirect inguinal hernia, whereas repair of the fascia transversalis or posterior wall of the inguinal canal, is an important step in case of direct inguinal hernia.

Reconstruction (repair or strengthening) of the inguinal floor is necessary in all adult hernias, irrespective of its type, to prevent recurrence.

HERNIOTOMY

Definition

It consists of identification and dissection of the hernial sac from the cord structures to the deep inguinal ring followed by opening the sac, reducing the contents within it in the abdominal cavity if present, and ligation and transfixation of the neck of the sac as high as possible (at the deep inguinal ring) and removing the remaining sac.

Anesthesia

Under caudal block or general anesthesia in infants and younger children and in regional anesthesia like spinal anesthesia in older children.

Position of the Patient on the Operation Table

Supine position.

Incision

Small transverse or skin crease incision directly over the internal inguinal ring (Fig. 7).

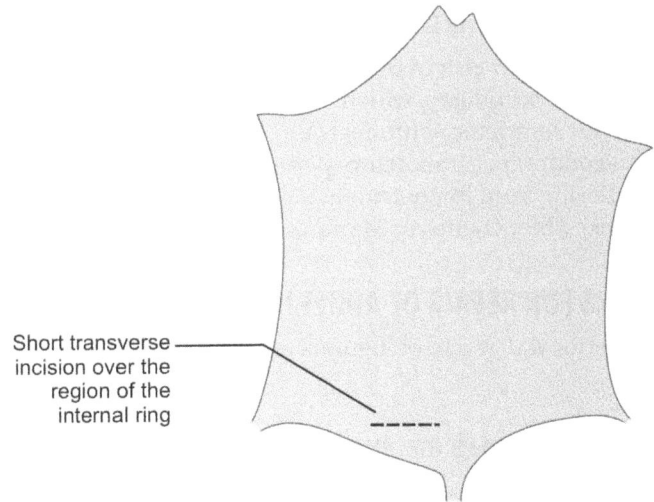

Fig. 7: Incision for herniotomy.

Steps of the Procedure

- Parts are painted with antiseptic solution and draped with sterile sheets
- Skin crease incision is given as described above
- Incision is deepened to incise the outer Camper's fascia and inner Scarpa's fascia
- External oblique aponeurosis is incised
- Ilioinguinal nerve safeguarded
- Cord is identified, elevated and its coverings like layers of external spermatic fascia, cremasteric fascia and internal spermatic fascia are opened to reveal the hernia sac
- Sac is identified by its pearly white color
- After dissecting out the sac from the rest of the cord structures, it has to be opened at its fundus
- Opened sac is examined for the peritoneal contents
- If peritoneal contents are present within the sac, they are reduced into the peritoneal cavity
- After reducing the contents into the abdominal cavity, ligation and transfixation of the neck of sac is done with absorbable suture (Vicryl 3-0, on round body needle) as high as possible, near the deep inguinal ring in the retroperitoneum, after twisting and rotating the sac and the remaining sac is excised
- Reposit the cord back into the wound
- External oblique is sutured with continuous absorbable suture (Vicryl 3-0, on round body needle)
- Subcutaneous tissue is sutured with interrupted absorbable suture (Vicryl 3-0, on round body needle)
- Skin is sutured with interrupted or in subcuticular fashion with non-absorbable suture (Nylon or silk 3-0, on cutting needle)
- Sterile adhesive dressing is applied.

Children having higher risk of recurrence should undergo herniorrhaphy/hernioplasty, which includes:

- Children with ventriculoperitoneal (VP) shunt
- Patient on continuous ambulatory peritoneal dialysis (CAPD)
- Patient suffering from malnutrition, growth failure and connective tissue disorders like Ehler Danlos or Marfan's syndrome.

OPERATIONS FOR REPAIR OF ADULT INGUINAL HERNIA

In adults, posterior wall repair of inguinal canal can be done by the following methods:

Three Categories of Repair are Available

1. Primary tissue repair (Herniorrhaphy)
2. Anterior tension free mesh repairs (Hernioplasty)
3. Preperitoneal repairs: Open and laparoscopic approach.

1. PRIMARY TISSUE REPAIRS (INGUINAL HERNIORRHAPHY)

In this, inguinal floor reconstruction is done primarily by natural tissue within the inguinal floor.

Definition

It consists of excision of the hernial sac (herniotomy) along with repair of the stretched internal inguinal ring (in case of indirect inguinal hernia) or simple invagination of the sac with repair of fascia transversalis (in case of direct inguinal hernia), with further reinforcement of the posterior wall of the inguinal floor by approximating the natural tissue present in the posterior wall of the inguinal floor by nonabsorbable sutures, which must be achieved without tension.

Indications

Direct or indirect inguinal hernia in adults.

Anesthesia

Usually done under regional anesthesia like spinal anesthesia (most commonly employed) or epidural or inguinal nerve block and rarely under general anesthesia.

Position of the Patient on the Operation Table

Supine position.

Incision

Incision is placed 1.25 cm above and parallel to the medial 2/3rd of the inguinal ligament, from the pubic tubercle to or beyond the deep (internal) inguinal ring (Fig. 8).

Steps of the Procedure

- Parts are painted with antiseptic solution and draped with sterile sheets
- Skin incision is given as described earlier
- Subcutaneous tissue and superficial fascia, i.e. inner scarpa and outer campa are incised along the line of skin incision
- External oblique aponeurosis and superficial (external) inguinal ring is identified
- External oblique aponeurosis is incised along line of its fibers (parallel to its fibers) to open the superficial inguinal ring and the inguinal canal, with due care not to injure the ilioinguinal nerve

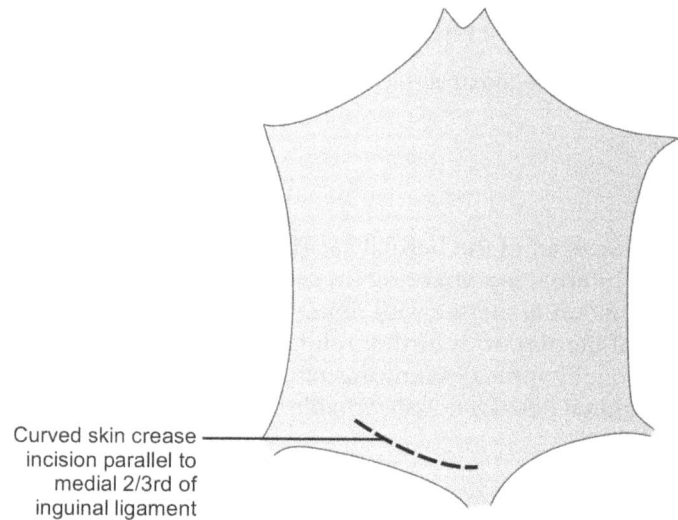

Fig. 8: Incision for repair of hernia by inguinal approach (herniorrhaphy/hernioplasty).

Curved skin crease incision parallel to medial 2/3rd of inguinal ligament

- After opening the inguinal canal, the inferior aspect of the upper portion of external oblique is separated from the internal oblique cranially and medially by blunt dissection
- Inferior aspect of lower portion is separated from the contents of the inguinal canal, until the inner aspect (upgoing part) of the inguinal ligament is seen
- Cremasteric muscle fibers are divided to display the spermatic cord
- Spermatic cord is identified and brought into the wound
- Skeletonization of the spermatic cord is done to identify the sac
- Sac is identified by its pearly white color
- Sac is freed till the deep inguinal ring within the inguinal canal from the rest of the cord structures taking care not to damage the vas deferens and the spermatic artery
- The sac is cut circumferentially in the inguinal canal at its fundus
- In case of sac adherent to the cord structures, which is difficult to separate and also in dissecting sac in infants and children, sac is dissected free from the cord by injecting saline under the posterior wall of the inguinal canal from within (hydrodissection)
- It is essential to open the sac before cutting or invaginating it into the abdominal cavity to ensure that no peritoneal contents like bowel or omentum, is adherent to the neck of the sac
- Contents of the sac are reposited back into the peritoneal cavity
- If omentum is adherent to the neck of the sac, it is freed and returned into the peritoneal cavity, and if adherent to the fundus of the sac, then it may be transfixed and ligated between the hemostatic forceps and cut across a suitable point

- If the sac is obviously empty in case of indirect hernia and in case of the direct hernia, where the sac has a too broad base for ligation and is small, then simply invert or invaginate the sac back into the peritoneal cavity, after it has been dissected and freed from the surrounding structures without opening, ligating and excising it
- Whatever type of the sac is encountered, it is necessary to free it till its neck by blunt dissection until parietal peritoneum is seen circumferentially from all sides of the sac, i.e. till or beyond the deep inguinal ring, where the retroperitoneal (preperitoneal) fat is seen
- Care must be taken not to injure the inferior epigastric vessels, which lie near the deep inguinal ring while dissecting the sac near the deep inguinal ring
- If the sac is opened, the contents of the sac are reduced into the abdominal cavity and the neck of the sac is ligated and transfixed as high as possible beyond the deep inguinal ring (high ligation of sac) with absorbable suture material (Vicryl 2-0, on round body needle) in the retroperitoneum after rotating and twisting it, before excising it
- Remaining redundant sac is excised
- Inferior epigastric artery is the important landmark for differentiating direct and indirect hernia intraoperatively. If the sac is lateral to the inferior epigastric pulsations, then it is an indirect sac, and if the sac is medial to inferior epigastric pulsations then it is the direct sac
- When the deep inguinal ring is weak, stretched and patulous, narrow the ring just to admit the tip of the little finger by plicating it (**Lytle repair:** When the deep inguinal ring is patulous, the fascia transversalis is plicated by suture narrowing the deep ring)
- Posterior wall repair or reconstruction of the inguinal floor is done by one of the method described below
- After posterior wall repair, spermatic cord is reposited back into the wound
- External oblique is sutured in front of the spermatic cord leaving a new external (superficial) ring that should only accommodate the tip of the little finger, and also due care must be taken to avoid excessive narrowing of the new external inguinal ring which could jeopardize the vascular supply and the venous return of the testis.

In primary tissue repair (herniorrhaphy), repair of the posterior wall of the inguinal canal is done by the following methods:

Commonly Performed Primary Tissue Repairs

- Bassini's repair
- Shouldice's repair
- Darn repair
- Halsted repair
- McVay (Cooper ligament) repair

Bassini's Repair

* Lateralization of the cord is done to keep it away from the operating field
* Fascia transversalis is opened from the pubic tubercle beyond the deep inguinal ring
* Conjoined tendon along with fascia transversalis above is sutured to the fascia transversalis below and to the undersurface of the inguinal ligament and to the pubic tubercle with nonabsorbable synthetic monofilament suture material (Polypropylene or polyamide no. 1, on round body needle).

Modified Bassini's Repair

* Commonly performed procedure rather than original Bassini's repair
* Lateralization of the cord is done to keep it away from the operating field
* In this, tendinous aponeurotic arch of the internal oblique and transversus abdominus (conjoined tendon) from above is sutured (approximated) to the undersurface (inward part) of the inguinal ligament and to the pubic tubercle below with nonabsorbable synthetic monofilament suture material (Polypropylene or polyamide no. 1, on round body) (Fig. 9).

In both the repairs, approximation of the tissue should be done without tension on the approximated tissue and on the suture line.

For releasing tension over the tissue approximated or anchored sutures, rectus-relaxing incision can be given over the anterior rectus sheath (Halsted Tanner incision).

Comments: No longer acceptable because of high recurrence rate (up to 15%) due to tension on sutures and approximated tissue and slow rehabilitation of the patient due to fear of recurrence.

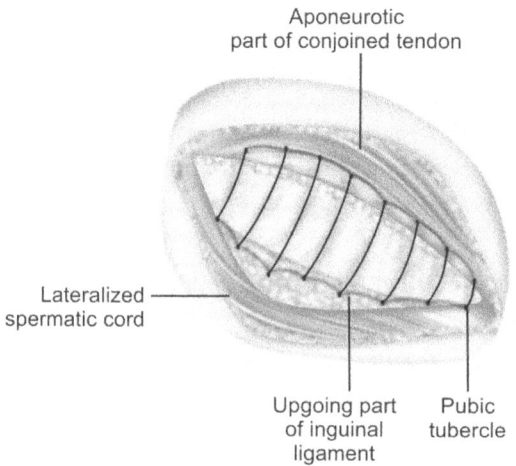

Fig. 9: Modified Bassini's repair.

Shouldice's Repair

- Popular tensionless repair wherein only local tissues are used
- Lateralization of the cord is done to keep it away from the operating field
- Fascia transversalis is incised and opened from the pubic tubercle beyond the deep inguinal ring and then it is freed from the extraperitoneal fat and inferior epigastric vessels
- An overlapping repair of the lower flap behind the upper flap is done by 'double breasting' of fascia transversalis, which forms a new posterior wall of the inguinal floor
- In 'Shouldice's repair, only 2 layer repair is done, 3rd and 4th layer repair not done
- In the 'Classic Shouldice's', 3rd and 4th layer repair also done by placing tension free sutures between the internal oblique aponeurosis arch and the inguinal ligament.

Layer by Layer Repair of Shouldice's

First layer: Edge of the lower flap of the fascia transversalis is sutured behind the posterior aspect of the upper flap of the fascia transversalis, posterior aspect of the rectus sheath and aponeurosis of the transversus abdominis, in medial to lateral fashion.

Second layer: Free edge of the upper flap of the fascia transversalis is sutured to the anterior surface of base of the lower flap and the inguinal ligament from deep inguinal ring to the pubic tubercle, in lateral to medial fashion.

Third layer: Suturing the inguinal ligament to the posterior surface of the conjoined tendon (transversus abdominis), in lateral to medial fashion.

Fourth layer: Suturing the anterior rectus sheath and conjoined tendon from front to the inner surface of the lower flap of the external oblique, in medial to lateral fashion.

Upper and lower flaps of the external oblique can also be superimposed on each other by suturing edge of the lower flap to the posterior aspect of the upper flap and edge of the upper flap to the anterior surface of the lower flap

Comment: As in this double breasting is done, rate of recurrence is very less (<2%) as compared to the Bassini's repair.

Lotheissen's Repair or McVay or Cooper's Ligament Repair

- Lateralization of the cord is done to keep it away from the operating field
- Fascia transversalis is incised from the deep inguinal ring to the pubic tubercle and then it is freed from the extraperitoneal fat and inferior epigastric vessels
- Cooper's ligament is dissected by dividing the iliopubic tract

- Repair is done by suturing the conjoined tendon and the lower edge of the fascia transversalis to the iliopectineal line. i.e. pectineal or cooper's ligament, starting from the pubic tubercle up to the medial margin of femoral vein below to form a shutter with interrupted nonabsorbable sutures
- In the lateral part of the repair, conjoined tendon and fascia transversalis is opposed to the inguinal ligament with interrupted nonabsorbable sutures
- Femoral ring is also closed by interrupted nonabsorbable sutures opposing the cooper's ligament to the anterior femoral fascia and the inguinal ligament
- It is classically recommended for strangulated femoral and recurrent inguinal hernia where inguinal ligament is destroyed.

Comment: It is advantageous, due to repair of femoral as well as inguinal ring and floor defects.

Darn Repair (Abrahamson's Nylon Darn Repair)

- One of the tensionless repairs like mesh repair
- Gets its name from the way, as a long nylon suture repeatedly passed between the tissues in the inguinal floor to create a weave that one might consider similar to an artificial mesh
- In this, the posterior wall of the inguinal canal is reinforced by forming a darn between the musculoaponeurotic arch of the conjoined tendon above and the inguinal ligament below with simple lattice of monofilament suture without tension, on which fibrous tissue develops
- In this, continuous monofilament polypropylene or nylon is used to approximate the conjoined tendon to the inguinal ligament from laterally to medially and then continuous suture passing medially from the pubic tubercle, through the rectus sheath and conjoined tendon above to the inguinal ligament below ending beyond the deep inguinal ring
- In this way, three runs of sutures are created on the posterior wall of the inguinal floor, thus providing a lattice of suture in the inguinal floor like an artificial mesh
- Collagen tissue lay down through the interstices of the weave, so material is incorporated into healthy new tissue to form a new posterior wall
- The sutures are not tied too tightly like Bassini's repair, but they are kept loose (Fig. 10).

Comment: As in this, there are less tension on the suture line as well as on the tissue approximated, rate of recurrence is very less, as compared to the Bassini's repair.

After herniorrhaphy patient can start his routine activities after suture removal, but he should avoid strenuous activities for at least a period of six months, to prevent recurrence.

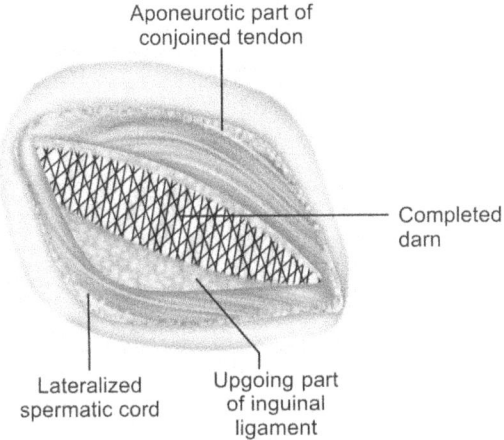

Fig. 10: Abrahamson's nylon darn repair.

2. ANTERIOR TENSION FREE MESH REPAIR (HERNIOPLASTY)

Definition

It consists of excision of the hernial sac (herniotomy) along with repair of the stretched internal inguinal ring (in case of indirect inguinal hernia) or simple invagination of the sac with repair of fascia transversalis (in case of direct inguinal hernia), with further reinforcement of the posterior wall of the inguinal floor by the mesh implants.

In this synthetic mesh prosthesis made up of non-absorbable material (Polypropylene) is used, to bridge the defect in the posterior wall of the inguinal floor.

Previously natural tissue was used to bridge the defect in the posterior wall of the inguinal floor like pedicled strips of external oblique aponeurosis, tensor fascia lata strips and fascial grafts from the thigh. But all of them are difficult to harvest in human tissue and tend to get absorbed causing recurrence.

Nowadays, monofilament polypropylene (prolene) is most commonly used material for repair of hernia. It is extremely smooth and inert and elicits very little tissue reaction and is indestructible in human tissue. Polytetrafluoroethylene (PTTE) and monofilament polyamide can also be used. But due their high price and poor incorporation into the tissues, PTEE is not used routinely.

Lichtenstein Tension Free Hernioplasty (Mesh Repair)

- Approximately 16 × 8 cm polypropylene mesh is kept as an extra lamina (on lay graft) anterior to the posterior wall of the inguinal canal (over the fascia transversalis)
- It is overlapped generously in all directions, including medially over the pubic tubercle and secured it by nonabsorbable sutures (polypropylene

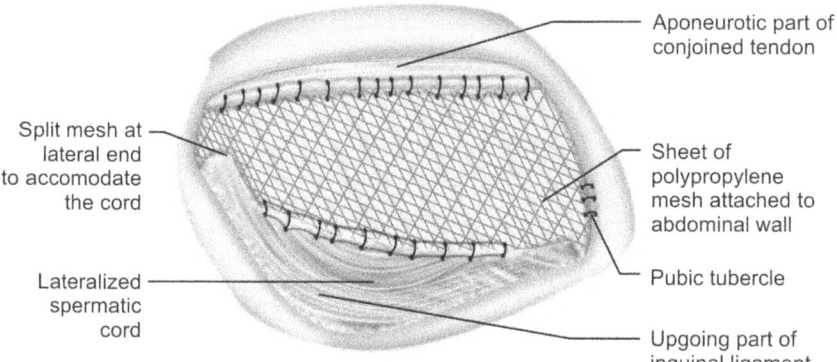

Fig. 11: Lichtenstein tension-free hernioplasty.

no. 2-0/3-0, on round body) to the inguinal ligament, lacunar ligament and the pubic tubercle below and to the conjoined tendon and the anterior rectus sheath above

❖ The lateral edge of the mesh is split around the cord at the deep inguinal ring and the two tails are brought around the cord, which are crossed over each other and sutured down to the inguinal ligament to create a snug new deep inguinal ring (Fig. 11).

Opinion: As it is a 'tensionless repair', recurrence rate is quite low (<2%) with this technique. It is the best tensionless repair, preferred by most of the surgeons nowadays.

Patch and Plug Technique

A plug of mesh is inserted into the hernial defect, i.e. in the deep inguinal ring in case of indirect inguinal hernia and in the Hesselbach's triangle in case of direct inguinal hernia, which expands by unwinding and blocks the anatomically and functionally defective deep inguinal ring or Hesselbach's triangle. Another piece of mesh is placed over the posterior wall of the inguinal canal (inguinal floor) which may/may not be sutured to the adjacent tissue as in Lichtenstein mesh hernioplasty.

3. PREPERITONEAL REPAIRS

❖ Recorded by ancient hindus for strangulated hernias
❖ In this, after reduction of the hernial contents and dealing with the sac, a large piece of mesh is kept in the preperitoneal space to cover the entire inguinal floor and the myopectineal orifice
❖ This procedure can be performed transperitoneally (by opening the peritoneum through lower midline laparotomy) or extra-peritoneally (without opening the peritoneum)
❖ Peritoneum is separated from the anterior abdominal wall and the bladder, transection of the sac is done in the retroperitoneum, and then the repair

of the deep inguinal ring is done from above, by keeping mesh in the preperitoneal space.

Rive's Preperitoneal Prosthetic Mesh Repair

- Through inguinal incision, after dealing with the sac, fascia transversalis is slit open from the deep inguinal ring up to the pubic tubercle and dissected all around widely to create plain in the preperitoneal space
- Mesh is kept in the preperitoneal space, i.e. space between the fascia transversalis and the peritoneum deep to the fascia transversalis
- Mesh is sutured with nonabsorbable suture material (Polypropylene no. 2-0/3-0, on round body needle) to the undersurface of the musculo-aponeurotic part of the transversus abdominis and the internal oblique and the upper portion of fascia transversalis above and the inguinal ligament and the lower protion of fascia transversalis below
- Superolateral edge of the mesh is split to accommodate the spermatic cord
- Mesh is covered by suturing the musculoaponeurotic part of the transversus abdominis and internal oblique and the upper portion of fascia transversalis above and the inguinal ligament and lower portion of the fascia transversalis below
- Indicated for very large hernias and for recurrent inguinal hernias with large defects of anterior abdominal wall
- It can be done by subumbilical lower midline incision, in which mesh is kept in the preperitoneal space in the inguinal region, through the approach above the inguinal canal which directly accesses the preperitoneal space without opening the inguinal canal (mesh kept between the peritoneum and the fascia transversalis, i.e. in the inner aspect of anterior abdominal wall on the side of hernia)
- Indicated for difficult recurrent inguinal hernias, in which inguinal ligament and anatomy of inguinal region has been destroyed and scared.

Stoppa's Great or Giant Prosthetic Reinforcement of Visceral Sac (GPRVS)

- In this, through the lower midline abdominal incision, large sheet of prosthetic mesh is kept between the peritoneum and the anterior, inferior, posterior and lateral anterior abdominal walls to close all the potential hernial orifices
- Mesh stretches in the lower abdomen and pelvis from one end to the other enveloping the lower half of parietal peritoneum
- It does not require any anchoring suture, or may be sutured by single suture to the umbilical fascia only
- Commonly indicated for bilateral inguinal hernias, large hernias, patient with collagen disease, Ehler's Danlos syndrome or Marfan's syndrome,

recurrent inguinal hernias, where tissue is scared, weakened and normal anatomy is completely destroyed.

KUNTZ OPERATION (Inguinal Orchidectomy)

In this, the spermatic cord is divided at the deep inguinal ring and removed with the testis, so that the deep inguinal ring can be permanently closed.

Indications for Kuntz Operation

- In elderly patients, with recurrent hernia with poor abdominal muscle tone
- If cord cannot be dissected free from the scar tissue in case of recurrent hernia
- If blood supply of the testis gets compromised, due to injury to the testicular artery while dissecting sac from the cord structures
- If cord has been damaged during dissection of the sac.

HERNIORRHAPHY VERSUS HERNIOPLASTY

Regarding Herniorrhaphy

- Herniorrhaphy is pure tissue repair, simple to perform and no foreign body is kept in the body
- In herniorrhaphy, there is tension on the suture line as well as on the anchored tissue, which results in breakage of the sutures or giving way by the tissue leading to higher recurrence rate of hernia (up to 15% cases) and slower return to unrestricted physical activity
- Herniorrhaphy is not physiological, as the inguinal ligament and the conjoined tendon are not in the same anatomical plane.

Regarding Hernioplasty

- In hernioplasty, synthetic nonabsorbable mesh has been used to reinforce the posterior wall of the inguinal canal which is anchored to the adjacent tissue without tension. Being a tensionless repair chances of recurrence are very rare (<2%)
- In hernioplasty, mesh being a foreign material it can be rejected by the human body which is revealed as wound infection or chronic sinus formation, however these complications are rare.

Comparatively tension free mesh hernioplasty is considered as a better alternative than herniorrhaphy due to lower recurrence rates, and hence, it is a dominant method of inguinal hernia repair and widely used nowadays in clinical practice.

In above-mentioned different procedures, rate of recurrence vary between 0.2 to 15%.

Any operative procedure can be done for repair of hernia, provided the recurrence rate is below 1%.

Complications of Hernia Surgery

- Recurrence of hernia
- Intraoperative bleeding due to injury to femoral or inferior epigastric vessels
- Injury to the vas deferens
- Postoperative hydrocele due to interference with the lymphatics of the testis of that side
- Injury or rupture of the bowel if present in the sac, while dissecting sac without reducing the contents
- Osteitis pubis in case of herniorrhaphy where stitch is taken from the periosteum of the pubis
- Hyperesthesia over the medial side of the inguinal canal due to injury to the ilioinguinal nerve
- Wound infection.

Causes of Recurrence

- Most recurrences occur within 1 year of repair
- Repair under tension: Excessive tension on the sutures resulting in breaking of the sutures or excessive tension on the tissues resulting in their giving way to the sutures or necrosis of the tissues
- Use of the absorbable suture rather than nonabsorbable sutures
- Faulty technique on the part of surgeon in identifying the anatomy and repair
- Failure to identify the sac properly and cutting it improperly in the inguinal canal rather than its high ligation
- While repairing the direct inguinal hernia, an indirect sac may be overlooked or vice-versa, in case of pantaloon type or dual hernia causing false recurrence
- Wound infection
- Hematoma formation
- Postoperative continuous and persistent increase in the intra-abdominal pressure due to strenuous work or due to chronic cough, straining while micturition due to benign hypertrophy of the prostate or stricture urethra, constipation, ascites, etc.

LAPAROSCOPIC HERNIOPLASTY

- Laparoscopic hernia repair is based on the technique of 'Stoppa's preperitoneal repair'

- ❖ The preperitoneal space is reached either by transabdominal preperitoneal laparoscopic approach (TAPP) or by totally extraperitoneal repair (TEP)
- ❖ Both the techniques are similar in actual repair, but differ in the manner by which the preperitoneal space is reached.

Indications of Laparoscopic Hernia Repairs

- ❖ Mostly indicated in cases of bilateral and recurrent inguinal hernias
- ❖ Can also be indicated for primary unilateral inguinal and femoral hernias for small cosmetic scar.

Anesthesia

Mostly done under general anesthesia and rarely under regional anesthesia like spinal or epidural anesthesia.

Position of the Patient on the Operation Table

Supine position.

Incision

Three incisions for 3 ports: 1 cm subumbilical incision for 10 mm port for telescope, 0.5 cm incision for 5 mm port midway between the symphysis pubis and the umbilicus, and 1 cm incision for 10 mm port through right or left iliac fossa, according to right or left side of hernia, respectively (Fig. 12).

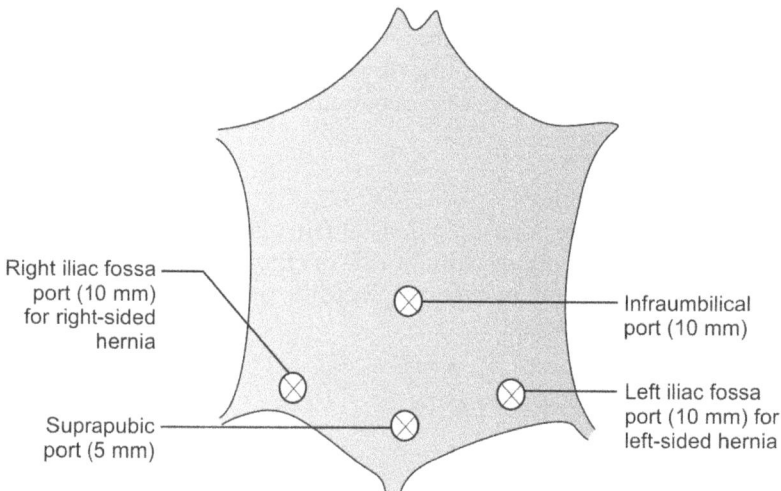

Fig. 12: Port sites for laparoscopic hernia repair.

TECHNIQUES

Transabdominal Preperitoneal Approach (TAPP)

Steps of the Procedure

- Pneumoperitoneum is created by insufflating carbon dioxide by Veress needle or by Hasan's cannula, and the peritoneal space is reached as by conventional laparoscopy
- Sac is dissected out from the hernia orifice (deep inguinal ring) from above
- Peeling of the peritoneum from the anterior abdominal wall is done by dissecting the parietal peritoneum of all hernia orifices and plane created between them
- Synthetic mesh is placed in the preperitoneal space, between the peritoneum and fascia transversalis, i.e. in the inner aspect of the anterior abdominal wall. Peritoneum is closed with absorbable suture (Vicryl 2-0, on round body needle) over the mesh.

Opinion: This procedure is having higher complications than TEP due to violation of the peritoneal cavity.

Preperitoneal Approach (TEP)

Steps of the Procedure

- This procedure is completely preperitoneal by insufflating carbon dioxide into the preperitoneal space via paraumbilical incision without entering the peritoneal cavity
- Preperitoneal space created either by balloon dissection or by direct dissection
- After dissecting the sac and dealing it with, mesh placed in the preperitoneal space
- Recurrence rate is less than 1% for TEP.

Opinion: This procedure is technically difficult and needs expertise, but is much safer than TAPP.

Advantages of Laparoscopic Hernia Repair

- It is quick, relatively atraumatic
- Bilateral repairs can be done at the same operation
- Clinically unsuspected contralateral hernias can be identified and repaired at the same time
- Early ambulation and return to normal activities.

Disadvantages of Laparoscopic Hernia Repair

- General anesthesia is required
- There is violation of abdominal cavity in case of TAPP, which leads to risk of adhesions in future leading to postoperative adhesive obstruction

❖ New hernias can develop at the site of introduction of the ports (port site hernias).

SURGERIES FOR HYDROCELE

REPAIR OF ADULT (ACQUIRED) HYDROCELE

Indication
Adult acquired vaginal hydrocele.

Anesthesia
Done under regional anesthesia like spinal anesthesia or can be done under local or rarely under general anesthesia.

Position of the Patient on the Operation Table
Supine position.

Incision
Pararaphian incision on the scrotum on the side of the hydrocele, lateral and parallel to the median raphae (Fig. 13).

Techniques

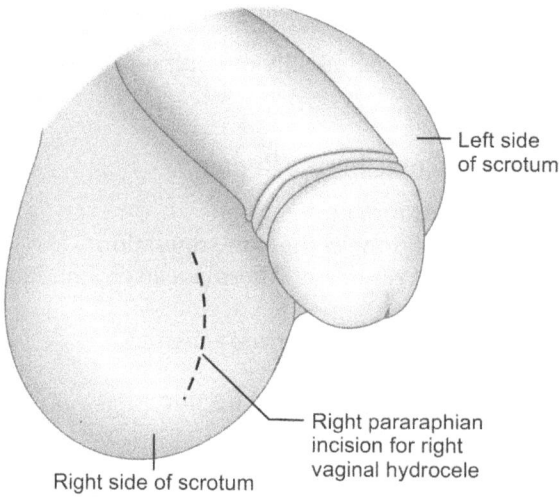

Fig. 13: Incision for repair of hydrocele.

LORD'S PLICATION OF THE SAC

Definition
Plication of the sac (tunica vaginalis) after draining the hydrocele fluid from the sac (Fig. 14).

Indication
For mild to moderate sized vaginal hydrocele with thin-walled sac.

Steps of the Procedure
- Parts are painted with antiseptic solution and draped with sterile sheets
- Pararaphian incision is given over the scrotal skin on the side of the vaginal hydrocele

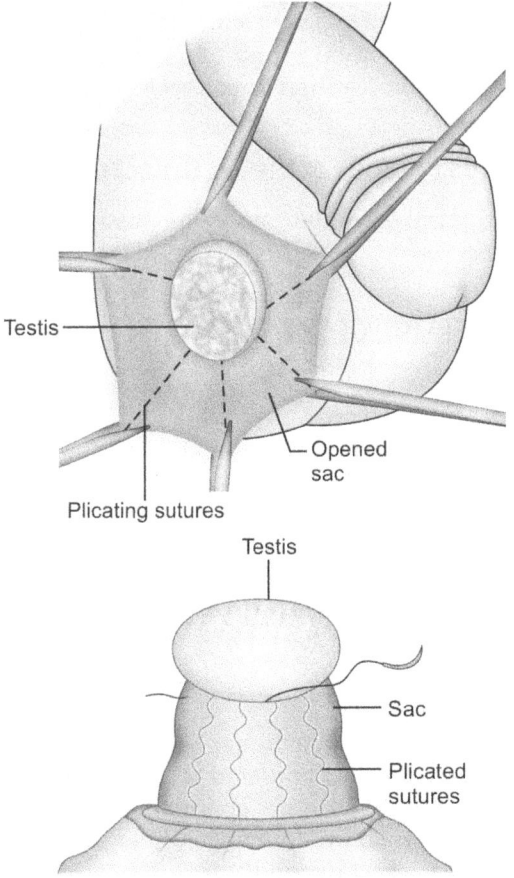

Fig. 14: Lord's plication.

- Incision is deepened to cut the dartos muscle, external spermatic fascia, cremasteric fascia, internal spermatic fascia to reach the sac (parietal layer of tunica vaginalis)
- Sac is opened without separating it from the layers of the scrotum
- Hydrocele fluid is drained in a sterile kidney tray after opening the sac
- Testis is delivered out into the wound from the sac
- Cut margins of the sac are plicated by series of interrupted absorbable sutures (Catgut or vicryl 1-0, on round body needle) to plicate the redundant opened sac, from the periphery of the opened sac to the testis where it is attach to it
- When these interrupted sutures are tied, sac is bunched up into a 'ruff' at the periphery of the testis
- Testis with plicated sac (tunica vaginalis) is reposited back into the scrotum
- Wound is closed in layers with absorbable sutures (Catgut or vicryl 1-0, on round body needle)
- Skin is sutured with interrupted nonabsorbable sutures (Nylon or silk 2-0, on cutting needle)
- Sterile dressing is applied and a coconut bandage is applied to the scrotum to give postoperative scrotal support for compression and hemostasis, which also prevents the scrotum from hanging.

Advantage of Lord's Plication of the Sac Over Eversion of the Sac

Chances of postoperative hematoma is less, as in this there is minimal dissection of tissue.

JABOULAY'S EVERSION OF THE SAC

Definition

Eversion of the sac around the testis after draining the hydrocele fluid from the sac (Fig. 15).

Indications

For moderate to large sized vaginal hydrocele with thin-walled sac.

Steps of the Procedure

- Steps of the procedure to reach the sac is same as that of Lord's plication
- After reaching the sac, it is separated all around from the layers of the scrotum (dartos muscle, external spermatic fascia, cremasteric fascia, internal spermatic fascia) by blunt finger dissection and testis along with the sac brought outside the wound

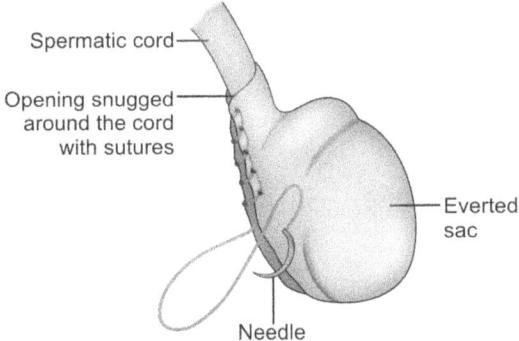

Fig. 15: Jaboulay's eversion of the sac.

- An incision is made over the sac (tunica vaganilis) in an avascular area anteriorly away from the testis, epididymis and cord structures and hydrocele fluid is drained in a sterile kidney tray
- Incision over the sac is extended and the testis is delivered out of the sac
- The cut margins of the fully opened sac from both sides are everted around the testis, i.e. eversion of the sac done around the testis and the everted cut margins of the sac are sutured together behind the testis with continuous absorbable interlocking sutures (Chromic catgut or vicryl 1-0, on round body needle) from one end to another, and the opening is snugged around the cord
- Testis with the everted sac is reposited back in the fascial plain of the scrotum by making pouch in the dartos muscle (subdartos pouch) or can be directly placed in the scrotal sac
- Corrugated rubber drain (CRD) can be kept below the dartos muscle or scortal sac for postoperative drainage of serous fluid or blood, as dissection of tissue is more than that of Lord's plication
- Wound is closed in layers with absorbable sutures (Catgut or vicryl 1-0, on round body needle)
- Skin is sutured with interrupted nonabsorbable sutures (Nylon or silk 2-0, on cutting needle)
- Sterile dressing is applied and a coconut bandage is applied to give the postoperative scrotal support for compression and hemostasis, which also prevents the scrotum from hanging.

Disadvantage of Jaboulay's Eversion of the Sac

As in this blind dissection of the sac is done for separating it from the layers of scrotum, chances of postoperative hematoma are more than that of Lord's plication.

Sharma and Jhawer's Technique

After evacuation of the fluid from the sac, the sac with the testis is placed in a newly created pocket between the fascial layers of the scrotum (subdartos pouch, space between dartos muscle and scrotal skin).

SUBTOTAL EXCISION OF THE SAC

Definition

Excision of the sac after draining the hydrocele fluid from the sac.

Indication

For moderate to large sized vaginal hydrocele with thick walled or calcified sac.

Steps of the Procedure

- Steps to drain the hydrocele fluid are the same as that of eversion of the sac
- The fully opened sac is excised circumferentially from all around the testis flushed to its attachment to the testis and the margin of the cut sac is sutured with continuous absorbable interlocking sutures (Chromic catgut or vicryl 1-0, on round body needle) all around the testis
- Testis reposited back in the scrotal sac
- Corrugated rubber drain (CRD) can be kept below the dartos muscle or scrotal sac for postoperative drainage of serous fluid or blood, as dissection of tissue is more in this procedure
- Wound is closed in layers with absorbable sutures (Catgut or vicryl 1-0, on round body needle)
- Skin is sutured with interrupted nonabsorbable sutures (Nylon or silk 2-0, on cutting needle)
- Sterile dressing is applied and a coconut bandage is applied to give the postoperative scrotal support for compression and hemostasis, which also prevents the scrotum from hanging.

Postoperative Complications

- Scrotal hematoma
- Wound infection
- Pyocele.

Temporary Methods of Repair of Hydrocele

- Drainage of hydrocele fluid by aspiration can be done, but the condition recurs within a week and only suitable for elderly infirm men who are unfit for surgery

- ❖ Primary sclerosants such as tetracyclines, streptomycin, talc are effective if installed in the layers of tunica vaginalis after aspirating the hydrocele fluid, as all of them causes aspetic inflammation between the opposing secreting surfaces of the tunica vaginalis.

Treatment of Congenital Hydrocele

Treatment of choice is herniotomy, which is described in the operative repair of hernia.

VASECTOMY

Definition

Division of the vas deferens.

Indication

Family planning (parents should have two healthy children).

Anesthesia

Under local anesthesia, by infiltrating 2% lignocaine with adrenaline in the skin and dartos muscle.

Position of the Patient on the Operation Table or Bed

Supine poisition.

Incision

Small vertical skin incision to the root of the scrotum on the median raphe.

Steps of the Procedure

- ❖ Parts painted with antiseptic solution and draped with sterile sheets
- ❖ Vas is felt at the root of the scrotum between index finger and the thumb
- ❖ Skin, dartos, external and internal spermatic fascia are incised along the skin incision
- ❖ Allie's forceps is introduced through the incision and cord is held with it
- ❖ Thick, firm, cord like vas dissected out and confirmed by its white color
- ❖ Division of vas done by three clamp method
- ❖ Vas is cut in two places, so that piece of vas is removed, which can be sent for histopathology to confirm it. As a piece of vas is removed, reunion of the cut edges will not occur
- ❖ The cut edges are doubly ligated with silk or thread

- The procedure repeated on the other vas deferens of the other side
- The skin edges sutured with silk or thread
- Sterile coconut bandage dressing is applied to give the postoperative scrotal support.

Postoperative Complications
- Scrotal hematoma
- Hematocele
- Pyocele
- Wound infection
- Sperm granuloma
- Recanalization of vas deferens.

Postoperative Advice
To avoid sexual contact or to use contraception for 2–3 months after the procedure, as some sperms may present in the distal end of the vas and seminal vesicles.

SUPRAPUBIC CYSTOLITHOTOMY

Definition
Removing of the stone (vesical calculus) from the bladder by suprapubic approach.

Indications
Large bladder stone which cannot be removed by the endoscopic methods.

Anesthesia
Done under regional anesthesia like spinal anesthesia and can be done under general anesthesia in case of pediatric patients.

Position of the Patient on the Operation Table
Supine position.

Incision
- Vertical or transverse skin incision over the lower abdomen in the suprapubic region
- Pfannenstiel incision is preferred, as it is cosmetic skin crease incision, which is situated 2.5 cm above the pubic symphysis (Fig. 16).

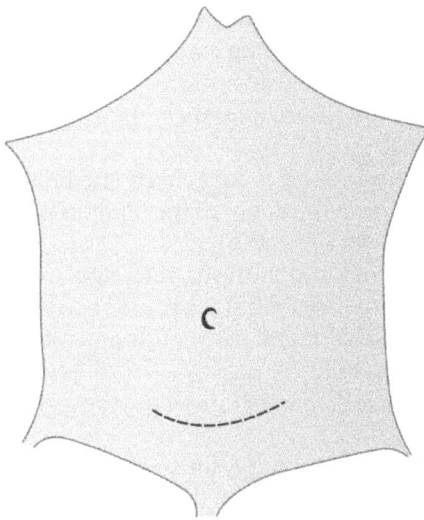

Fig. 16: Pfannenstiel (transverse suprapubic) incision.

Steps of the Procedure

- Before stating the procedure, bladder should be distended with normal saline by perurethral catheter or by urine, by asking patient not to pass the urine 4–5 hours prior to proposed time of surgery, to distend the bladder preoperatively
- Parts are painted with antiseptic solution and draped with sterile sheets
- Transverse pfannenstiel skin incision is given and subcutaneous tissue and fat are incised as that of the skin incision, to reach the anterior rectus sheath
- Anterior rectus sheath is incised transversely and freed from the underlying rectus and pyramidalis muscle
- Both rectus abdominis and pyramidalis muscle are separated in the midline by curved hemostatic forceps and then retracted laterally from the midline by Langenbach's right angled retractors
- Extraperitoneal fat and the peritoneum is stripped upwards, to expose the bladder wall, which is identified by thin-walled vertical veins on its surface
- Bladder opened vertically (mostly) or transversely between the two stay sutures taken through the serosa of the bladder
- Urine or normal saline is sucked out with the suction cannula from the bladder
- Stones are identified by palpating them with the index finger and removed with the cystolithotomy forceps
- Confirm the number of stones removed as per preoperative X-ray KUB or USG of the bladder

- Bladder is closed with interrupted or continuous absorbable sutures (Vicryl 2-0, on round body needle) taking care not to penetrate the mucosa of the bladder (Serosa to submucosal sutures are taken, to prevent recurrent stone formation, as the suture may act as a foreign body for the formation of future stones)
- Second layer closure is done to invaginate the first layer, taking only the bites of serosa from both the edges of the bladder with absorbable sutures (Vicryl 2-0, on round body needle)
- Retractors are removed and both the recti approximated in the midline with absorbable suture (Vicryl 2-0, on round body needle)
- Anterior rectus sheath is sutured with continuous absorbable suture (Vicryl 2-0, on round body needle)
- Retropubic (perivesical) space drained postoperatively with malecots or Foley's catheter
- Perurethral Foley's catheter kept, for postoperative free drainage of the urine from the bladder
- Suprapubic catheter can also be kept to drain the bladder, if required
- Subcutaneous tissue and fat approximated with absorbable suture (Vicryl 2-0, on round body needle)
- Skin sutured with interrupted nonabsorbable suture (Silk or nylon 2-0, on cutting needle)
- Sterile adhesive dressing applied.

Postoperative Complications

- Hemorrhage from the cut edges or from the overlying veins of the bladder
- Postoperative urinary leak, from the suture line of the bladder causing vesicocutaneous fistula.

MODIFIED RADICAL MASTECTOMY: MRM (PATEY'S MASTECTOMY)

It is most commonly performed surgery for operable carcinoma breast, nowadays than Halsted's radical mastectomy.

Definition

The whole breast tissue (mammary fat) along with the overlying skin over the breast is removed, including nipple and aerola complex, with excision of all level of axillary lymph nodes up to level III (level I, II and III) along with removal of pectoralis minor and preservation of pectoralis major. Pectoralis major is only retracted and not excised in MRM, to get access for clearance of levels III group of axillary lymph nodes.

Indications of MRM

Stage I, II and III a (Operable) of carcinoma breast.

Anesthesia

Under general anesthesia or regional anesthesia like thoracic epidural anesthesia.

Position of the Patient on the Operation Table

Supine with small pillow placed below the shoulder blade of the side to be operated to elevate the breast of that side with arm of that side supported on arm table.

Incision

Transverse or oblique elliptical incision encircling the nipple and areola, encompassing 3–5 cm margins all around the palpable tumor to ensure complete histological clearance of the tumor (Fig. 17).

Steps of the Procedure

- Parts are painted with antiseptic solution and draped with sterile sheets
- Skin incision is given as described earlier
- 7–8 mm thick flaps are raised between the subcutaneous and the mammary fat

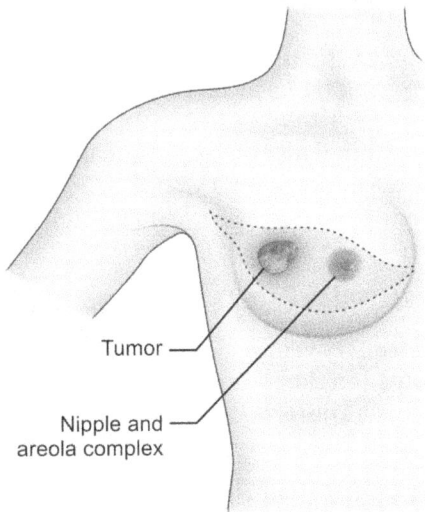

Fig. 17: Transverse or oblique elliptical incision.

- ❖ They should not be too thin to cause postoperative flap necrosis due to ischemia or not to be too thick to harbor the residual malignant cells from the tumor mass
- ❖ Superior flap is raised up to the clavicle or subclavius muscle and inferior flap is raised up to the upper quadrant of rectus sheath, 2–3 cm below inframammary folds
- ❖ Dissection should be carried out medially up to the midline of sternum and laterally up to the anterior margin of latissimus dorsi
- ❖ After dissection of the entire breast tissue along with the underlying pectoral fascia from the chest wall, dissected breast is allowed to hang laterally keeping axillary tail of breast in continuity with the axillary lymph nodes, which helps in removal of all levels of axillary lymph nodes by applying gentle traction on the dissected breast tissue
- ❖ Lateral border of pectoralis major is cleared of loose areolar tissue (axillary fat removed) and level-I group of lymph nodes are removed
- ❖ Pectoralis minor is dissected and divided from its insertion from the coracoid process of the scapula, rest of the lymphatics of the axilla (Level II and level III group of lymph nodes) and loose areolar tissue are cleared from the axillary vein and removed
- ❖ Wound is drained using a wide bore suction tube, one tube in the axilla and another one underneath the breast flaps
- ❖ Subcutaneous tissue is approximated with absorbable suture (Vicryl 2-0, on round body needle)
- ❖ Wound is closed with interrupted non absorbable sutures (Silk or nylon 2-0, on cutting needle) or with skin staplers.

Postoperative Complications

- ❖ Wound infection
- ❖ Wound gape due to excessive tension on the suture line, because of excision of too much of overlying skin which is required in case of large malignant tumor
- ❖ Flap necrosis due to thin flaps compromising their blood supply
- ❖ Postoperative seroma or hematoma
- ❖ Hemorrhage.

Structures to be Preserved in Patey's MRM

- ❖ Cephalic vein and axillary vein
- ❖ Nerves to the serratus anterior (Long thoracic nerve: Bell's nerve) and nerve to the latissimus dorsi (Thoracodorsal nerve).

Advantages of Patey's MRM Over Halsted Radical Mastectomy

- ❖ Survival rate of patients treated by MRM is equivalent to that of patient treated by Halsted's radical mastectomy

- ❖ Cosmetically better accepted as axillary fold is maintained
- ❖ Function of the shoulder is better as it gives a stronger and more useful arm
- ❖ By preserving pectoralis major, it provides a good vascular bed for skin grafting.

OTHER TYPES OF MASTECTOMY

Simple Mastectomy

- ❖ The whole breast tissue (mammary fat) along with the overlying skin over the breast is removed, including nipple and areola complex, along with the axillary tail. No dissection of any level of axillary lymph nodes are done in this
- ❖ It has to be followed by radiotherapy to the chest wall and axilla to prevent recurrence.

Extended Simple Mastectomy

It involves simple mastectomy + removal of level-I group of axillary lymph nodes.

Halsted and Meyer's Radical Mastectomy (Halsted Radical Mastectomy)

- ❖ The whole breast tissue (mammary fat) along with the overlying skin over the breast is removed, including nipple and areola complex, with excision of all level of axillary lymph nodes up to level III (level I, II and III) along with removal of pectoralis major and minor muscles
- ❖ This procedure is no longer indicated as it causes excessive morbidity with no survival benefit more than MRM.

Disadvantages of Halsted Radical Mastectomy

- ❖ Mutilating surgery
- ❖ Poor cosmetic results.

Extended Radical Mastectomy

Radical mastectomy + removal of internal mammary group of lymph nodes.

Super Radical Mastectomy

Radical mastectomy + removal of internal mammary lymph nodes + mediastinal lymph nodes + supraclavicular lymph nodes.

Auchincloss Procedure

- The whole breast tissue (mammary fat) along with the overlying skin over the breast is removed, including nipple and areola complex, with excision of axillary lymph nodes up to level II (level I and II) with preservation of both pectoralis major and minor muscles and they are only retracted to get access to the axillary lymph nodes
- Usually removal of level I and level II group of lymph nodes is done and if possible level III are removed, but usually not possible. As this procedure restricts dissection of apical (level III) group of lymph nodes, nodal recovery is less than modified radical mastectomy (MRM) due to the incomplete dissection of level III lymph nodes.

Levels of Axillary Lymph Nodes to be Removed in Carcinoma Breast

- Level I: Lymph nodes from the axillary tail of the breast to the lateral border of the pectoralis minor
- Level II: Lymph nodes behind the pectoralis minor
- Level III: Lymph nodes medial to the medial border of pectoralis minor situated at the apex of the axilla.

SURGERIES FOR THYROID GLAND

Emil Theoder Kocher is the first surgeon to do thyroid surgery and received noble prize for that.

Indications for Operations in Case of Thyroid Swelling

- Neoplasia (FNAC positive, clinical suspicion)
- Recurrent cyst
- Toxic adenoma (solitary nodular goiter)
- Pressure symptoms due to goiter
- Cosmetic reason
- Patient's preference
- Retrosternal prolongation of goiter with compressive symptoms.

Preoperative Treatment

- Good preoperative preparation of the patient, good anesthetic and surgical techniques and good postoperative care will reduce the complications of surgery
- Patient should be biochemically and clinically euthyroid before operation by assessing serum T_3, T_4, TSH and assessing improvement in symptoms like weight gain, decrease pulse rate, etc.
- Antithyroid drugs like carbimazole 30–40 mg/day is the drug of choice for preparation of the patient till he/she become euthyroid (about 8–12 weeks)

and then 5 mg TDS till the day of surgery (continued up to the evening before the day of surgery)
- Clinical manifestation of toxic state can be abolished using beta-blockers, which acts on target organs and not on the gland itself, which results in rapid control of symptoms and operation may be arranged within 1 or 2 weeks
- Tablet propranolol (inderal) 40 mg TDS to upto 80 mg TDS or preferably longer acting Nadolol 160 mg once daily dose increases up to 320 mg
- Important to continue the drug for 7 days postoperatively also
- Iodine may be given as Lugol's iodine solution (3 drops twice daily) for 10 days before operation
- Preoperative treatment with iodine produces transient remission and also reduces vascularity of the gland, thereby marginally improving safety
- All these measures decreases the risk of thyroid storm which can be precipitated by surgery in unprepared patients.

Preoperative Investigations

- Serum T_3, T_4 and TSH
- Laryngoscopy for vocal cord assessment and knowing involvement of recurrent laryngeal nerve (RLN) in diseased process before operative procedure has to be undertaken
- Thyroid antibodies titer
- Serum calcium estimation
- Isotope scan: In patients with toxic nodular goiter, to know which nodules if anyone is autonomous and active, to ensure their reduction by doing appropriate surgery. No value in diffuse toxic goiter as uptake is uniform.

Types of Surgeries to be Done in Case of Benign Thyroid Swelling

- **For solitary nodule:** Hemithyroidectomy
- **For multinodular goiter:** Near total thyroidectomy: Hemithyroidectomy on the more affected side and subtotal lobectomy on the other side, leaving 4–5 g of thyroid tissue in less affected lobe (Hartley-Dunhill procedure). The purpose of this surgery is to preserve at least one RLN and one prarathyroid gland
- **For large goiter:** Bilateral subtotal thyroidectomy: In this, 4–8 g of thyroid tissue left on both sides or near total thyroidectomy can be done
- Young patients with small gland are at greater risk of recurrence, so total thyroidectomy with lifelong thyroxine replacement is the treatment of choice.

Anesthesia

Mostly done under general anesthesia (GA), but can be done under cervical epidural anesthesia.

Patient's Position on the Operation Table

- Supine with table tilted up 15° at the head end to reduce venous engorgement (reverse Trendelenburg)
- Sandbag should be placed transversely under patients shoulders and head supported by the ring with neck extended, to make the thyroid gland more prominent and to apply tension to the skin, platysma and the strap muscles, which makes dissection easier.

Incision

Kocher's skin crease transverse incision, midway between the notch of thyroid cartilage and the suprasternal notch, about 1 cm below the cricoid cartilage which is carried through platysma muscle (Fig. 18).

Steps of the Procedure

- After giving skin incision as described above, flaps of skin and platysma are raised upwards to the superior thyroid notch and downwards to the suprasternal notch
- Upper flap dissection is done in an avascular subplatysmal plane anterior to anterior jugular veins and deep to platysma to the level of the thyroid cartilage
- Lower flap is mobilized till the suprasternal notch
- Deep cervical fascia is divided in midline between strap muscles of both sides to the plane of thyroid capsule
- Thyroid gland is exposed by midline incision through the superficial layer of deep cervical fascia between sternohyoid and sternothyroid muscles
- Muscles are retracted laterally and gland is reached
- Strap muscles are dissected from thyroid gland and retracted laterally
- In rare cases, strap muscles may be divided to get accesses in case of large thyroid tumor
- Middle thyroid veins are divided and ligated laterally from thyroid surfaces

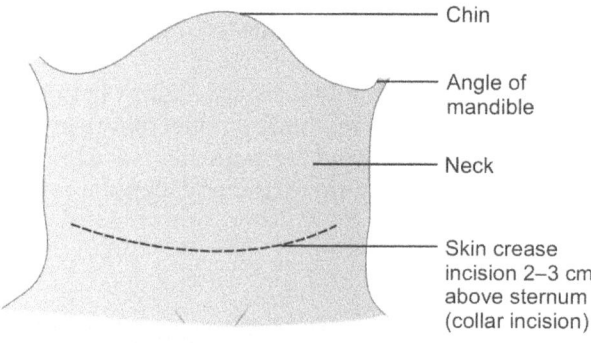

Fig: 18: Kocher's skin crease neck incision.

- Superior pole of thyroid is mobilized and superior thyroid vessels are then individually identified and ligated doubly near to the thyroid gland to save external laryngeal nerve
- RLN enters larynx at the level of cricoid cartilage passing under or through ligament of belly
- Similarly inferior thyroid pole is mobilized and inferior thyroid vessels ligated away from the gland to save RLNs
- When hemithyroidectomy has to be performed, isthmus is divided flush with contralateral lobe to be removed and oversewn
- In subtotal thyroidectomy, subtotal lobectomy on both sides leaving about 4–8 g of thyroid tissue in both tracheoesophageal grooves is done
- In case of near total thyroidectomy, total lobectomy on one side and subtotal lobectomy on other side leaving about 4–5 g of thyroid tissue in the tracheoesophageal groove is done
- Removing all thyroid tissue on one side has the advantage of obviating need to reoperate on one side in cases in which reoperation is necessary and possibility of damage to RLN and parathyroid on that side during future surgery is reduced
- If parathyroid gland is inadvertently or unavoidably excised or devascularized, it should auto transplanted immediately within the adjacent sternocleidomastoid muscle
- Suction drain kept, strap muscles reapproximated with absorbable sutures, platysma sutured, skin closed with subcuticular absorbable skin sutures or skin clips or staplers.

Postoperative Care

- Postoperative IDL or direct laryngoscopy in OT by anesthetist to see movements of vocal cord postoperatively, to know whether RLN is damaged or normal
- To screen parathyroid insufficiency, serum calcium estimation should be done after 4–6 weeks of operation
- Thyroxine should be withheld during the first 6 months after surgery, even when there are clinical features of thyroid failure.

Postoperative Complications and their Management

1. **Hemorrhage**
    - May be early or late
    - Mostly presents as reactionary hemorrhage and is dangerous
    - Occurs within 6–8 hours after surgery most commonly due to slipping of ligature of superior thyroid artery
    - Hemorrhage may occur from thyroid remnant or thyroid vein
    - Due to hemorrhage, tension hematoma may occur deep to cervical fascia causing compression of trachea and larynx.

Treatment: Patient should be taken to the operation theater in emergency, to relieve tension by removing the sutures and opening the layers of the wound. Bleeding vessel can be ligated if found during re-exploration of the neck, under general anesthesia.

2. **Respiratory obstruction**
   - Due to collapse or kinking of trachea (tracheomalacia) and larynx (laryngomalacia) due to removal of goiter
   - Most commonly, it occurs due to laryngeal edema, due to trauma to the larynx by anesthetic intubation and due to surgical manipulation
   - Most important cause of respiratory obstruction is a tension hematoma
   - May occur due to bilateral RLN palsy, but not cause immediate respiratory obstruction unless laryngeal edema is also present.

   Treatment: Intubation with endotracheal tube or needle tracheostomy should be done, to relieve obstruction in emergency. Steroids given to reduce edema.

3. **Laryngeal nerve palsy**
   - Injury to RLN (1% cases) postoperatively revealed as hoarseness of voice, non-occlusive cough
   - Injury to the external branch of the superior laryngeal nerve results in paralysis of cricothyroid muscle causing difficulty in shouting, singing high notes
   - May be unilateral or bilateral
   - May be transient or permanent
   - In case of bilateral RLN palsy also known as bilateral abductor paralysis, both the vocal cords lie in the median position and the airway may get obstructed causing dyspnea and stridor
   - Recovery occurs in 3 weeks to 3 months
   - May require tracheostomy if airway get obstructed in case of bilateral RLN palsy.

4. **Cervical sympathetic trunk injury** causes Horner's syndrome.

5. **Thyroid insufficiency:** Occurs within 2 years of thyroid surgery. Incidence higher than previously and rates of 20–45% at 10 years have been reported.

6. **Parathyroid insufficiency (Hypoparathyroidism)**
   - Occur due to accidental removal of the parathyroid glands during surgery or infarction of parathyroid due to vascular injury, due to damage to the parathyroid end arteries
   - Vascular injury is more common than inadvertent removal causing parathyroid ischemia due to interruption of its blood supply rather than their removal
   - Revealed within 2–5 days after operation as tingling numbness around lips (circumoral) and fingers presents as carpopedal spasm
   - Sometimes symptoms may get delayed up to 2–3 weeks.
   - If removed accidentally at the time of surgery, it should be cut into 1 mm cubed pieces and implanted into the ipsilateral sternocleidomastoid muscle
   - Incidence of permanent hypoparathyroidism is less than 1%.

Treatment: Oral calcium (1 g 3 or 4 times daily) and vitamin D supplements given for mild hypocalcemic symptoms (<8 mg/dL), and intravenous calcium gluconate 10 mL of 10% is given, if associated with severe symptoms of hypothyroidism.

7. **Thyrotoxic crisis (Thyroid storm)**
   - Life-threatening condition
   - Acute exacerbation of hyperthyroidism
   - It occurs in patients of primary thyrotoxicosis, who are not properly treated preoperatively and not made euthyroid before the thyroid surgery
   - During surgery due to handling of the gland, sudden release of thyroxine into the systemic circulation occurs, resulting in this condition
   - Rarely thyrotoxic patient presents in crisis and this may follow an unrelated operation or precipitated by infection such as pharyngitis, pneumonia, etc. or acute illnesses like stroke, trauma, diabetic ketoacidosis or administration of iodine or after I^{131} treatment.

   Symptoms: Tachycardia, fever (hyperpyrexia >105°F), severe sweating, gross dehydration due to vomiting, diarrhea, hypovolemic shock, confusion, overt mania, coma, seizures and delirium.

   Treatment

   Prophylaxis: To make the patient euthyroid before operation.

   Symptomatic and supportive treatment
   - Intensive monitoring, identification and treatment of the precipitating causes
   - Dehydration should be treated by administration of intravenous fluids by rapid fluid replacement
   - Hyperpyrexia managed by cooling the patient with ice packs
   - Restlessness, agitation and hyperactivity treated by sedating the patient
   - For cardiac failure oxygen, diuretics should be administrated
   - For uncontrolled atrial fibrillation digoxin should be given
   - Intravenous hydrocortisone can also be given.

   Specific treatment:
   - Antithyroid drugs carbimazole 10–20 mg 6 hourly or propylthiouracil can be given
   - Lugol's iodine (5% iodine in 10% potassium iodide solution) 10 drops 8 hourly by mouth or sodium iodide 1 g intravenously or sodium iodate solution is given which inhibits thyroid hormone release from the thyroid gland
   - Beta-blockers: Propranolol 40 mg 6 hourly orally or may be given intravenously in a dose of 1–2 mg. It reduces tachycardia and other adrenergic manifestations
   - In extreme cases, peritoneal dialysis or hemofiltration is effective in lowering T_3, T_4.

8. **Wound infection**
9. **Hypertrophic scar and keloid formation:** Most common in dark skinned individuals.
   Treatment: Injection of corticosteroid intradermally and repeated monthly, if necessary.
10. **Stitch granuloma:** With or without sinus formation, due to use of non-absorbable suture material like silk. Absorbable ligatures and sutures must be used throughout the thyroid surgery.

CHAPTER 35

Minor Operative Procedures

INCISION AND DRAINAGE OF AN ABSCESS

Definition
Incising the wall of an abscess cavity to drain pus inside it.

Indications
Abscess.

Anesthesia
Mostly done under general anesthesia or nerve block or regional anesthesia like spinal anesthesia in case of extremity abscess.

Position of the Patient on the Operation Table
As per the site of the abscess and its easy accessibility to the operating surgeon to drain the abscess.

Techniques
1. Free or liberal method
2. Hilton's method.

Free or Liberal Method

Incision
- ❖ Incision is given on the most prominent (pus pointing part) and most dependent part (dependent in respect to gravity) of the abscess for free drainage of pus

❖ Stab incision is given with stab knife (11 number blade) in a single stroke penetrating the skin, subcutaneous tissue and deep fascia, to reach the abscess cavity and drain the pus.

Counter Incision

When the most prominent part of the abscess is not the most dependent part, free drainage of the abscess is not possible with single incision given at the most prominent part. In such cases, another incision (counter incision) is necessary to the most dependent part of the abscess to facilitate its drainage by gravity. For example, breast abscess situated in upper quadrant of the breast.

Steps of the Procedure

- ❖ Parts are painted with antiseptic solution and draped with sterile sheets
- ❖ Skin incision is given as described above
- ❖ Pus is drained in a kidney tray, and sends for culture and sensitivity
- ❖ Index finger is then introduced into the abscess cavity to explore the cavity and all the loculi are broken
- ❖ All loculi should be broken to form one single cavity for complete drainage of the abscess, as if any loculus remains, it leads to recurrence or chronicity
- ❖ After complete drainage of the pus from the abscess cavity, it is washed with hydrogen peroxide, antiseptic solution like povidone, iodine and then normal saline
- ❖ Magnesium sulfate and antiseptic soaked roller gauze is packed in the abscess cavity, to obliterate the dead space and prevent bleeding from the raw area of the cavity
- ❖ Intravenous antibiotics, elevation and rest to the affected part, daily dressing should be done postoperatively
- ❖ Counter incision is given as described above if required
- ❖ Corrugated rubber drain (CRD) can be kept for free drainage of pus between the two incisions, and also not to allow the tract between the two incisions to obliterate, to keep the tract open for free drainage
- ❖ Sterile dressing is applied.

Hilton's Method of Abscess Drainage

- ❖ If important structures like nerve or vessels are present in the area of abscess, then incision should be parallel to them or it should be incised and drained by Hilton's method
- ❖ Abscess is drained by Hilton's method, when abscess is situated at an important site, where major blood vessels and nerves are situated, which are liable to be injured during incision and drainage of the abscess, if adequate care not taken
- ❖ Mostly employed in cases of abscesses situated in neck, axilla and groin.

❖ Skin and subcutaneous tissue is incised with stab knife (11 number blade), on the most prominent and most dependent part of the abscess as described in liberal method above.

Steps of the Procedure
- ❖ Parts are painted with antiseptic solution and draped with sterile sheets
- ❖ Skin and subcutaneous tissue is incised with stab knife (11 number blade), on the most prominent and most dependent part of the abscess
- ❖ In this case, deep fascia is not incised with the blade
- ❖ Tip or point of the curved hemostatic forceps or preferably sinus forceps is forced through the deep fascia into the abscess cavity
- ❖ Blades of sinus forceps are gradually opened and pus extruded out
- ❖ Sinus forceps is taken out with its jaws opened, to enlarge the opening in the deep fascia for easy drainage of pus
- ❖ Index finger is then introduced into the abscess cavity, to explore the cavity and all the loculi are broken
- ❖ All loculi should be broken to form one single cavity for complete drainage of the abscess, as if any loculus remains, it leads to recurrence or chronicity
- ❖ After complete drainage of the pus from the abscess cavity, it is washed with hydrogen peroxide, antiseptic solution like povidine, iodine and then normal saline
- ❖ Magnesium sulfate and antiseptic soaked roller gauze is packed in the abscess cavity, to obliterate the dead space and prevent bleeding from the raw area of the cavity
- ❖ Sterile dressing is applied
- ❖ Intravenous antibiotics, elevation and rest to the affected part, daily dressing should be done postoperatively.

Incision and Drainage of Neck Abscess
- ❖ Occurs due to suppuration of regional lymph nodes
- ❖ Skin crease incision or incision parallel to the anterior border of the sternocleidomastoid of the affected side is given and abscess drained by Hilton's method.

Incision and Drainage of an Axillary Abscess
- ❖ Occurs due to suppurative lymphadenitis or boil affecting many hair follicles or sweat glands of the axilla
- ❖ Incision given half inches behind the anterior axillary fold, and abscess drained by Hilton's method.

Postoperative Complications
- ❖ Bleeding from the abscess cavity
- ❖ Injury to the adjacent important structures if due care not take while draining it.

INSERTION OF AN INTERCOSTAL DRAIN

Definition

Insertion of an intercostal drain (ICD) in the pleural cavity through the intercostal space (ICS).

Indications

- Traumatic hemothorax
- Traumatic pneumothorax
- Traumatic hemopneumothorax
- Drainage of empyema or pleural effusion
- Following thoracotomy for postoperative drainage.

Anesthesia

Under local anesthesia by infiltrating 2% lignocaine with adrenaline around the marked site in the selected intercostal space by infiltrating skin, subcutaneous and parietal pleura.

Position of the Patient on the Operation Table or Bed

Supine position with backrest lifted to 45° (Propped up position).

Incision

- 1–1.5 cm incision is given at the following sites as per the indication of ICD insertion
- **In case of pneumothorax:** ICD is inserted through the incision in the 2nd intercostals space, anteriorly (anterior axillary line) or through triangle of safety, which is located between anterior and midaxillary line. Triangle of safety is bounded by anterior border of latissimus dorsi (anterior to midaxillary line), posterior border of pectoralis major (below and lateral to the pectoralis major muscle) and superior border of the 5th rib (above the level of nipple), this will ideally find the 5th intercostal space
- **In case of hemothorax:** ICD is inserted through the incision in the 7th or 8th ICS in the midaxillary or in the posterior axillary line
- **In case of hemopneumothorax:** ICD is inserted through the incision in the 7th or 8th ICS in the midaxillary or in the posterior axillary line, with the tip of the tube in an upward direction towards the apex of the lung or directing towards the opposite shoulder.

Steps of the Procedure

- Parts are painted with antiseptic solution and draped with sterile sheets

- Skin incision with stab knife (11 number blade) is made at the level of upper border of the rib in the selected intercostals space as per the indication of ICD insertion
- Using long curved hemostatic forceps, the intercostals muscles are split, separated and the parietal pleura reached
- Blunt dissection completed with the index finger to reach the parietal pleura
- The tract should be oblique, so that the skin incision and the hole in the parietal pleura do not overlie each other and the drain is in a short tunnel, which reduces chances of entering atmospheric air
- Drain is held by the hemostatic forceps and inserted into the pleural cavity through the split intercostals muscles, by piercing it through the pleura
- The drain should pass over the upper edge of the rib to avoid injury to the neurovascular bundle that lies beneath the rib
- A drain for pneumothorax and hemopneumothorax should directed towards the apex of the lung, whereas the drain for pleural effusion or empyema should be nearer the base of the lung
- Intercostal tube may be inserted by using stylet or trocar, to puncture the pleura
- Outer end of the tube is clamped with the hemostatic forceps, while inserting the tube and then opened and connected to a underwater seal drainage bag, which has to be kept below the chest level
- Drain is fixed to the skin with nonabsorbable sutures (Nylon or silk no. 1, on cutting needle)
- Another stitch in a purse string fashion is given around the drain and kept untied, which has to be tied during removal of the chest tube to seal the skin incision
- Sterile dressing is applied, to fix the tube to the skin, so that the drainage bag should not hang
- After completion of the procedure, chest radiograph should be taken to confirm the position of the drain.

Intra- and Postoperative Complications

- Hemorrhage from the muscles and the subcutaneous tissue
- Damage to the intercostals vessels and nerves
- Lung and mediastinal injury, while piercing the tube inside the pleural cavity
- Pulmonary infection.

TRACHEOSTOMY

Definition

Making an opening in the trachea.

Indications

Emergency indications
- In head, neck and facial injuries, where tracheal intubation is difficult or not possible
- Chocking of the larynx due to dentures, foreign bodies, fish bones, etc.
- Stridor due to laryngeal spasm as in diphtheria, tetanus, etc.
- Tracheomalacia after thyroidectomy.

Elective indications
- Carcinoma larynx
- Major head and neck surgeries
- ICU ventilation after 4-5 days in comatose intubated patients.

Anesthesia

Under local anesthesia, by infiltrating 2% lignocaine with adrenaline in the skin and subcutaneous tissue along the line of skin incision.

Position of the Patient on the Operation Table or Bed

Supine position with extended neck by keeping a sandbag or pillow under the shoulders.

Incision

Transverse skin crease curved incision at the level of 2nd cricoid cartilage.

Steps of the Procedure

- Parts are painted with antiseptic solution and draped with sterile sheets
- Skin crease incision is given and deepened through the subcutaneous tissue and deep fascia
- Strap muscles are reached and retracted laterally from the midline
- Isthmus of the thyroid is separated, divided or retracted below
- A circular opening is made in the 2nd tracheal cartilage by holding the cartilage with Allie's tissue forceps, and the cut cartilage is removed
- A suitable size tracheostomy tube is introduced through the opening
- The cuff of the tube is inflated with 2-5 mL of air, and the tube is held in place by passing a tape around the neck or by anchoring sutures
- Skin is sutured with interrupted silk or nylon sutures (3-0, on cutting needle)
- Sterile adhesive dressing is applied.

Postoperative Complications

- Tracheal stenosis
- Air leakage with surgical emphysema in the neck

- Bleeding
- Aspiration
- Wound infection.

Postoperative Advice

- Regular suctioning and cleaning of the tube to prevent its blockage
- Humidification of the inspired air.

VENESECTION

Definition

It involves exposure of the vein, venotomy (cutting half the circumference of the vein) and introducing a wide bore cannula inside the vein, under direct vision.

Indications

- In a patient with hypovolemic shock, where all the peripheral veins are collapsed and venepuncture or insertion of intravenous cannula is not possible
- Patient requiring rapid infusion of intravenous fluid in short-time
- For prolonged period of intravenous fluid therapy
- For giving intravenous parenteral nutrition
- For measurement of central venous pressure (CVP), by passing long cannula down through the vein up to the superior vena cava through basilic or cephalic vein.

Anesthesia

Under local anesthesia, by infiltrating 2% lignocaine with adrenaline in the skin and subcutaneous tissue across the selected vein.

Position of the Patient on the Operation Table or Bed

Supine position.

Incision

Small transverse skin incision given across the selected vein (Fig. 1).

Sites where Venesections are Usually Done

- Great saphenous vein at the ankle (most common site)
- Basilic vein in the arm
- Cephalic vein in the deltopectoral groove.

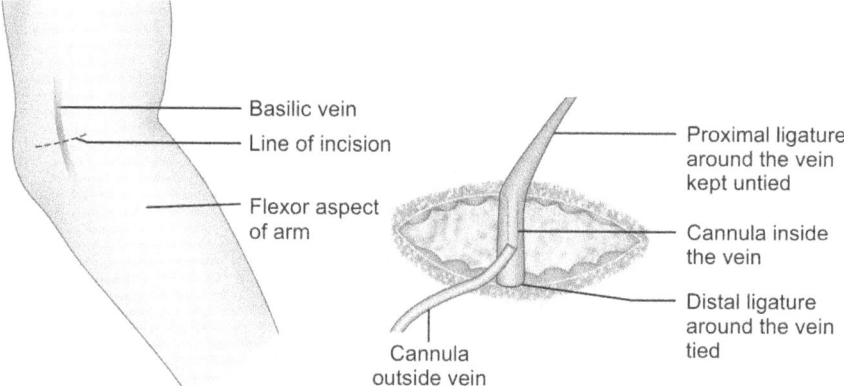

Fig. 1: Incision for venesection in the arm for basilic vein.

Steps of the Procedure

* Parts are painted with antiseptic solution and draped with sterile sheets
* Skin crease incision is given as per selected site and deepened through the subcutaneous tissue
* Vein is identified by its blue color isolated from the subcutaneous tissue
* Two ligatures are passed around the vein
* Distal ligature is tied and held by a hemostatic forceps and traction given to the vein distally to make it straight and taught
* A needle is passed through the middle of the circumference of the vein in between the proximal and distal ligatures, and the vein incised over the needle on its anterior wall only (half of its circumference)
* Number 6 to 9 number of infant feeding tube or tubing of scalp vein set after cutting its needle, is introduced through the venotomy incision and advanced in the vein proximally as far as possible
* After advancing the cannula proximally, the proximal ligature is tied along with the cannulated vein to fix the cannula within the vein
* Outer end of the cannula is connected to the intravenous tubing and then fixed to the skin
* Skin incision closed with interrupted nonabsorbable sutures (Silk or nylon 3-0, on cutting needle)
* Adhesive sterile dressing is applied.

Complications

* Wound infection
* Ascending infection in the vein through the outer end of the cannula
* Injury to the surrounding structures like tendon, nerve, etc.
* Chances of deep vein thrombosis, if patient does not walk because of the venesection cannula in case of venesection done in lower limb

- Accidental incision over the brachial artery, by mistaking it as a basilic vein while performing venesection in the upper arm.

EXCISION OF THE CYST (SEBACEOUS OR DERMOID CYST)

Definition
Removing the cyst from the body along with its wall.

Indication
Cyst (sebaceous or dermoid cyst).

Anesthesia
Done under local anesthesia after infiltrating 2% lignocaine with adrenaline all around the cyst in the skin and subcutaneous tissue.

Position of the Patient on the Operation Table
As per the site of the cyst and its easy accessibility to the operating surgeon.

Incision
An elliptical skin crease incision is given over the cyst centring over the punctum in case of sebaceous cyst (Fig. 2).

Steps of the Procedure
- Parts are painted with antiseptic solution and draped with sterile towels
- Skin incision is given as described above and deepened through the subcutaneous tissue taking care not to puncture the cyst wall as puncture of the cyst wall causes difficulty in its complete excision

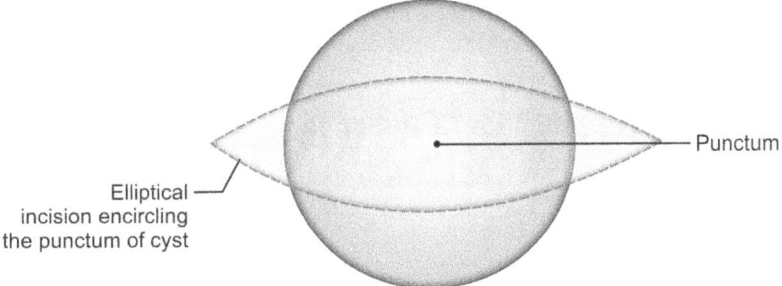

Fig. 2: Skin crease elliptical incision centring over the punctum.

- Skin incision should be equal or larger than the size of the cyst, to prevent its rupture during dissection for its complete removal along the wall, to prevent recurrence
- Skin flaps are raised through the plane between the subcutaneous tissue and the cyst wall
- Cyst wall is dissected free from the surrounding tissue all around with a fine curved scissor or by blunt dissection with curved hemostatic forceps
- After complete dissection of the cyst wall from the surrounding tissue, cyst is excised completely from the body along with the overlying elliptical skin
- Skin incision is sutured with interrupted nonabsorbable sutures (Silk or nylon 3-0, on cutting needle)
- Adhesive sterile dressing is applied.

Postoperative Complications
- Wound infection
- Wound gape
- Hemorrhage
- Hematoma or seroma if the dead space not obliterated properly. After excision of the cyst
- Injury to the underlying vessels or nerves
- Recurrence if cyst along with its wall not excised completely.

EXCISION OF THE LIPOMA

Definition
Removing of the lipoma from the body.

Indication
Lipoma.

Anesthesia
Done under local anesthesia after infiltrating 2% lignocaine with adrenaline all around the lipoma, in the skin and subcutaneous tissue.

Position of the Patient on the Operation Table
As per the site of the lipoma and its easy accessibility to the operating surgeon.

Incision
- Linear skin crease incision parallel to the Langer's line

❖ Skin incision may be slightly smaller than the size of the lipoma, as the lipoma may be shelled out from one side by finger dissection and the remaining part dissected similarly.

Steps of the Procedure

- ❖ Parts are painted with antiseptic solution and draped with sterile sheets
- ❖ Skin crease incision is given and deepened through the subcutaneous tissue
- ❖ Skin flaps are raised after reaching the plane between the subcutaneous tissue and the capsule of lipoma, if capsulated
- ❖ Lipoma is dissected out all around from the surrounding tissue with a fine curved scissor or by blunt dissection with curved hemostatic forceps or by blunt dissection with a finger
- ❖ Small vessels supplying the lipoma are ligated and divided
- ❖ After complete dissection of the lipoma from the surrounding tissue, it is excised
- ❖ Hemostasis secured
- ❖ If lipoma is large enough to leave dead space after its excision, it has to be obliterated with absorbable suture (Catgut or vicryl no. 2-0, on round body needle), otherwise it leads to postoperative seroma or hematoma
- ❖ Skin is sutured with interrupted non-absorbable sutures (Silk or nylon 3-0, on cutting needle)
- ❖ Sterile adhesive dressing is applied.

Postoperative Complications

- ❖ Wound infection
- ❖ Wound gape
- ❖ Hemorrhage
- ❖ Hematoma or seroma, if the dead space not obliterated properly after excision of the lipoma
- ❖ Injury to the underlying vessels or nerves.

LYMPH NODE BIOPSY

Definition

Excision of the lymph node from the body for histopathological examination.

Indications

Generalized or isolated lymphadenopathy.

Anesthesia

Done under local anesthesia after infiltrating 2% ligocaine with adrenaline all around the lymph node, in the skin and subcutaneous tissue.

Position of the Patient on the Operation Table

As per the site of the lymph node and its easy accessibility to the operating surgeon.

Incision

Linear skin crease incision parallel to the Langer's line.

Steps of the Procedure

- Parts are painted with antiseptic and draped with sterile towels
- Skin crease incision is given and deepened through the subcutaneous tissue and fat
- Skin flaps are raised through the plane between the subcutaneous tissue and the capsule of lymph node
- Lymph node is dissected out all around from the surrounding tissue with a fine curved scissor or by blunt dissection with curved hemostatic forceps
- After complete dissection of the lymph node from the surrounding tissue, it is excised and send for histopathological examination
- Skin is sutured with interrupted nonabsorbable sutures (Silk or nylon 3-0, on reverse cutting needle)
- Sterile adhesive dressing is applied.

Postoperative Complications

- Wound infection
- Wound gape
- Hemorrhage
- Hematoma or seroma, if the dead space not obliterated properly. After excision of the lymph node
- Injury to the underlying vessels or nerves.

Section 9

Bedside Procedures

Section Outline

36. Bedside Procedures

CHAPTER 36

Bedside Procedures

■ PERIURETHRAL CATHETERIZATION

Definition
Insertion of the catheter perurethrally.

Indications
- To relieve acute retention of urine by catheterization in case of benign hyperplasia of prostate, in case of unconscious or comatose patient unable to pass urine
- To measure urine output in postoperative patient or patient of renal failure
- To diagnose upper and midurinary urinary tract injuries (except urethral). If catheterization of the bladder reveals hematuria, it indicates presence of injury to the kidney, ureter, bladder, etc.
- For administration of intravesical chemotherapy for treatment of bladder carcinoma
- 3-way Foley catheter is mostly used after open prostatectomy or transurethral resection of the prostate for benign prostatic hyperplasia, for postoperative irrigation of the bladder
- 3-way catheter also used in case of hematuria due to injury to upper and midurinary tract or in case of hematuria due to malignant growth of the bladder, to prevent formation of clots in the bladder which may block the catheter and subsequently bladder drainage.

Anesthesia
Under local anesthesia, after introducing 2% lignocaine jelly in the urethra through the external urethral meatus.

Position of the Patient on the Bed
Supine with legs apart.

Steps of the Procedure

- Clean the genital area, lower abdomen and upper thigh with antiseptic solution and draped with sterile sheets
- In case of male patients, clean the glans penis and the urethral meatus by retracting preputial foreskin, and in case of female patients clean the urethral meatus by separating the labia
- Take 10 mL of 2% lignocaine jelly in a syringe and introduce it into the urethra through the external urethral meatus and press the meatus for sometime, to prevent the jelly from spilling out
- Massage the undersurface of penis to allow the jelly to go further down in to the proximal urethra
- Wait for 10 minutes for the anesthetic effect of jelly
- Penis is held vertically upwards by the nondominant hand by encircling it with a sterile gauge around the base of the penis, to straighten the penile urethra
- Lubricate the tip of the catheter with jelly or liquid paraffin and insert it through the external urethral meatus
- The catheter advanced gradually, slowly, smoothly till it reaches the bladder, which is confirmed by observing urine from the outer end, main channel
- Catheter is advanced little further, and about 3–15 mL (depending upon capacity of the balloon) of distilled water is introduced through the side channel of the catheter to inflate the balloon, to make the catheter self-retaining
- After the balloon is inflated, catheter is gently pull outward just to confirm that the balloon is properly inflated
- Main drainage channel is then connected to drainage (urosac) bag
- Hugely or grossly distended bladder should be emptied slowly to prevent vasovagal attack
- In males, preputial skin to be replaced back to cover the glans penis, to prevent paraphimosis.

Causes of Failure to Pass Catheter

- Tight phimosis
- Meatal stenosis
- Stricture urethra
- Bladder neck stricture
- Severe BHP causing complete obstruction of the prostatic urethra
- Catheter too large as compared to patients urethra and external urethral meatus
- Due to inadequate anesthesia, patient may resist while inserting the catheter.

Complications:
- Bleeding
- False passage

- Urinary tract infection
- Rupture urethra if balloon inflated in the urethra without properly placing and confirming it that it is in the bladder
- If patient is irritable, he can accidently pull the catheter with inflated balloon, causing rupture urethra.

■ RYLES TUBE (NASOGASTRIC) INSERTION

Definition

Insertion of the nasogastric tube from one of the nostril into the stomach.

Indications

- To decompress the stomach in intestinal obstruction, gastric outlet obstruction (GOO)
- To decompress the stomach in perforation peritonitis, to limit the peritoneal contamination by aspirating gastric contents through the tube
- Decompression of the stomach preoperatively in surgeries of upper gastrointestinal tract to prevent intraoperative contamination from the gastric or intestinal contents
- Decompression of the stomach in comatose patient of head injury to avoid aspiration of gastric contents into the trachea causing aspiration pneumonitis
- To monitor gastric bleeding and to give stomach wash in case of bleeding peptic or malignant ulcer
- To aspirate the gastric contents and giving gastric lavage in case of suspected oral poisoning, drug overdose, etc.
- For giving nasogastric feeding to a comatose patients who are on intravenous fluids and parenteral nutrition for long time or patients who are not able to feed themselves properly.

Anesthesia

Under local anesthesia, after applying 2% lignocaine jelly in one of the nostril and also over the tip of the tube. It lubricates the tube as well.

Position of the Patient on the Bed

Supine with neck slightly fixed.

Steps of the Procedure

- In conscious patients, explain the procedure to the patient, that this tube has to be inserted through one of his/her nostril and when it reaches the oropharynx, he/she should swallow it

- Introduce the tip of the tube through one of the nostril by holding its tip in the dominant hand and rest of the tube coiled on fingers in non-dominant hand
- When the tube reaches the oropharynx, ask the patient to swallow or sips of water can be given if the patient is conscious, so that patient will swallow and the tube will enter the esophagus
- Tube is further advanced till its 2nd mark lying at the level of nostril and secured to the nose with an adhesive tape
- Stomach contents aspirated with syringe or it can be attached to the drainage bag.

How to Confirm that Tube is in the Stomach and not in the Trachea

- While passing the tube in a conscious patient, if the patient coughs, tube must have entered the trachea and has to be removed immediately
- Aspirate the tube, aspiration of greenish gray fluid confirms that tube is in the stomach
- Inject about 50 mL of air through the tube and listen the sound with the stethoscope kept over the epigastrium. Audible gurgling sound will confirm the tube, that it is in the stomach
- Put the outer end of the tube in a kidney tray containing water, if air bubbles seen, then tube must be in the trachea
- Listen to the outer end of the tube. Sound of moving air will confirm that the tube is in the trachea
- Chest X-ray with upper abdomen can be taken, to know the position of tip of the tube.

Complications

- Bleeding due to trauma to the nostril, nasopharynx and oropharynx
- Insertion of the tube in the trachea.

PROCTOSCOPY/ANOSCOPY

Definition

To examine and visualize the anal canal and lower 1/3rd of the rectum, with the 'anal speculum' or 'anoscope' or 'proctoscope'.

Indications

- For various diagnostic and therapeutic purposes affecting anal canal and lower rectum
- For diagnosis of piles (hemorrhoids), rectal polyps, rectal ulcer, carcinoma of the anal canal or lower rectum, internal opening of the perianal fistula, etc.

- For therapeutic uses like injection of sclerosant in the piles, during excision of polyp, anal dilatation, drainage of pelvic and prostatic abscess in males, etc.
- For taking biopsy from anal or rectal growth, to rule out malignancy.

Anesthesia

Under local anesthesia. 2% lignocaine jelly should be applied at the tip of the obturator and also perianally for lubrication of the instrument and anal canal and also to anesthetise the anal mucosa for painless insertion of the anal speculum.

Position of the Patient on the Bed

Left lateral (Sim's position) or knee elbow position.

Steps of the Procedure

- Per rectal digital examination with gloved index finger lubricated with 2% lignocaine jelly should be done prior to the insertion of the anal speculum, to rule out any painful pathological conditions like anal fissure or abscess
- Anal speculum is introduced within the anal canal directing it first upwards and forwards towards the umbilicus, and then pushed upward and backward towards the sacrum with obturator inside the sheath, then the obturator withdrawn from the sheath and the sheath is steadily withdrawn from the anal canal
- The examination of lower rectum and anal canal is carried out by throwing light inside the sheath from a torchlight, while withdrawing the sheath slowly, as the pathologies of the anal canal has tendency to prolapse into the sheath, whereas it get compressed between the rectal wall and the sheath while introducing the instrument.

Complications

Bleeding from the anal mucosa due to injury to it, if not inserted gently.

INTRAVENOUS CANNULA INSERTION

Definition

Inserting a wide bore cannula inside the vein.

Indications

- In a patient of hypovolemic shock
- For giving intravenous fluids pre- and postoperatively
- For giving intravenous drugs like antibiotics, analgesics, antiacids, etc.

Anesthesia

No anesthesia given, as it is a simple needle puncture.

Position of the Patient on the Bed

Supine and as per easy accessibility of the selected vein to the operating surgeon.

Steps of the Procedure

- Apply tourniquet above the selected vein, mostly above the elbow when the cannula has to be inserted in the forearm or dorsum of the hand
- Ask the patient to close and open the fist repeatedly to make the veins prominent on the dorsum of the hand
- Selected site should be cleaned with spirit swab
- Vein to be punctured is steadied with nondominant hand and the cannula should be held in the dominant hand with bevel of the needle within the cannula pointing upwards
- Needle inserted through the skin and subcutaneous tissue into the selected vein
- As the cannula enters the vein, blood will be seen into the distal end of the cannula
- Stylet withdrawn slightly, keeping it inside the cannula to avoid counter puncture of the vein and then the cannula along with the needle advanced further inside the vein
- After making the cannula steady, needle withdrawn and cannula secured to the skin by adhesive tape
- Outer end of the cannula is attached to the tubing of the intravenous set to start the intravenous fluid bottle.

Complications

- Counter puncture of the vein, causing bleeding and extravasations of the fluid in the subcutaneous tissue
- Thrombophlebitis (Inflammation of the vein).

Section 10

Advanced Techniques in General Surgery

Section Outline

37. Laparoscopy Surgery and Instruments
38. Robotic Surgery

CHAPTER 37

Laparoscopy Surgery and Instruments

INTRODUCTION

Nowadays, most of the patients want to get operated by minimal invasive surgery. One of that is laparoscopic surgery. The main advantage of laparoscopic surgery is that instead of operating patients through large incisions, patients get operated through small incisions with less trauma to the tissue. There is less postoperative pain, fast recovery, and shorter hospital stay with sooner return to work. The chances of wound infection are less because of less handling of tissue and better and acceptable cosmetic scar than traditional open surgery. Also, there are less chances of postoperative adhesions and incisional hernia than seen in traditional open surgeries.

Laparoscopy is the word derived from Greek word lapara, means "the soft part of the body between ribs and hip, loin, and flank" and skopein means to "look".

IMAGING SYSTEM

Imaging system consists of laparoscope, i.e. telescope, camera, light source, light cable, and monitor.

Laparoscopes

In 1952, British physicist Hopkins invented telescope. Laparoscopes may be rigid or fiber optics (Figs. 1 to 3). Commonly used are rigid ones having angle 0°, 30°, and 45°. Diameter of telescope varies. It may be 10 mm, 5 mm, and 3 mm. 10 mm scope is routinely used in adult practice while 3 mm scope is used in pediatric practice. The scope provides attachment to light cable. Fogging of lens occurs intraoperatively due to increased temperature in abdomen which is prevented or cleared by dipping tip in warm water. After its use, telescope eye piece, light cable slot, and its patient end must be cleaned with warm water. It is sterilized with chemical sterilizers.

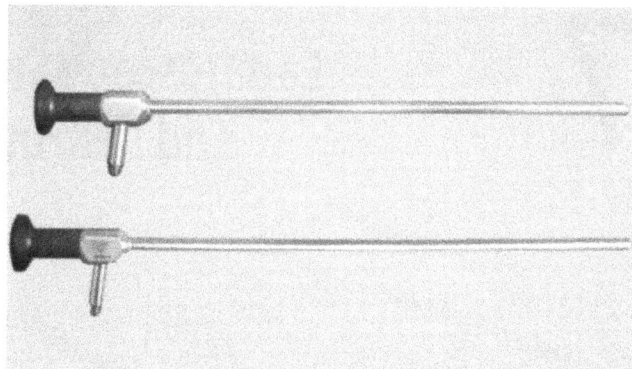

Fig. 1: 0° and 30° telescopes.

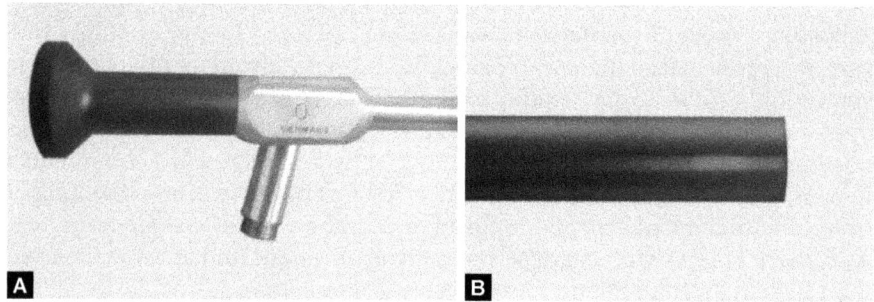

Figs. 2A and B: 0° telescope with oval end.

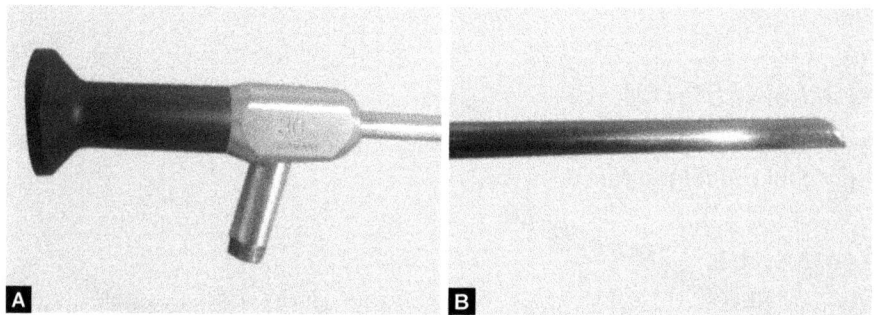

Figs. 3A and B: 30° telescope with oblique end.

Cameras

It is the most important part of the imaging system. It allows all members in the operation theater to view the operative field simultaneously. It also permits the type of coordinating movements required for complex operations. The sensor called charged-coupled device (CCD) has small pieces of silicon called pixels, arranged in rows and columns. Nowadays, high resolution with good optical sharpness and light weight cameras are available. It may be single chip

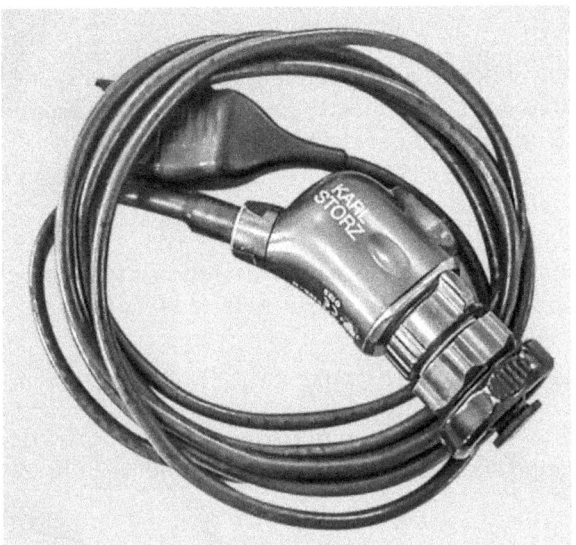

Fig. 4: Camera.

or three chips. A single chip camera has resolution of point 450–600; while the three chip cameras has more than 750 horizontal lines which give better visual clarity. Usually, single chip cameras are used for routine laparoscopic surgeries. It has white balancing and zoom option (Fig. 4).

Light Source

Three types of light sources are routinely used: halide, halogen, and xenon. Most common type of light source used is halogen bulb. The halogen lamp of 250 watt with a condenser system is economical and is routinely used. Xenon lamp of 175–300 watt gives better visual clarity and is natural, but is expensive. The intensity of light can be regulated manually or automatically. For obtaining natural color, a proper white balancing before start of the operation is necessary (Figs. 5A and B).

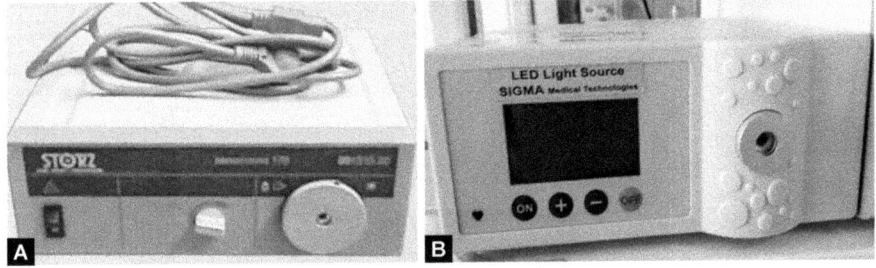

Figs. 5A and B: Light source.

Light Cable

Light cable may either be a fluid filled (liquid crystal gel) or fiberoptic. The cable is available at different lengths and diameters. Fiberoptic cable is user friendly than fluid-filled cable (Fig. 6).

Monitors

The video monitor should produce high resolution image after connection. 20 inches and above large video screen is preferred (Fig. 7).

■ GAS FOR PNEUMOPERITONEUM

Initially air was used to create pneumoperitoneum, but not used nowadays. The main complication of using air is the risk of air embolism. The ideal insufflating

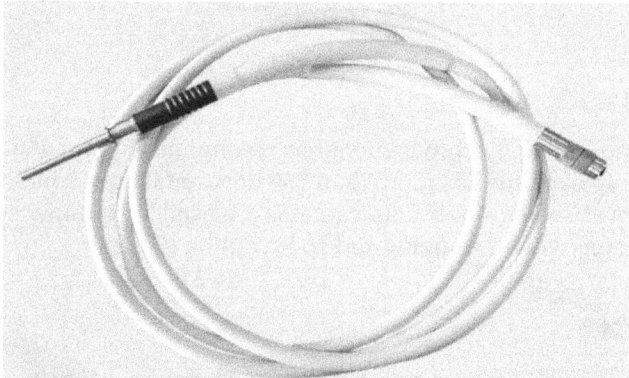

Fig. 6: Light cable.

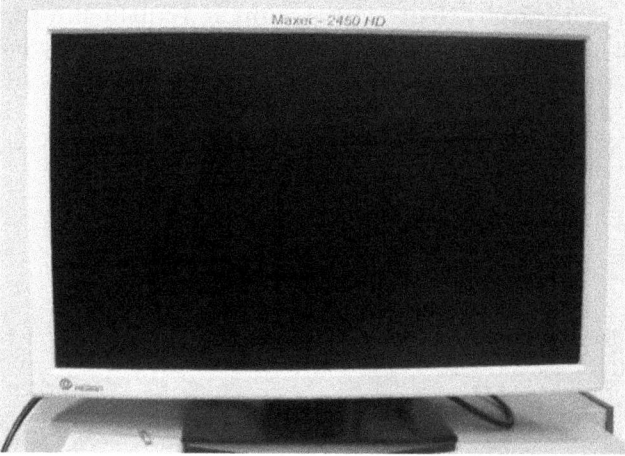

Fig. 7: Monitor.

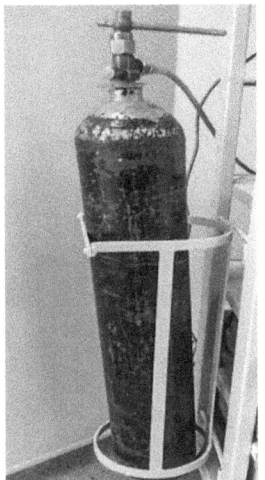

Fig. 8: Carbon dioxide cylinder attach to instrument trolley.

agent for laparoscopic procedures should be physiologically inert, colorless, and nonexplosive. It should be inexpensive, readily available, and nontoxic. It should be highly soluble in blood.

Carbon Dioxide

It is most commonly used in laparoscopic procedures. Risk of venous gas embolism is low and is nonexplosive. Hypercarbia and acidosis are the complications after using carbon dioxide. Decreased cardiac contractility, systemic vasodilation, and pulmonary hypertension are potential complications of using carbon dioxide (Fig. 8).

Other gases that are used in laparoscopy are nitrous oxide (NO), helium (He), and argon.

INSUFFLATOR

Generally used insufflator in laparoscopic surgery is electronic CO_2 insufflator (Figs. 9A and B). Insufflating peritoneal cavity allows the necessary work space for laparoscopic surgery by distending the abdominal wall and depressing the

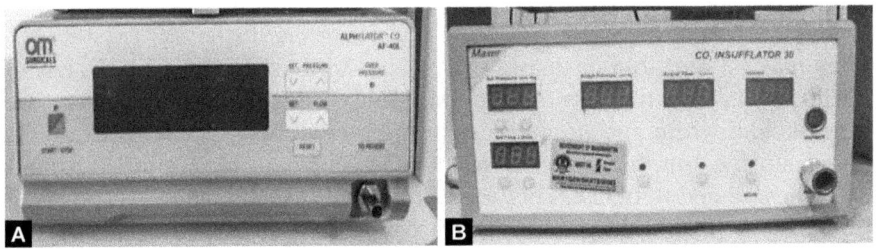

Figs. 9A and B: Insufflators.

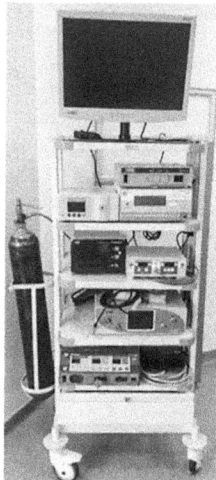

Fig. 10: Instrument trolley.

hollow organs. Two types of insufflators are in use, automatic and manual. In automatic insufflators, the surgeon presets the insufflating pressure and it supplies gas until the required intra-abdominal pressure is reached. The insufflator automatically starts and delivers gas when the intra-abdominal pressure falls because of gas leakage from the ports. Insufflation pressure can vary from 0 mm Hg to 30 mm Hg.

INSTRUMENT TROLLEY

All the imaging system instruments has to be arranged in instrument trolley (Fig. 10). It makes it easy to shift the trolley in other operation theater whenever required.

SUCTION IRRIGATION MACHINE

It is used for cleaning and flushing the abdominal cavity and cleaning during operations. It is used routinely at the time of laparoscopy to make the field of vision clear. For irrigation, mostly normal saline is used.

OPERATIVE HAND INSTRUMENTS

They may be reusable or disposable. Disposable instruments have better performance and higher safety on single use. Some surgeons reuse the disposable instruments after sterilization. Most of the reusable instruments are expensive, but they are cost-effective in long run use and need proper cleaning and maintenance. They are dismountable so easy to wash and clean properly. The disposable instruments are difficult to sterilize properly as they does not get dismantled.

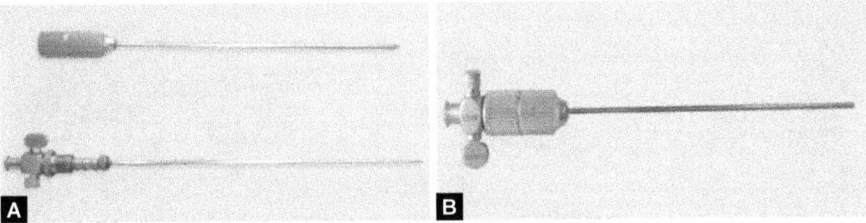

Figs. 11A and B: Veress needles.

■ INSUFFLATION CANNULAS

1. Veress Needle

Veress needle consists of an outer cannula with a beveled needle point for cutting through tissues (Figs. 11A and B). Inside the cannula, there is an inner stylet, which is loaded with a spring. This spring springs forward in response to the sudden decrease in pressure encountered during crossing the anterior abdominal wall and entering the peritoneal cavity. The lateral hole on this stylet enables CO_2 gas to be delivered intra-abdominally. Veress needle is used for creating initial pneumoperitoneum so that the trocar can enter safely and the distance of abdominal wall from the abdominal viscera should increase. Veress needle technique is the most widely practiced way of intra-abdominal access. It is important to check its potency and spring action every time before using it. It is available in three lengths: 80 mm, 100 mm, and 120 mm. In obese patient, 120 mm is preferred and in very thin patient with scaphoid abdomen 80 mm Veress needle is preferred. Disposable needles can also be used.

2. Hassan Cannula

It is less commonly used than Veress needle. It carries less risk of hollow visceral and vascular injury. It is safer than Veress needle to enter the abdomen, especially in those patients having previously history of intra-abdominal operations. It consists of three pieces: a cone-shaped sleeve, a metal or plastic sheath with a flap valve, and a blunt tipped obturator. On the sheath, there are two struts for affixing fascial sutures. The sutures are then wrapped tightly around the struts, which creates an effective seal to maintain pneumoperitoneum (Figs. 12A and B).

■ TROCARS

Trocars and cannulas used to pierce the anterior abdominal wall for placement of laparoscope and surgical instruments. Trocar is a stylet which is introduced through the cannula. The trocars are available with different type of tips (Figs. 13A to G). Tips can be pyramidal, conical, blunt tipped, or may have optical access. Conical-tipped trocars are less traumatic to the tissue. Risk of herniation or hemorrhage is less with conical-tip trocars. Cannulas may be

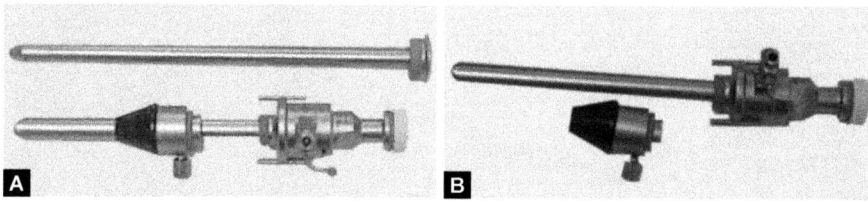

Figs. 12A and B: Hassan cannula.

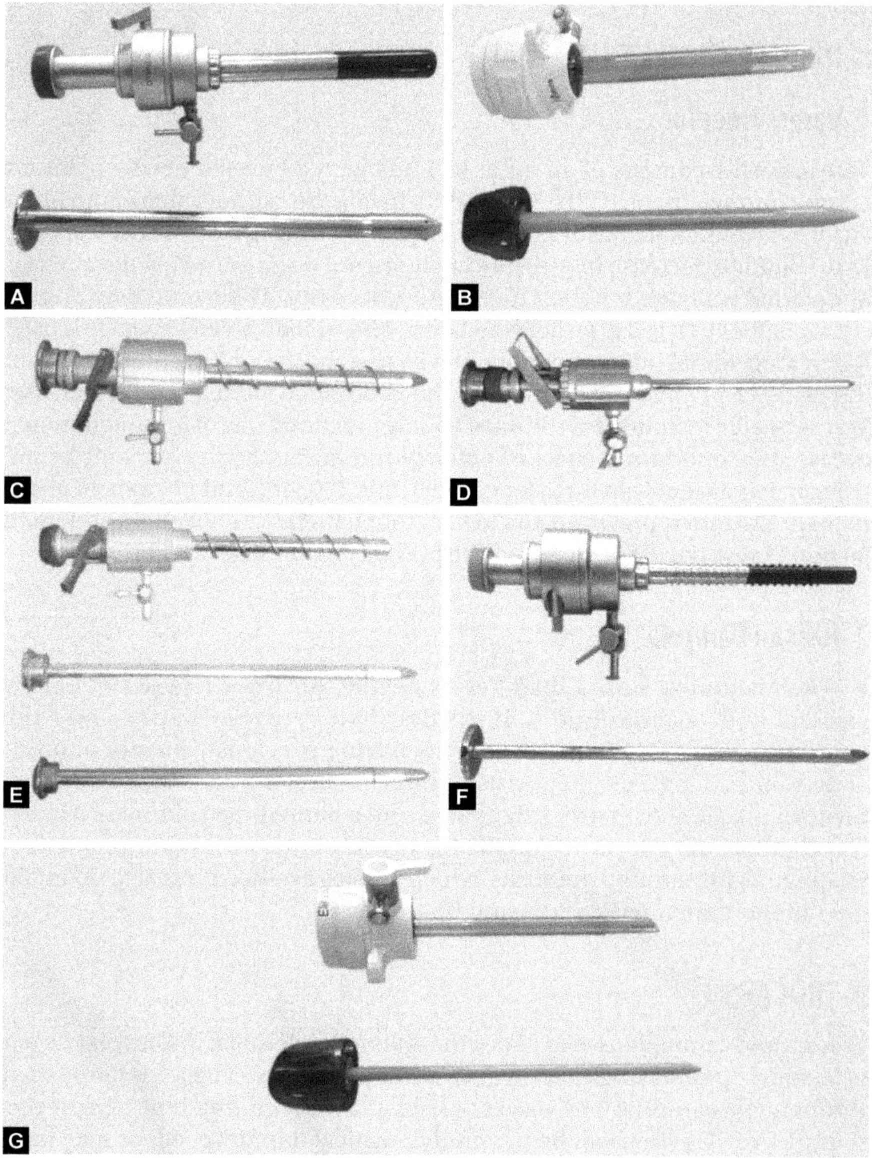

Figs. 13A to G: Different sizes of trocars and stylets: (A) 10 mm metal trocar and cannula; (B) 10 mm plastic trocar and cannula; (C) 10 mm trocar within cannula; (D) 5 mm trocar within cannula; (E) 10 mm trocar with conical and blunt tip stylets; (F) 5 mm metal trocar and cannula; (G) 5 mm plastic trocar and cannula.

of metal (reusable) or plastic. Reusable and disposable trocars are made by a combination of plastic and metal. Many of the disposable plastic trocars have spring loaded mechanism which withdraws the sharp tip immediately after it penetrates the abdominal wall reducing chances of injury to viscera. Trocar and cannula are of different sizes and diameter depending upon the instrument. The diameter of cannula ranges from 3 mm to 10 mm. The most common size is 5 mm and 10 mm (Figs. 13A to G).

All the cannulas have a valve mechanism at the top to avoid leakage of pneumoperitoneum. The sharp trocars are good than blunt trocars as they need less force to introduce inside the abdominal cavity which reduces the chances of forceful entry of full length of trocar. The end of the cannula may be straight or oblique.

■ REDUCING SLEEVE

It is used to reduce the size of the port from 10 mm to 5 mm or from 5 mm to 3 mm, so that pneumoperitoneum is maintained whenever surgeon changes the instrument from larger diameter to smaller diameter (Figs. 14A and B).

■ OPERATIVE HAND INSTRUMENTS (FIGS. 15 TO 20)

Types of Instruments:

1. Atraumatic forceps
2. Grasping forceps
3. Needle holder
4. Scissors
5. Monopolar instruments
6. Bipolar forceps
7. Loop applicator
8. Clip applicator
9. Retractors
10. Suction and irrigation instrument
11. Trackers.

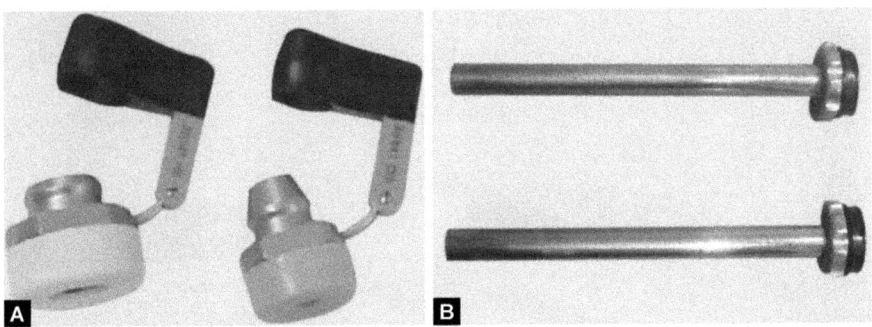

Figs. 14A and B: Reducing sleeves.

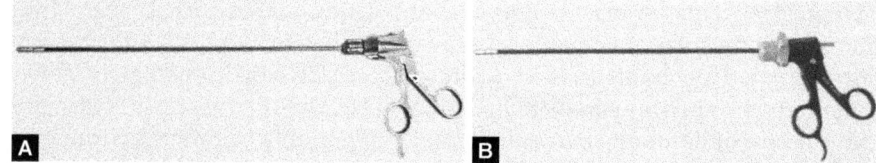

Figs. 15A and B: Typical hand instruments with tip, shaft with insulator, and handle.

The instruments vary in lengths from 18 cm to 45 cm. Mostly, it is of 36 cm in length in adults and 28 cm in pediatric practice. Their diameter varies between 18 mm and 12 mm, but most of them pass through 10 mm and 5 mm of cannulas.

The main parts of hand instruments are handle, shaft with insulation, and tip (Figs. 15A and B). Many laparoscopic instruments like graspers and scissors have opening and closing function. Some instruments have ratchet for locking. Laparoscopic hand instruments are design for sharp and blunt dissection. Most of the instruments are hold in palm grip hand position with the pistol handle, i.e. thumb outside the ring with the palm resting on the thumb ring.

GRASPERS

Graspers are used to grasp or hold the bowel and intra-abdominal viscera during operations. Graspers may be traumatic or atraumatic.

Traumatic Grasping Forceps

They are used to hold the tissue firmly. They hold the tissue firmly without slipping it for long time if ratchet is closed but causes trauma to tissues (Figs. 16A to D).

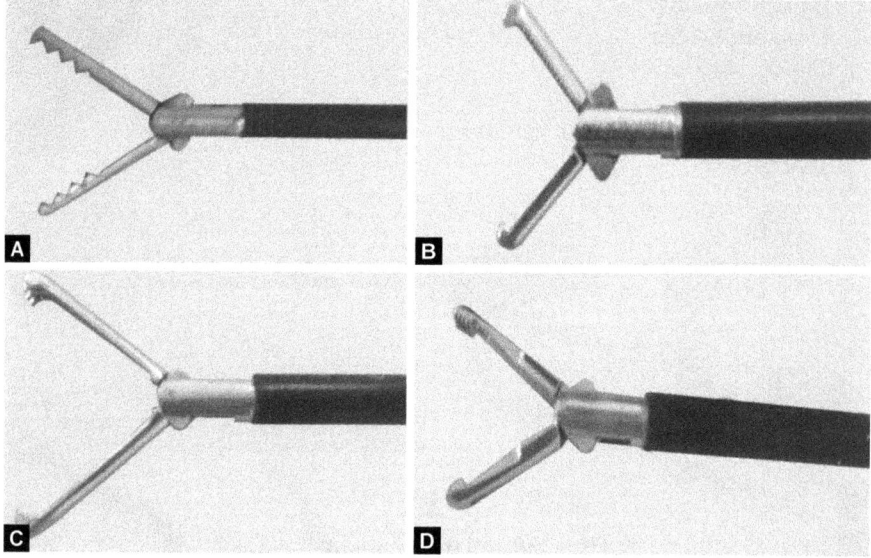

Figs. 16A to D: Different tips of traumatic forceps.

Atraumatic Grasping Forceps

These are used to hold the tissue without causing trauma to it (Fig. 17). These are mostly used to hold appendix, bowel, etc.

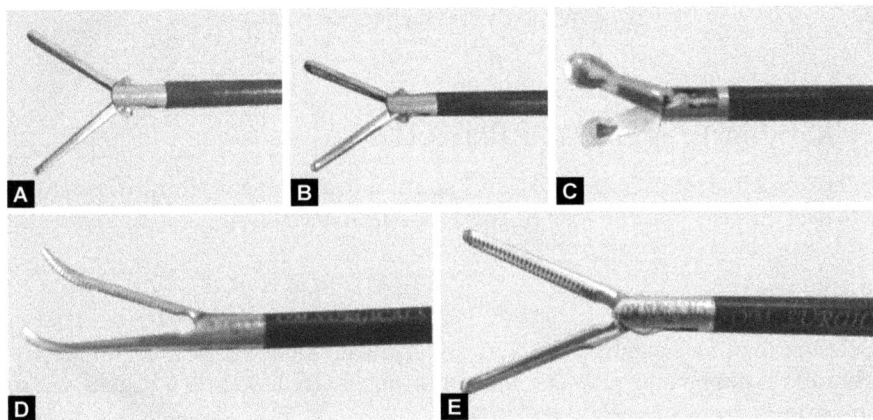

Figs. 17A to E: Different tips of atraumatic forceps.

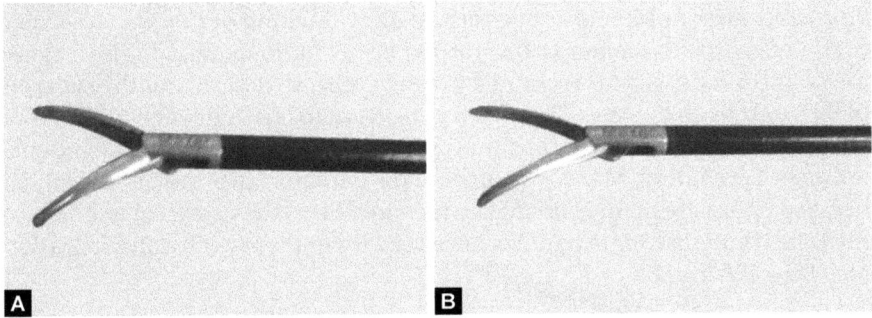

Figs. 18A and B: Fine tip dissector for fine dissection.

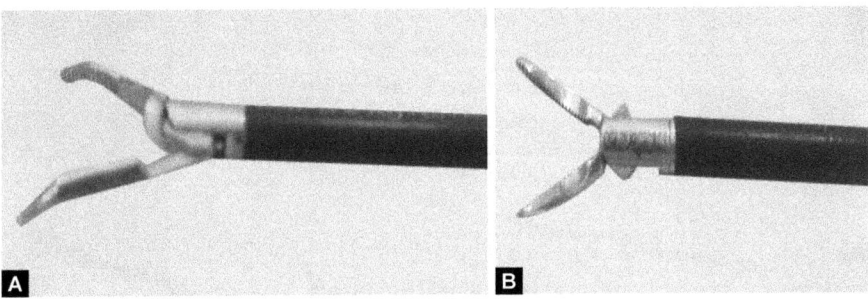

Figs. 19A and B: Maryland forceps.

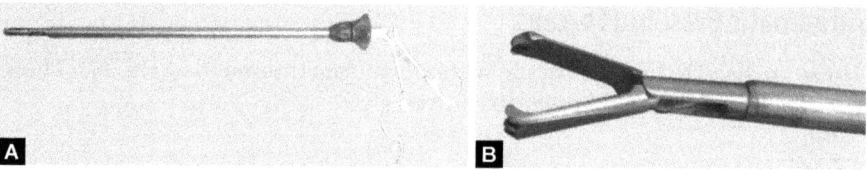

Figs. 20A and B: Specimen removal forceps.

■ INSTRUMENTS FOR SHARP DISSECTION

Scissors, electrosurgery hook, and spatula are used for sharp dissection. Electrocautery knife can also be used for sharp dissection.

Scissors

Scissors may be straight or curved. In laparoscopic surgeries, use of scissor should be done cautiously because of unnecessary bleeding and damage to important structures (Figs. 21A and B).

■ DIFFERENT HANDLES OF HAND INSTRUMENT

Some instrument handles have lock to allow locking of the jaw. It is very useful when the tissue has to be grasped firmly for long period. The locking mechanism is usually incorporated in the handle, so it is easy for the surgeon to lock or release the jaws. The locking instruments has ratchet which allows jaws to be closed in different positions. Many of the handles have attachments for unipolar cautery. Many instruments have rotator near the handle which helps to rotate the tip in 360° angle which increases the degree of freedom of these instruments. Some handles have attachment for suction and irrigation too (Figs. 22A and B).

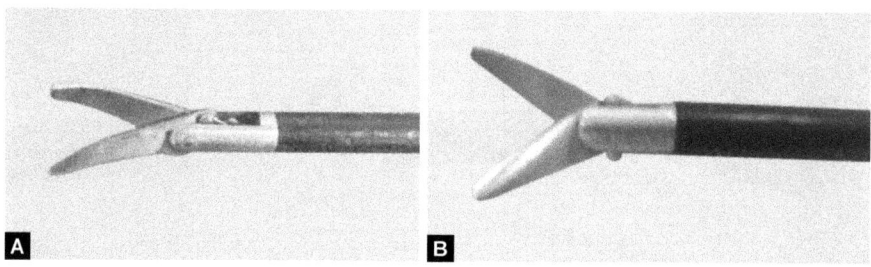

Figs. 21A and B: Scissors.

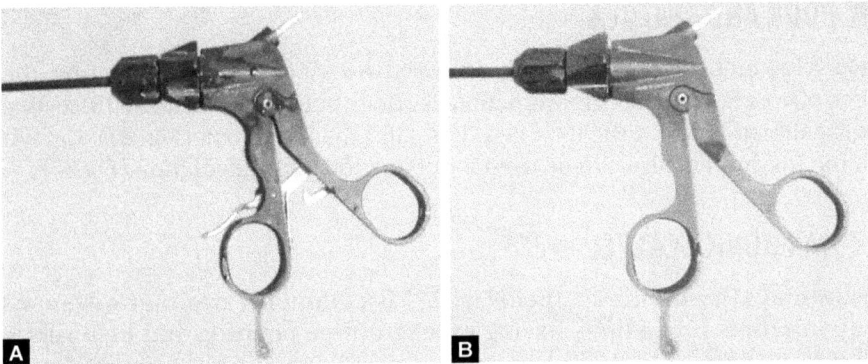

Figs. 22A and B: Different types of handles of hand instruments: (A) Handle with ratchet or lock; (B) Handle without ratchet or lock.

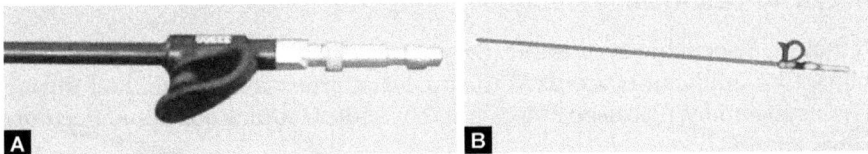

Figs. 23A and B: Outer sheath.

INSULATED OUTER TUBE

The insulation covering of outer sheath is designed to prevent accidental electric burn to bowel or other intra-abdominal viscera. The covering may be of plastic or silicon (Figs. 23A and B).

NEEDLE HOLDERS

Laparoscopic needle holders are available with straight or curved tips. Endo-suturing is done with needle holder and a grasper (Figs. 24A to C).

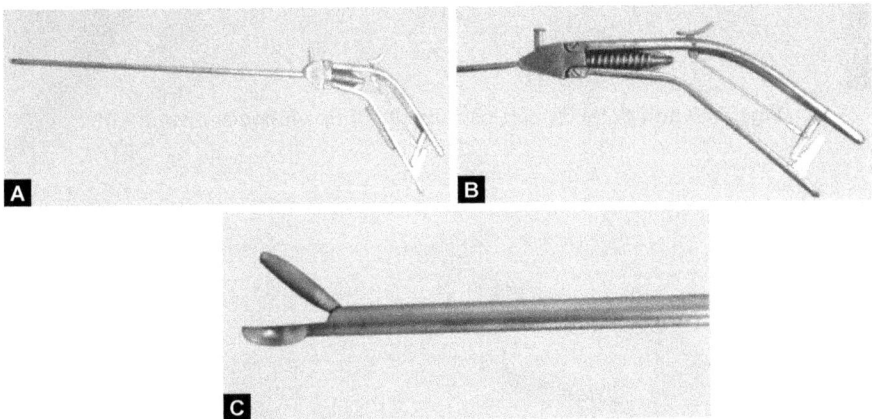

Figs. 24A to C: Needle holder: (A) Typical needle holder; (B) Handle of needle holder; (C) Tip of needle holder.

HOOK AND SPATULA

Hook has an L-shaped tip. Mostly, it is used to dissect the gallbladder from the bed of liver. Spatula has same function like hook but having flat tip for dissecting the gallbladder from the liver bed. It is safer than the hook (Fig. 25). Bipolar hand instrument also can be used for dissection and coagulation (Fig.26).

HARMONIC SCALPEL

Nowadays, harmonic scalpel (Fig. 27) is commonly used for advanced laparoscopic procedures having excellent tissue cutting and hemostatic function.

CLIP APPLICATOR

It may be disposable or reusable. Disposable clip applicators have preloaded clips. Clip applicators are used to clip cystic artery and cystic duct during cholecystectomy. Also used at appendix base before cutting it in appendectomy (Figs. 28A to D).

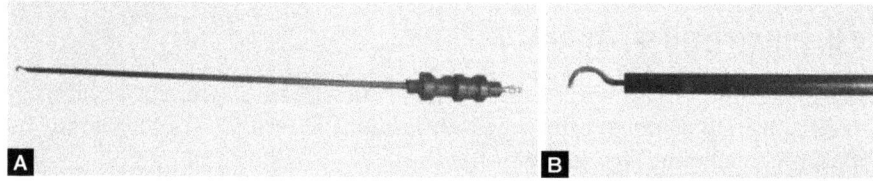

Figs. 25A and B: (A) Hook having attachment for monopolar cautery; (B) Tip of hook.

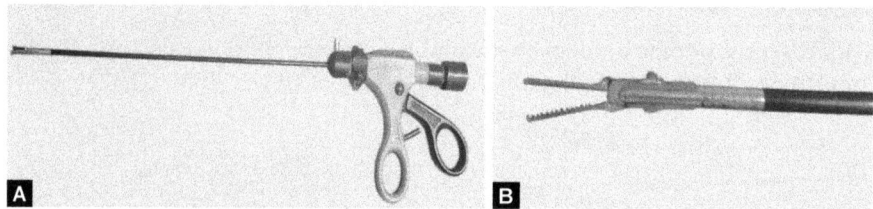

Figs. 26A and B: (A) Bipolar instrument; (B) Tip of bipolar instrument.

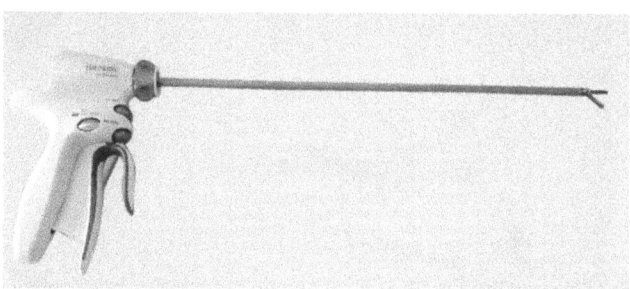

Fig. 27: Harmonic scalpel.

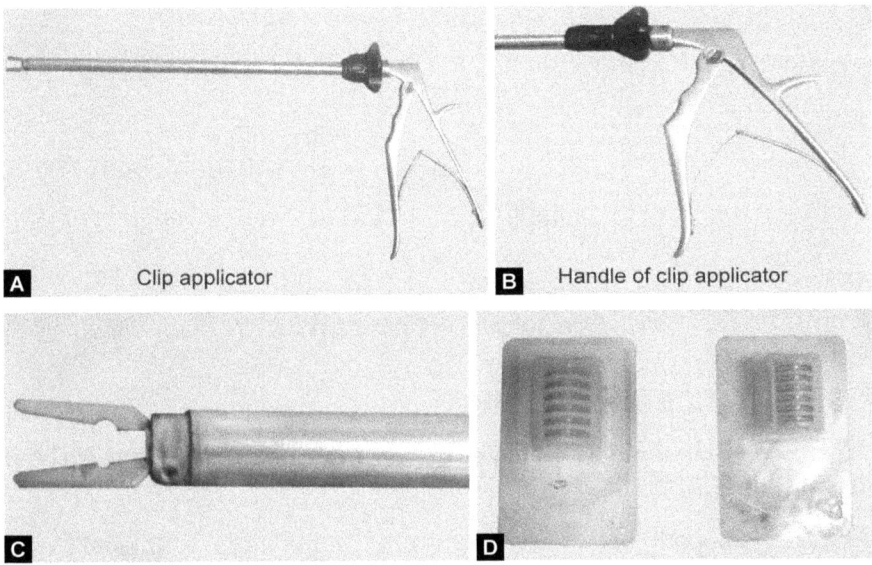

Figs. 28A to D: (A) Clip applicator; (B) Handle of clip applicator; (C) Tip of clip applicator; (D) Clips of clip applicator.

SUCTION AND IRRIGATION HAND APPARATUS

Irrigation and suction are very important during laparoscopic surgeries to maintain clear operative field. It comes in 5 mm and 10 mm reusable sizes (Figs. 29A and B). The suction tip is useful for intermittent suction and also used as blunt dissecting instrument. Suction or irrigation tubes are thoroughly cleaned with running tap water before autoclaving them.

PORT CLOSURE INSTRUMENT

These are hand instruments to close the to close the laparoscopic port sites, especially 10 mm or more port sites, which has to be closed to prevent port site hernia in future. Cobbler needle is commonly used (Figs. 30A and B).

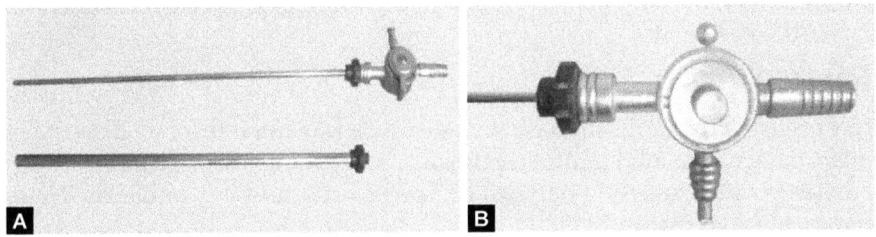

Figs. 29A and B: Suction irrigation hand apparatus.

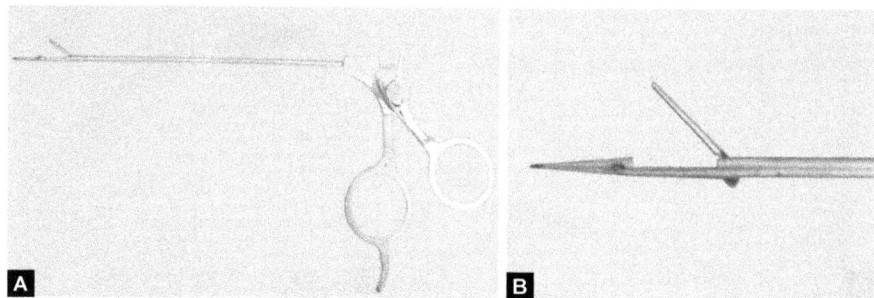

Figs. 30A and B: Cobbler needle.

STERILIZATION OF INSTRUMENTS

Laparoscopic instruments should be sterilized by sterilization or by high level disinfection (HLD).

Cleaning and Sterilization

Laparoscopic instruments can easily dismantle. Instruments which are difficult to dismantle should be used to harbor blood/tissue within their shafts. With a sterile sponge, visible blood and tissue should be wiped off. All contaminated instruments should be placed and soaked for 10 minutes in a container containing a disinfectant solution. Because of fear of damage, instruments should not be left in this solution for longer period. Laparoscopic instruments are best rinsed in running water to clear the particulate matter and residues of chemicals used for cleaning. The instruments should be dried at the end of the cleaning before they are packed for sterilization.

There are three sterilization processes available: steam, ethylene oxide, and peracetic acid.

Steam Sterilization

Steam sterilization is one of the most common forms of sterilization in general practice. Autoclaving at 121°C for 15 minutes is ideal for all reusable metal instruments. It is cheap alternative and effective too. Before sterilization, all the instruments, tubing, and cords should be wrapped doubly in a cloth to prevent contact with the hot metallic container which are then placed in the autoclave.

Gas Sterilization

Gas used for gas sterilization is ethylene oxide. It is suitable for all disposable instruments, insulated hand instruments, and tubing. Gas sterilization with ethylene oxide causes no damage to instruments, and it is noncorrosive to optics, but it is costly.

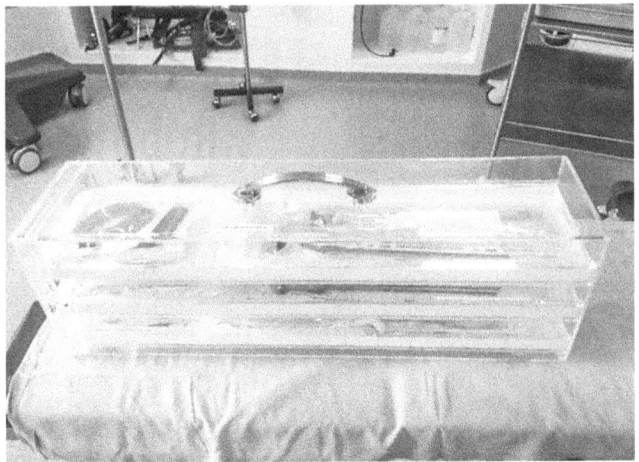

Fig. 31: Formalin chamber containing formalin tablets.

High Level Disinfection

When sterilization is not available, high-level disinfection is used for sterilizing the instruments.

The agents used are 2% glutaraldehyde, peracetic acid, and 6% stabilized hydrogen peroxide.

Fiberoptic light cords, camera, and telescopes are soaked in 2% glutaraldehyde for at least 10 minutes.

Soaking must not more than 20 minutes. Soakage of metallic instruments like trocars and hand instruments are recommended for 60 minutes. Formaldehyde also can be used. But its use for sterilizing instruments and other items is not recommended nowadays (Fig. 31).

STERRAD® is one of the newer sterilizer systems. It takes about 75 minutes for sterilization.

After sterilization or HLD, items should be properly stored immediately to avoid contamination.

CHAPTER 38

Robotic Surgery

INTRODUCTION

It is advanced technique in surgery. It is a type of minimally invasive surgery.

It is robot (computer)-assisted surgery. In this, surgeon decides and gives commands and the robot performs.

The main advantage of robotic or minimal invasive surgery is that instead of operating patients through large incisions, patient get operated through small incisions with less trauma to the tissue. There is less pain and shorter hospital stay with sooner return to work.

Most commonly used surgical robot is of "Da Vinci system". It consists of surgical console, patient side cart and instruments, and imaging processing equipment (Fig. 1). The surgeon controls the instruments and the camera from a console located in the operating room. Placing his fingers into the master controls, he is able to operate all four arms of the Da Vinci simultaneously while looking through a stereoscopic high definition monitor that places him inside the patient, giving him a better and more detailed 3-D view of the operating site more than the human eye.

The robot system is very costly, costing around 12–20 crores (in Indian rupees) (Figs. 2 to 5).

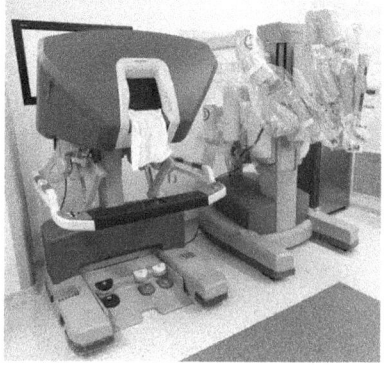

Fig. 1: Robotic Surgery Equipments.

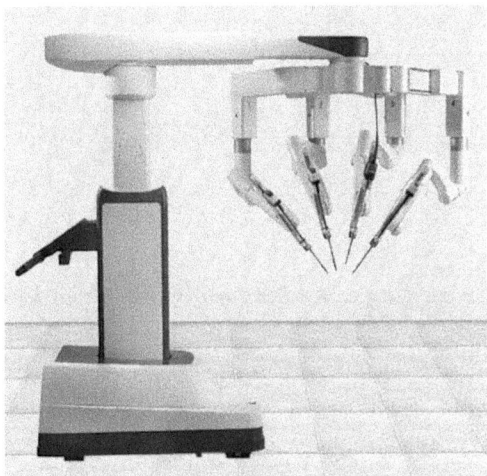

Fig. 2: Surgical cart.

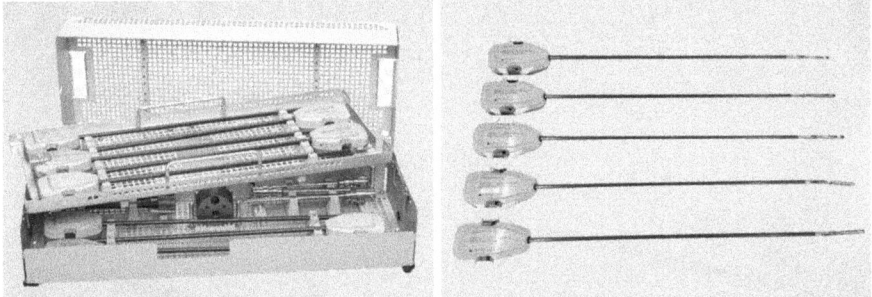

Fig. 3: Different ports used in robotic surgery.

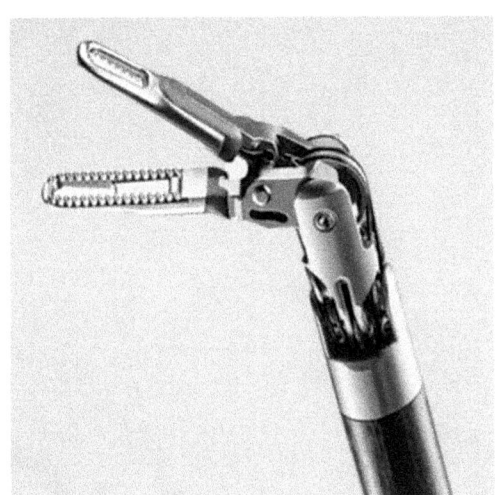

Fig. 4: Tip of port.

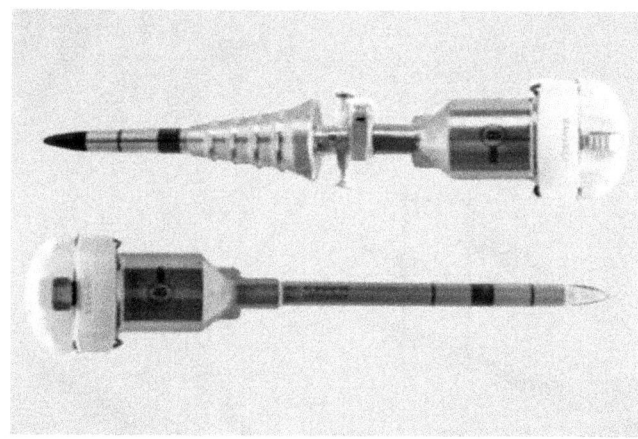

Fig. 5: Port with trocar.

Section 11

Energy Sources in Surgery

Section Outline

39. Energy Sources in Surgery

CHAPTER 39

Energy Sources in Surgery

Energy sources are used in surgery to cut, coagulate, and evaporate tissue. Energy sources are classified as radiofrequency electrosurgery, laser, ultrasonic, and argon beam coagulation. The majority (85%) of surgeons use monopolar electrosurgery. The electrosurgical effect on the tissue causes cutting, coagulation, and/or fulguration and desiccation.

Monopolar circuits have a pencil-like instrument, the active electrode which is placed in the entry site and used to cut the tissue and coagulate bleeding (Fig. 1). The return electrode pad is attached to the patient. It is simple to use but causes more tissue damage than bipolar. Hemostasis is not good in unipolar as compared to bipolar.

In bipolar instruments, which are like a forceps, electrons flow between two adjacent electrodes and the tissue between the two electrodes is heated and desiccated. A bipolar instrument shows a reduction in the amount of tissue damage and is best for coagulation. Another obvious advantage of bipolar electrosurgery over monopolar electrosurgery is the absence of a return electrode on the patient, which eliminates the possibility of ground pad and alternate site burns reducing risk of patient burn (Figs. 2 and 3).

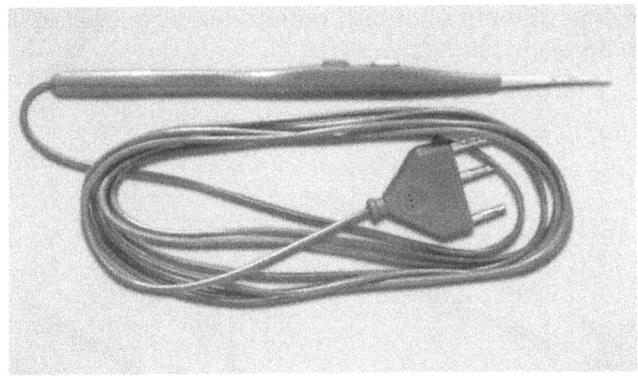

Fig. 1: Monopolar cautery cord.

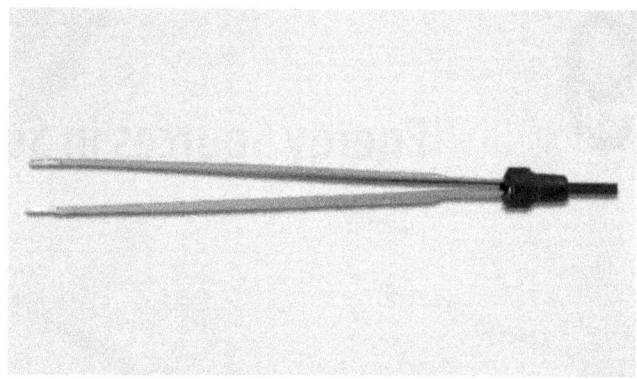

Fig. 2: Bipolar cautery forceps.

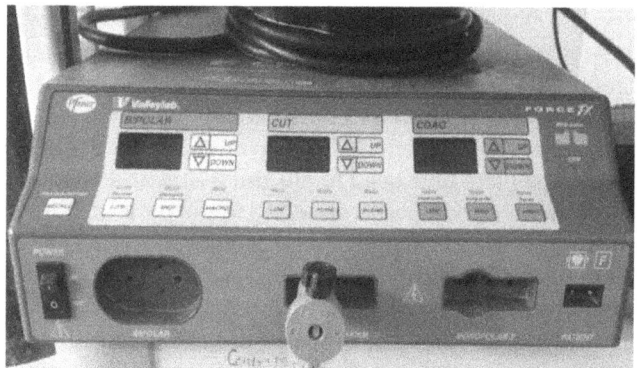

Fig. 3: Cautery machine.

Bipolar is controlled by foot pad, whereas monopolar can be controlled by foot or hand switch.

Recent advanced technologies in electrosurgery are argon beam coagulator, ultrasonic energy like harmonic scalpel, laser (light amplification through stimulated emission of radiation), radiofrequency ablation, microwave ablation, cryotherapy, etc.

Section 12

Approach to Surgical Patients in Emergency Room

Different types of surgical patients attend emergency room for treatment. In this section, we are mentioning some of the common emergencies to be attended by duty doctor in emergency room, their diagnosis, and subsequent treatment in brief.

Section Outline

40. Approach to Trauma Patients in Emergency Room
41. Approach to Patient of Acute Abdominal Conditions in Emergency Room
42. Approach to Patients of Genitourinary Emergencies in Emergency Room

CHAPTER 40

Approach to Trauma Patients in Emergency Room

▞ INTRODUCTION

A patient presenting with history of trauma due to assault or road traffic accident (RTA) or fall has to be evaluated thoroughly in the emergency ward. It may be blunt trauma (car bonnet), penetrating trauma (knife), blast injury (bomb) or crush injury (building collapse), or thermal. Accordingly, patient has to evaluated and treated.

Advanced Trauma Life Support (ATLS) system is now used globally for trauma patients. The primary survey of ATLS encourages the identification and treatment of life-threatening conditions.

Triage is an important concept to divide the patients according to the seriousness of trauma and presence of life-threatening conditions. In mass casualty, triage is used to decide who is most urgently in need of care, those who have a chance of survival but who would die without immediate treatment, and whose injuries are less severe and must wait for medical care. In triage, patients are divided into four categories according to their injuries and condition—*Red tag (immediate):* Those who cannot survive without immediate treatment but whom have a chance of survival if treated. *Yellow tags (observation):* Their condition is stable for the moment and they are not in immediate danger of death but they need observation in hospital and treated accordingly. *Green tags (wait):* Healthy having minor wounds requiring treatment. *Black:* Dead or expectant whose injuries are so extensive that they will not able to survive even after immediate treatment.

Primary survey starts with ABCDE: A—airway maintenance and cervical spine protection; B—breathing and ventilation; C—circulation and control of bleeding; D—disability; and E—exposure.

Airway can be assessed by checking verbal response. Clear mouth and airway with large bore sucker. Protection or maintenance of airway by turning patient to one side, mouth suction and intubation or pharyngeal airway to prevent tongue bite, and maintaining patency of airway. Endotracheal tube (ETT) can be inserted if respiratory distress and patient is in gasping. Oxygen must be administered to all trauma patients.

The patient must be fully exposed and examined from front and back using a carefully controlled log roll. Spinal alignment must be maintained during this procedure with inline traction.

Accurate clinical assessment of neurological status and exclusion of other surgical injuries like intra-abdominal and intrathoracic injuries should be done. Explore local wounds to assess depth of involvement.

Secure neck and spine, 30º head up with neck in neutral position.

Along with primary survey, blood should be sent for cross match and full blood count. ECG can be done. Two wide bore cannulas need to be inserted for intravenous fluids. Urinary and gastric catheters inserted. Radiographs of cervical spine and chest can be taken.

Secondary survey from head to toe has to be done after resuscitative measures completed.

Evaluate head and face for maxillofacial fractures, ocular injury, open head injury, and evidence of bleeding or discharge from the ears suggestive of basal skull fracture. See for midfacial injury and potential airway compromise.

Inspect and palpate cervical spine anteriorly and posteriorly for tenderness. Spine should be mobilized with a hard collar or sandbag.

The chest should be palpated and auscultated thoroughly for crepitus and any decease in breath sounds. Distended neck veins, distant heart sounds, and narrow pulse pressure suggest cardiac tamponade.

Examine Glasgow Coma Scale (GCS) repeatedly (in every 15 minutes).

Inspect abdomen and pelvis for distension. Inspect perineum for bleeding and ecchymosis. Palpate iliac crests to detect significant fractures. Per rectal examination is needed to asses tone, prostate level, and to look for bleeding.

Palpate the upper and lower extremity. Move the relevant joints to exclude dislocations.

APPROACH TO PATIENT SUSTAINING HEAD INJURY

Patients of head injury present in emergency room with antecedent history of road traffic or vehicular accident, fall from height, or assault. The term "head injury" includes injury to scalp, skull, or brain associated with loss of consciousness for some time. Such patients present in casualty with history of loss of consciousness or altered sensorium or sometime irritability, convulsions, ear/nose/throat bleed, and vomiting. Fracture of anterior cranial fossa presents with hemorrhage from nose (epistaxis) and escape of cerebrospinal fluid (CSF) from nose (CSF rhinorrhea). Hemorrhage in orbital cavity in lower and upper eyelids presents as periorbital edema or ecchymosis, seen in subgaleal trauma (Black eye, Panda sign, Raccoon sign). Subconjunctival hemorrhage may be seen. Fracture of middle cranial fossa presents with hemorrhage and CSF escapes from ear (otorrhea). Fracture of posterior cranial fossa presents with extravasation of blood in suboccipital region and swelling at back of upper part of neck and ecchymosis near tip of mastoid process (Battle sign).

Injury to brain divided into two parts. Primary brain injury occurs at the time of impact of injury and includes injuries, such as brainstem and hemispheric contusions, diffuse axonal injury, and cortical lacerations. This is due to diffuse neuronal (axonal) lesion (injury) called "concussion" associated with momentary loss of consciousness. Secondary brain injury occurs sometime after the moment of impact, due to subsequent or progressive brain damage and is often preventable. In the second part due to brain swelling (cerebral edema) or intracranial hemorrhage, resulting from initial trauma to the head (primary brain injury), patient again gradually loses consciousness a few hours after the injury or trauma. Principle causes of secondary brain injury are hypoxia, hypotension, raised intracranial pressure (ICP), reduced cerebral perfusion pressure, and pyrexia.

To assess the prognosis of head injury patients, GCS is used. It is composed of three components—eye (E), verbal (V), and motor (M). Best possible score is 15/15 and the worst possible score is 3/15.

Eye opening:
- Spontaneous: 4
- To speech or verbal commands: 3
- To painful stimulus: 2
- None (do not open): 1.

Best motor response (limb movements):
- Obeys commands: 6
- Localizes pain: 5
- Withdrawal/flexion: 4
- Abnormal flexion (decorticate): 3
- Extensor response (decerebrate): 2
- None (no motor response): 1.

Verbal response:
- Oriented: 5
- Confused: 4
- Inappropriate words: 3
- Incomprehensive sound: 2
- None (no sounds): 1.

Minor head injury: GCS 15 with no loss of consciousness (LOC)
Mild head injury: GCS 14 or 15 with LOC
Moderate head injury: GCS 9-13
Severe head injury: GCS 3-8.

Investigations

- Any patient having history of loss of consciousness, convulsion, ear/nose/throat (ENT) bleed, headache, and vomiting should be send to computed tomography (CT) scan of head
- Plain CT head is gold standard
- It should be performed after stabilization of patient and if normal can be repeated after 24–48 hours, if patient deteriorates
- It will provide information about an intracranial hematoma, intracerebral contusions, scalp soft tissue injury, skull fracture, etc.

Management of Patient of Head Injury

- Emergency room management will be same as above as described in management of any trauma patient
- Principle aim of treatment is the prevention of secondary brain injury, by avoidance of hypoxia and hypotension
- To reduce ICP, elevate head end of the bed to 20–30° (reverse Trendelenburg, head up)
- Intravenous isotonic or hypertonic saline (NS) should be given until nasogastric tube (NGT) feeding is started.
- Five percent dextrose and dextrose-containing fluids should be avoided as they raise the intracranial tension (ICT)
- Osmotic diuretics like 20% mannitol is used, 0.5–1 g/kg. Adult volume: 250 mL over 20–30 minutes TDS or QID (0.25–1 g/kg body weight), furosemide: 40–80 mg IV (20–40 mg/TDS)
- Prophylactic anticonvulsants, like injection phenytoin 100 mg IV TDS, reduce chances of seizures
- Antibiotics can be given if associated with open head injury or CSF leak.
- Scalp wounds bleed profusely. Hemostasis should be achieved by ligation and suturing in one or two layers
- Surgical management of head injury patients consists of evacuating intracranial hematomas by craniotomy, if causing significant mass effect. In case of skull fracture with depressed fragments, elevation of significantly depressed fragments is recommended.

APPROACH TO PATIENTS SUSTAINING CHEST INJURY

Injuries of the chest may be open or closed. Most of them are closed and occur due to blunt trauma chest due to road traffic accidents (RTAs) or assault or penetrating injuries by gunshot and stab wounds. Chest injuries which need urgent attention and treatment itself in casualties are pneumothorax, hemothorax, and cardiac tamponade.

Pneumothorax

Air in the pleural cavity, commonly due to trauma, due to fracture ribs, is called as "traumatic pneumothorax". In majority of cases of trauma, air in the pleural cavity is associated with blood called as "hemopneumothorax".

There are three types of pneumothorax:

1. **Closed pneumothorax:** Air comes out in the pleural cavity through small rent in the underlying lung due to fracture ribs and rent closed subsequently.
2. **Open pneumothorax:** Air enters pleural cavity through wound in the chest wall, in which full thickness segment of chest wall is destroyed. They are of two types—sucking and nonsucking. With every respiration, if air is sucked in the pleural cavity, it is called as "sucking pneumothorax". Due to negative

intrapleural pressure, air sucks directly through the chest wall, rather than through trachea into alveoli. Most commonly, it occurs after shotgun blasts explosion with flying debris.
3. **Tension pneumothorax:** When lacerated lung communicates with branch of bronchial tree, which permits air to enter in the pleural cavity during inspiration, but not permitting air during expiration to go out, as leak in lung become closed and rent becomes valvular. Intrapleural pressure causes collapse of lung and displaces mediastinum and causes compression of large veins resulting in decrease cardiac output. Clinical features are dyspnea, pain, shock, cyanosis, hyper-resonance on percussion, and absence of breath sounds on auscultation.

Investigations

X-ray chest: It shows shift of trachea to the opposite side due to pneumothorax, air in the pleural cavity with collapse of underlying lung.

Management of Patient with Pneumothorax

- **In case of closed injury:** Air steadily absorbed, if distress increasing, air evacuated by wide bore needle aspiration or intercostals drain (ICD) with underwater seal inserted in 2nd intercostals space (ICS) anteriorly in midclavicular line.
- **In case of open injury:** Patient stabilized by mechanically covering the open wound. Water tight dressing should be placed and ICD inserted in the pleural cavity. Early debridement and formal closure of the wound of chest wall should be done.
- **In case of tension pneumothorax:** It is a lifesaving emergency. Wide bore needle inserted through 2nd ICS followed by urgent insertion of ICD in triangle of safety which is bonded anteriorly by latissimus dorsi, posteriorly by pectoralis major, and superiorly bounded by 5th rib.
- **If associated with hemopneumothorax:** One chest tube is inserted in the 2nd ICS for evacuation of air and another through 7th or 8th ICS to drain the blood from the pleural cavity.

Hemothorax

Hemothorax is the accumulation of blood in the pleural cavity due to contusion of lung or due to injury to heart or blood vessels. Most commonly occurs due to trauma to thorax. Patients present with dyspnea, chest pain, or cyanosis. Percussion reveals dullness due to presence of fluid in the pleural cavity.

Investigations

- **X-ray chest posteroanterior (PA) supine or lateral view (decubitus):** 400–500 mL blood required for blunting of cardiophrenic (CP) angle.

- Subpulmonary trapping of blood will be better seen on lateral decubitus X-ray

Management of Patient with Hemothorax
- Blood transfusion
- In case of minimal hemothorax: Repeated aspiration by wide bore needle
- In case of moderate hemothorax: ICD inserted (tube thoracotomy) through 7th or 8th ICS in midaxillary line or postaxillary line
- Open thoracotomy may needed in some cases.

Cardiac Tamponade

Cardiac tamponade is the accumulation of fluid in the pericardium in an amount sufficient to cause serious obstruction to inflow of blood to the ventricle. Clinical features are muffled heart sounds, distended or engorged neck veins due to rising venous, hypotension, pallor, and rapid pulse due to failing arterial pressure; pulsus paradoxus is important clue to cardiac tamponade.

Investigations
Echocardiography: Shows abnormal amount of pericardial fluid.

Management of Patient with Cardiac Tamponade
Pericardiocentesis or surgical pericardiotomy.

APPROACH TO PATIENT SUSTAINING ABDOMINAL INJURIES

Patient presents in casualty with history of blunt or penetrating injury to abdomen. Blunt trauma causes contusion, lacerations, and avulsion injuries of solid intra-abdominal organs. Penetrating injuries occur due to stab injury and gunshot wounds.

Patients who have suffered abdominal trauma can be classified into following categories based on their physiological condition after initial resuscitation.
1. **Hemodynamically normal:** All necessary investigations done and treatment planned accordingly.
2. **Hemodynamically stable:** Investigations limited and patient mostly managed conservatively. In some cases, surgery may be required.
3. **Hemodynamically unstable:** Immediate surgical correction of the cause responsible for bleeding is required.

Clinical Features
- Patient presents with generalized pain in the abdomen or pelvis
- Abdominal distension and tenderness is due to hemoperitoneum

- Respiratory distress may be present due to abdominal distension
- Patient may present with hypotension, shock, and tachycardia due to ongoing blood loss
- Patient may succumb rapidly due to heavy blood loss depending on the severity and rapidity of intraperitoneal hemorrhage
- Kher sign [after elevation of the foot end for 15 minutes, referred pain is felt at the tip of the left shoulder due to irritation of undersurface of left diaphragm with contact of blood through affected fibers of phrenic nerve (C3,4)] will be positive in case of splenic injury
- Ballance sign (mass or percussible area of fixed dullness in left upper quadrant) positive in case of splenic injury. Hematuria may be present in case of genitourinary injuries.

Investigations

- Investigations have to be done according to cardiovascular status of the patient.
- In stable patients, CT scan of the abdomen and pelvis with intravenous contrast is the gold standard and is the investigation of choice as it also assesses retroperitoneal injuries. In unstable patient, CT is generally not possibl.e
- **Diagnostic peritoneal lavage (DPL):** DPL is done to assess presence of blood in the abdomen. A cannula is inserted below the umbilicus directed caudally and posteriorly. The cannula is aspirated for the blood (more than 10 mL blood is considered as positive). One liter of warmed Ringer lactate solution is allowed to run into the abdomen and is then drained out. Presence of >100,000 red cells μL^{-1} or >500 white cells μL^{-1} is considered to be positive. Nowadays, DPL has been largely replaced by focused abdominal sonar for trauma (FAST), but it still remains the standard where FAST not available.
- **Focused abdominal sonar for trauma:** It is the ultrasound imaging to assess presence of blood in the abdominal cavity. It determines presence of free intra-abdominal or pericardial fluid. It focuses on four areas: pericardial, splenic, hepatic, and pelvic. FAST is rapid, portable, and noninvasive bedside investigation of use in casualty. It is accurate for the detection of >100 mL of free blood. It does not identify injury to hollow viscus, so of no use in penetrating injury of the abdomen.
- Diagnostic laparoscopy can be done in case of penetrating injury to detect or exclude peritoneal penetration. Also to exclude peritoneal penetration and diaphragmatic injury in abdominal or thoracoabdominal stab wound.
- Decreased hemoglobin or hematocrit due to continuing blood loss.
- USG abdomen and pelvis diagnostic if more than 200 mL blood in the abdominal cavity. If USG not available, four quadrant aspiration/tap can be done which reveals fresh or clotted blood.
- **X-ray chest and upper abdomen:** Reveals fracture of ribs left side, elevated left hemidiaphragm, obliteration of splenic and psoas shadow; ground glass appearance may be seen due to blood in peritoneal cavity.

Management of Patient with Intra-abdominal Injuries

❖ Emergency room management will be same as above as described in management of any trauma patient. Intravenous fluids and blood transfusion in emergency cases
❖ Penetrating injuries should be explored, whereas blunt injuries can be treated conservatively
❖ If ongoing blood loss continues and peritonitis develops, then laparotomy can be done to control the bleeding, and if required to repair or remove the traumatized bleeding organ.

APPROACH TO PATIENT SUSTAINING BURNS

Patients of burns present in casualty with history of accidental, suicidal, or homicidal burns. Most of the burns in today's practice are thermal burns. Others are scalds, chemical, and electric burns. Burn causes coagulative necrosis of tissue. Most common affected organ is skin. It can also damage the airways and lungs. Majority of burns in children are scalds by accidental fall of hot drinks, bath water, or due to steam. In older children and adults, burns occur due to flames as a result of house fire. Industrial accidents occur due to chemical and electrical burns. Size of burn associated with 50% survival rate has increased in recent years from 30% of total body surface area (TBSA) to over 80% in otherwise healthy young adults. It may lead to hypothermia due to heat loss because of evaporation of water from the burn wounds.

Assessing the size of burn or extent of burn (TBSA) is the single most important factor in predicating burn-related mortality. In case of smaller burns or patches of burn, best measurement is to cut a piece of clean paper to the size of patients whole hand (palmar surface of digits and hand), which represents 1% TBSA and match this to the burn area. Patients total hand accounts for 2.5% of TBSA, dorsal surface including fingers accounts for 1%, palmar surface including fingers accounts for 1%, and vertical surface for 0.5% of TBSA. Rule of nines invented by Alexander Wallace is most commonly used to assess size or extent of burn.

Rule of Nine

Anatomic area	% of body surface
❖ Each upper limb	9%
❖ Each lower limb	18%
❖ Abdomen and chest (anterior trunk)	18%
❖ Back (posterior trunk)	18%
❖ Head, neck, and face (HNF)	9%
❖ External genitalia (perineum)	1%

"Rule of 9" is applicable only to adults and does not apply strictly to infants and children as they have much larger surface area of heads and smaller surface area of thighs in proportion to body size than do adults. In infants, head accounts for nearly 20% of TBSA and each lower extremity represents 13% of TBSA.

Management of the Burn Patient

- ❖ Cool the burn wound by cold clean water at 15ºC for at least 10 minutes. It provides analgesia and slows down the delayed microvascular damage that can occur after burn injury.
- ❖ Person trapped in an enclosed space should be given oxygen with propped up position on bed.
- ❖ Burned airways create symptoms by swelling or edema of oropharynx and vocal cords and if not treated, can occlude the upper airway completely. Initially, secure the airway with an endotracheal tube (ETT) until the swelling has subsided for about 48–72 hours and not to remove the tube for 3 days once inserted, as reintubation technically becomes difficult after that. Also, delay in intubation makes its difficult later on because of swelling. If intubation is not possible because of delay, cricothyroidotomy or tracheostomy can be done. Warm, humidified 100% oxygen should be given. Continuous ventilatory support or intermittent positive pressure ventilation (IPPV) support is given, if needed.
- ❖ Intravenous fluid resuscitation should be started to any child having burn >10% of TBSA and any adult having burns >15% TBSA as soon as possible. Fluids used are preferably crystalloids on day 1 and colloids along with crystalloids from 2nd day. Ringer lactate, Hartmann solution, human albumin solution, or fresh frozen plasma (FFP) are routinely used. Some use hypertonic saline. Fluid mostly crystalloid, intravenous Ringer lactate should be administered at a rate of approximately 1 liter/hour in adults and 20 mL/kg in infants. Simplest and most widely used formula for calculating crystalloid solution in the first 24 hours is Parkland formula for fluid to be replaced in the first 24 hours. It recommends 4 mL/kg/% burn in the first 24 hours of burn, i.e. volume in mL = 4 × total percentage BSA × weight in kg. If >50% area is burned, BSA should be taken to 50% only. Half of this volume is given in first 8 hours and the second half in the subsequent 16 hours. Children required proportionately more fluid than adults, at the rate of 5.8 mL/kg/% of burn.
- ❖ Key to monitoring of resuscitation is urine output. Urine output should be between 0.5 mL/kg and 1 mL/kg body weight/hour in adults, i.e. 30–60 mL/hour in an average 60 kg man. If the urine output is below this, infusion rate should be increased by 50%. If urine output is inadequate and the patient is showing signs of hypoperfusion, then a bolus of 10 mL/kg body weight should be given. If urine output in excess of 2 mL/kg body weight/hour then decrease the rate of infusion.
- ❖ Acid-base balance and hematocrit can be measured and corrected.
- ❖ After stabilization of the patient in casualty, patient to be shifted to burn care unit where dressing and if require early excision and grafting can be done by a plastic surgeon.

CHAPTER 41

Approach to Patient of Acute Abdominal Conditions in Emergency Room

■ INTRODUCTION

Different surgical patients of acute abdomen attend emergency room. Following are the clinical diagnosis and treatment of patients presenting with acute pain in the abdomen.

■ APPROACH TO PATIENT WITH ACUTE APPENDICITIS

Appendicitis is the most common cause of acute abdomen in young adults presenting with acute onset of pain in the right iliac fossa.

Clinical Features

- ❖ Pain is the early symptom followed by vomiting. Pain is first poorly localized causing central colicky abdominal pain due to midgut visceral discomfort due to appendiceal inflammation and obstruction. Pain is first noticed in the periumbilical region and then shifts to the right iliac fossa. Later diffuse pain occurs corresponding to generalized peritonitis due to free perforation of appendix causing peritonitis. Pelvic appendix may produce suprapubic discomfort and tenesmus rather than producing pain in the right iliac fossa.
- ❖ Nausea/vomiting may follow the onset of pain
- ❖ Fever, tachycardia
- ❖ Limitation of respiratory movements in the lower abdomen
- ❖ Tenderness, muscle guarding, and rigidity in right iliac fossa.

Palpation of abdomen starts in left iliac fossa and moving anticlockwise to right iliac fossa, will demonstrate muscle guarding over the point of maximum tenderness, classically at McBurney point.

Pointing sign: Patient asked to point where the pain started and where it moves.

Blumberg sign: Asking patient to cough or gentle percussion over the site of maximum tenderness, will elicit rebound tenderness due to inflammation of parietal peritoneum.

Rovsing sign: Deep palpation of left iliac fossa may cause pain in right iliac fossa (RIF) because of displacement of colonic gas and small bowel coils impinging upon the inflamed appendix.

Psoas sign: In retrocecal appendix, inflamed appendix lies on the psoas muscle, so right hip is flexed by the patient for pain relief due to psoas spasm. Hyperextension of right hip joint induces abdominal pain.

Obturator test (Zachary cope): In case of inflamed appendix in contact with obturator internus, flexion and internal rotation of hip causes pain in hypogastrium due to spasm of the obturator internus muscle.

Dunphy sign: Any movement including coughing causes pain.

Cutaneous hyperesthesia can be demonstrated in Sherren triangle due to irritation of lower abdominal nerves which is formed by anterior superior iliac spine, umbilicus, and pubic symphysis.

In retrocecal appendix: Tenderness is slight and rigidity is often absent (silent appendix) due to distended cecum preventing pressure exerted by the hand from reaching the inflamed structure. Deep tenderness is often present in loin; psoas sign is also present.

Pelvic appendix (pelvic abscess): Tenderness in rectovesical pouch or pouch of Douglas especially on right side on rectal examination. Inflamed appendix in contact with the bladder may cause frequency of micturition and early diarrhea being in contact with the rectum due to their irritation.

In postileal appendix, which lies behind terminal ileum, diagnosis is difficult because pain may not shift, and diarrhea is a feature.

In case of generalized peritonitis due to rupture or perforation of appendix, abdomen is diffusely tender, rigid, and silent on auscultation.

If perforated appendix, walled off by surrounding structures into an appendix abscess, palpation reveals tender lump in right iliac fossa.

To confirm the diagnosis of acute appendicitis, Alvarado scoring system is used.

Symptoms

Migratory pain in RIF: 1; Anorexia: 1; Nausea, vomiting: 1.

Signs

Tenderness in RIF: 2; Rebound tenderness: 1; Elevated temperature: 1.

Laboratory Findings

Leukocytosis: 2; Shift to left of neutrophils: 1.

Total: 10

Sum of all scores are calculated and based on results, Patients are divided into three groups:

Aggregate Score

7–10: Strongly predictive of appendicitis
5–6: Equivocal
1–4: Appendicitis can be ruled out.
USG and CT are done to make diagnosis in equivocal cases.

Investigations

- Diagnosis of acute appendicitis is essentially made on clinical history, physical findings with assistance of laboratory, and radiological investigations. There is no laboratory or radiologic test that is 100% diagnostic of appendicitis.
- Increased total leukocytes count (TLC): TLC >12,000/mm^3 with polymorphonuclear leukocytosis (>75% neutrophils).
- **X-ray abdomen erect:** It shows localized ileus in right iliac fossa with dilated small bowel loop and gas in cecum, ascending colon, and terminal ileum. Fecalith may be seen at the base of the appendix. Free intraperitoneal gas may be seen suggestive of perforated appendix.
- **USG abdomen and pelvis:** To confirm the diagnosis of appendicitis. It shows dilated, noncompressible, aperistaltic tubular structure. Fecalith may be seen.
- **Contrast-enhanced CT abdomen:** Most reliable than USG. Most confirmatory in patients with diagnostic uncertainty, but rarely done due to high cost to diagnose this condition, but mostly done to rule out other the intra-abdominal pathologies.

Management of the Patient of Acute Appendicitis

- After diagnosing patient of acute appendicitis, patient should not be allowed anything to be taken by mouth. Intravenous fluids and broad-spectrum antibiotics should be started. Analgesics can be given if patient has severe pain.
- Appendicectomy is the treatment of choice and urgent operation is essential to prevent increased morbidity and mortality of peritonitis. Laparoscopic appendicectomy is treatment of choice nowadays. Appendicectomy should be done when patient comes within 24–48 hours of acute attack of appendicitis. If patient comes after 2–3 days of pain and lump is palpable, it is better not to operate at that stage. Appendicular lump should be treated conservatively by "Ochsner Sherren regimen" by keeping the patient nil by mouth (NBM) with intravenous fluid supplementation along with broad-spectrum intravenous antibiotics. Regime consists of observing and examining the patient regularly on hourly basis, to know whether the patient is responding to the conservative regime or not. Majority of appendix masses (90%) resolves by this regime. If patient responds to the conservative regime, "interval appendicectomy" should be done after 6–8 weeks in such cases.

APPROACH TO PATIENT WITH INTESTINAL OBSTRUCTION

Patient of acute intestinal obstruction as in a case of small bowel obstruction presents with sudden onset of severe colicky central abdominal pain, early vomiting, distension of abdomen, and constipation. It is mostly seen in case of postoperative adhesive obstruction, obstructed hernia, etc. In case of chronic obstruction which is seen in case of large bowel obstruction, patient presents with lower abdominal colic with absolute constipation and distension of the abdomen with late vomiting seen as seen in case of carcinoma colon. Incomplete obstruction is seen in case of tuberculosis of intestine. In simple obstruction, blood supply of obstructed bowel is intact whereas in strangulated obstruction, there is direct interference to blood supply of the bowel.

Clinical Features

- Diagnosis of intestinal obstruction is based on the classic quartet of abdominal pain, distension, vomiting, and absolute constipation.
- Small bowel obstruction presents with abrupt onset of symptoms. High small bowel obstruction occurs due to obstruction at jejunum or proximal ileum. It presents with early vomiting which is bilious and profuse with rapid dehydration and less abdominal distension. Low small bowel obstruction occurs due to obstruction at distal ileum. Patient has abrupt onset of symptoms, predominant pain, and central distension with delayed vomiting.
- Large bowel obstruction presents with early distension of abdomen, mild pain, with late vomiting and dehydration. Long history of obstructive symptoms may be present. Proximal colon and cecum are distended.
- Colicky abdominal pain in central abdomen, which is centered around the umbilicus, is seen in case of small bowel obstruction and in lower abdomen in case of large bowel obstruction. Initially, pain is diffuse and poorly localized, intermittent, or crampy in nature with onset of bowel ischemia pain and becomes constant. Constant pain, abdominal tenderness, rigidity, shock, tachycardia, fever, and leukocytosis are all signs of strangulation.
- More distal the obstruction, later the appearance of the symptoms like nausea and vomiting. As obstruction progresses, the character of the vomitus alters from digested food to feculent material.
- Other features like dehydration, oliguria, hypovolemic shock, pyrexia, hypokalemia, abdominal tenderness in case of impending or established gangrene or in case of peritonitis are due to infarction or perforation.
- In external hernia, if strangulation occurs the lump becomes tense, tender, irreducible, and no expansile cough impulse.

Investigations

- Increased hematocrit, blood urea, and total leukocyte count. Hypokalemia, hypochloremia, and metabolic alkalosis may be present.

- **Plain X-ray abdomen in erect or supine position:** It shows multiple air fluid levels (more than three is diagnostic). In case of small bowel obstruction, air fluid level is concentrated in the central abdomen and lie transversely, and no gas is seen in colon. In case of jejunal obstruction, valvulae conniventes is seen as transverse lines completely passing across the bowel and regularly placed giving concentric or step ladder pattern. Ileal obstruction is characterless as it does not show any characteristic feature like jejunum or large intestine. Large bowel obstruction shows haustral folds, which are spaced irregularly and indentations are not placed opposite to each other and are concentrated at the periphery of the abdomen. Number of fluid levels is directly proportional to degree of obstruction and to its site, number of air fluid level increases the more distal the level of obstruction. When fluid levels are pronounced, obstruction is advanced.
- In X-ray abdomen in infants less than 2 years of age, more than three air fluid levels in small intestine is physiological. In adults, two inconstant fluid levels, one at duodenal cap and other at terminal ileum is normal.
- Air fluid level may be seen in acute pancreatitis, inflammatory bowel disease, and intra-abdominal sepsis.

Management of Patient with Intestinal Obstruction

- Patient should not allow taking anything by mouth. Nasogastric decompression should be done with Ryle tube to prevent vomiting and to decrease abdominal distension. Electrolytes should be replaced, if needed. Intravenous broad-spectrum antibiotics should be given. Catheterize the patient to measure urine output.
- In case of adhesive intestinal obstruction, if there is no pain or tenderness, conservative management can be given in hope of spontaneous resolution.
- Immediate operation is needed in all patients with complete small bowel obstruction
- Incomplete small bowel obstruction with no signs of ischemic bowel can be safely treated for period of time, since resolution in this group is 80%.
- Most of these patients successfully treated nonoperatively, show definite signs of improvement within 24 hours and nearby all show improvement by 48 hours. This is the maximum period of observation, after that laparotomy is indicated.

APPROACH TO PATIENT WITH SIGMOID VOLVULUS

Most of the patients of sigmoid volvulus are elderly, with acute onset pain and distension of the abdomen.

Clinical Features

- Mostly seen in elderly patients around 60–70 years of age

- Presents with large bowel obstruction initially followed by passage of large quantity of feces and flatus
- Distension of abdomen, vomiting, and obsolete constipation are the presenting symptoms.

Investigations

Plain X-ray abdomen: It shows dilated bowel loop running diagonally across abdomen from right to left with two fluid levels one in each loop. The grossly dilated loop of colon are with/without haustrations. Air fluid level may be seen rising from pelvis and extends obliquely across spine to upper abdomen. Barium enema shows bent inner tube.

Management

- Flexible or rigid sigmoidoscopy and insertion of flatus tube to allow deflation of gut and derotation
- Effective in 80% cases, but recurrence is common
- In case of failure of derotation, emergency laparotomy with untwisting of loop with peranal decompression and sigmoidopexy (fixation of cecum to postabdominal wall) or sigmoidectomy can be done, if sigmoid gangrenous or otherwise also to prevent recurrence. Sigmoid colectomy with descendo-rectal anastomosis, or descending colostomy with Hartmann procedure are other alternatives.

APPROACH TO THE PATIENT WITH PERFORATION PERITONITIS

Patients of perforation peritonitis presents in emergency room as acute pain and distension of the abdomen. Most common cause of perforation peritonitis is peptic ulcer perforation. Less common causes are perforation of typhoid ulcer of small intestine, tuberculous ulcer, Crohn disease, perforation of gangrenous and obstructed bowel, and perforation of malignant ulcer of large intestine. Sometimes peroration of Meckel diverticulum and perforation of diverticulum in diverticulosis of colon are the other causes.

Clinical Features

- There is abrupt onset of epigastric pain in a known patient of peptic ulcer with or without radiation of pain to shoulders. Pain in epigastrium and right iliac fossa as fluid tract down the right paracolic gutter.
- Generalized peritonitis supervenes within hours causing severe generalized abdominal pain due to irritant effect of gastric acid on the peritoneum (stage of chemical peritonitis). There may be disappearance of abdominal wall rigidity and improvement of symptoms after few hours due to dilution of acid in peritoneal cavity as peritoneum reacts by secreting more peritoneal fluid.

This stage is stage of reaction and called as "stage of delusion" or "stage of illusion", which lasts for 3–6 hours. "Stage of bacterial peritonitis" supervene over a few hours, as peritoneal contents get contaminated with Gram-negative organisms from the organisms of the gastrointestinal tract.
- Patient severely ill, dehydrated, toxic with drawn in cheeks.
- Tongue is dry and coated (Hippocratic facies).
- Tachycardia with feeble thread pulse.
- Shallow respiration
- High-grade fever
- Cold extremities
- Persistent hypotension
- Gross abdominal distension
- Board like rigidity, guarding, tenderness all over abdomen suggesting generalized peritonitis
- On percussion, liver dullness gets obliterated and replaced by tympanic note, due to collection of free air (gas) under the right dome of diaphragm.
- Patient declined to move because of pain.
- Abdomen does not move with respiration.
- Bowel sounds is absent or diminished.

Investigations

- **Complete blood count [TLC, differential leukocyte count (DLC)]:** It shows polymorphonuclear leukocytosis
- **Erect plain X-ray chest and upper abdomen:** It shows free gas under both domes of diaphragm, especially right dome in 70–75% cases
- If patient is bed ridden and unable to stand, then left lateral decubitus X-ray is taken
- **CT scan of abdomen and pelvis:** More accurate but rarely done to diagnose perforation, but done to rule out other intra-abdominal pathology like pancreatitis
- Water soluble contrast swallow show free peritoneal leak and established diagnosis, if pneumoperitoneum absent on plain X-ray
- Diagnostic peritoneal lavage by peritoneal tapping can be done which may show fluid and food debris or frank pus.

Treatment

- Patient should be kept strictly nil by mouth
- Insertion of nasogastric tube, aspiration, and continuous drainage of gastrointestinal contents to limit further peritoneal contamination of the peritoneal cavity by leakage of gastric or bilious or fecal contents through perorated ulcer site
- Resuscitation with intravenous fluids and electrolytes to correct fluid and electrolyte imbalance

- Broad-spectrum intravenous antibiotics to control infection and further septicemia
- Adequate analgesia should be given
- Catheterize the patient to measure urine output in case of septicemic shock
- Emergency laparotomy almost always required in every case, for closure of the perforated ulcer and for giving peritoneal lavage to limit peritoneal contamination and septicemia.

APPROACH TO PATIENT WITH STRANGULATED OR OBSTRUCTED HERNIA

Patient presents with history of sudden irreducibility of hernial contents and swelling. Any hernia can obstruct and strangulate, but mostly indirect inguinal hernias strangulate more easily than other varieties of hernias. Constricting agents may be neck of the sac (most commonly) as it is most constricted part of the hernia sac or adhesions within the sac (rarely). Contents are usually small intestine and sometime omentum, but rarely large intestine. If obstruction is not relieved in specified time, then gangrene appears within 5–6 hours of the first symptoms of obstruction, and then the gangrene of the whole bowel occurs within the sac. Perforation of the wall of gangrenous intestine may occurs, either at the convexity of the loop or at the seat of constriction leading to peritonitis which spreads from the sac to the peritoneal cavity.

Clinical Features

- Sudden local pain first over the swelling followed by generalized colicky abdominal pain.
- Nausea and subsequently vomiting
- Abdominal distension and constipation
- Tense, extremely tender, and irreducible swollen swelling
- Overlying redness of the skin
- No expansile cough impulse
- General condition of the patient is poor with feeble pulse and hypotension
- Unless strangulation relieved by operation, spasms of pain continue until peristaltic contractions cease with the onset of ischemia, when paralytic ileus as a result of peritonitis and septicemia develops
- Spontaneous cessation of pain may be a sign of perforation.

Investigations

- **X-ray abdomen supine:** It shows abnormal air fluid levels like of intestinal obstruction.
- **USG abdomen and pelvis:** It shows contents of the sac, peristalsis of the contents if it is intestine, and vascularity of obstructed segment of the intestine.

Management

- Management depends upon length of time of strangulation and age of the patient
- Infants and children should be operated early without wasting any time for conservative management
- Treatment is by emergency operation
- Vigorous resuscitation of patient should be started with intravenous fluids to correct dehydration
- Patient has to be kept nil by mouth (NBM) with nasogastric tube aspiration to decompress the stomach to prevent vomiting and reducing abdominal distension
- Patient can also be catheterized to measure the urine output
- Broad-spectrum antibiotics should be started.

Conservative Treatment

Foot end of bed should be raised so that irreducible hernia may reduce by gravity.

In infants, analgesics and Gallows traction can be given to reduce the contents in case of congenital inguinal hernia.

Manual reduction of the hernial contents (taxis) can be tried if patient presents early with no signs of strangulation by manipulation under sedation (in cases of obstructed hernia only and not for strangulated). If hernia reduces, then patient can be operated electively.

Taxis has no place in modern surgery, as its dangers include: it can result in contusion or rupture of the intestinal wall, sliding of gangrenous contents into the abdominal cavity, reduction-en-masse may occur when sac together with the hernia contents is pushed forcibly back into the abdomen where strangulation continues as the bowel will still be strangulated by the neck of the sac, sac may rupture at its neck and the contents are reduced, not into the peritoneal cavity but comes to lie in the extraperitoneal space.

Urgent operative intervention is indicated if patient already presents late in emergency room after the features of obstruction or after failure of above conservative management. By inguinoscrotal incision, sac is opened to inspect the contents of obstructed/strangulated hernia. If contents are nonviable and gangrenous, then they are removed.

CHAPTER 42

Approach to Patients of Genitourinary Emergencies in Emergency Room

■ INTRODUCTION

Different surgical patients of acute genitourinary emergencies attend emergency room. Following are the clinical diagnosis and treatment of patients presenting with acute genitourinary emergencies.

■ APPROACH TO THE PATIENT OF TORSION OF THE TESTES

Patient presents in emergency room with complaints of severe pain in the testicle, groin, and lower abdomen. Torsion is the twisting of the testes on the spermatic cord. Torsion of the spermatic cord causes strangulation of blood supply to the testis, and unless it is treated within 3–4 hours, testicular atrophy or necrosis is inevitable due to infarction of the testes. It is uncommon in normally fully descended testes, as it is well anchored and cannot rotate. Straining at stools, lifting a heavy weight, and forceful coitus are all precipitating factors for sudden torsion of the testes. Torsion may develop spontaneously during sleep.

Clinical Features

- Most common in young adolescents between 10 years and 25 years of age, although few cases may occur in infancy
- Presents as sudden agonizing pain in the testicle, groin, and the lower abdomen
- Vomiting and nausea
- Testes lie high and thickened tender twisted cord can be palpated above it
- Elevation of the testes reduces pain of epididymo-orchitis, whereas it increases and becomes worse in torsion (Prehn sign: Pain on elevation of testis)
- Scrotum may be empty and a tender lump may be palpable at the superficial inguinal ring (Deming sign).

Investigations

- **Color Doppler USG scan of testis:** Confirm the absence or decreased blood supply to the affected testis and is the investigation of choice
- **^{99}mTc (Technetium pertechnetate) scan:** It demonstrates decreased blood flow to the testes.

Treatment

- It is a surgical emergency and requires urgent intervention.
- Within first hour if the patient presents, testes may be untwisted with gentle manipulation
- If manipulation is successful, then pain subsides and the testes are out of danger, but arrangement should be made for early operative fixation to avoid recurrent torsion
- If manipulation fails to correct the torsion or if patient presents after 1 hour of torsion, then immediate surgical exploration is performed through scrotal incision within 4–6 hours of onset of symptoms
- On exploration, if the testes are viable when the cord is untwisted, it should be prevented from twisting again by fixation with nonabsorbable sutures between the tunica vaginalis and the tunica albuginea
- Totally infracted, nonviable testes should be removed
- The opposite testes should also be fixed (orchidopexy of other side should be done simultaneously) in the same procedure, because the anatomical predisposition responsible for torsion of the involved side is likely to be bilateral.

APPROACH TO THE PATIENT WITH URINARY RETENTION

Patient presents in emergency room with complaints of no passage of urine for several hours. Bladder is visible, palpable, and tender on palpation and dull on percussion.

Causes of Acute Retention of Urine

In male:
- Bladder outlet obstruction (due to benign hypertrophy of prostate): Most common
- Urethral stricture
- Acute urethritis or prostatitis
- Phimosis.

In female:
- Retroverted gravid uterus
- Bladder neck obstruction.

Both:
- After spinal anesthesia
- Postoperatively
- Blood clot in the bladder
- Urethral calculus
- Rupture urethra
- Neurogenic: Injury or disease of the spinal cord
- Smooth muscle cell dysfunction associated with aging
- Fecal impaction
- Anal pain (after hemorrhoidectomy)
- Intensive postoperative analgesic treatment
- Some drugs like antihistamines, antihypertensive, anticholinergic, and tricyclic antidepressants.

Management of Patient with Acute Urinary Retention

Perurethral catheterization with 14 Fr plain red rubber catheter or Foley catheter should be done to drain the distended bladder.

Steps in Perurethral Catheterization
- Following through hand wash sterile gloves are worn
- External gentiles cleaned with antiseptic solution
- Local anesthetic lignocaine jelly inserted into the urethra
- Jelly should be massaged posteriorly, to anesthetize the sphincter region
- Place a penile clamp for 10 minutes
- A small Foley catheter should be passed, while the penis is held taut
- Once urine begins to drain, pass the catheter more into the bladder before the balloon is inflated, to avoid inflation of the balloon in the prostatic urethra
- If a catheter will not be able to pass, it may be due to poor technique, lack of anesthesia, traumatization of urethra or a stricture urethra, or may due to prostatic median lobe hypertrophy in adult males.

Suprapubic Puncture or Cystostomy (SPC)

In case of failed perurethral catheterization in BHP, stricture urethra, or rupture urethra, suprapubic catheter is inserted under local anesthesia, after infiltrating 0.5% lignocaine in skin, fascia, and retropubic space.

APPROACH TO THE PATIENT WITH PARAPHIMOSIS

Patient presents in emergency room with unable to retract back the prepucial skin over glans with swelling of the glans. A tight foreskin once retracted may be difficult to return and paraphimosis results. Prepuce becomes difficult to return or retract back in its normal position, causing tight ring of foreskin to cause stricturous ring around corona behind glans penis. This constricting band of phimotic prepuce causes obstruction of venous and lymphatic return from the glans penis and distal foreskin, leading to venous congestion causing edema and enlargement of glans. The glans swells leading to more difficulty in retracting back the prepuce. As the condition progresses, arterial occlusion and necrosis (gangrene) of glans may occur in neglected cases. It occurs due to forceful retraction or pulling of prepuce over the glans penis; it may get stuck behind the glans. It may occur due to nonpulling of prepuce in its original position, after perurethral catheterization. Sometimes, it may occur after a sexual intercourse.

Clinical Features

- Severe pain in the glans penis
- Gross swelling of retracted prepucial skin and edema of the distal glans penis.

Management

- Cold fomentation by applying ice bags to reduce edema of the glans and retracted prepucial skin
- Gentle manual compression or squeezing of the glans for 5 minutes to reduce edema and decrease size of the glans penis. Skin can be drawn forward over the glans after that
- Injection of a solution of hyaluronidase 250 units in 10–15 mL of NS injected into the constriction ring may help to reduce the swelling
- If not managed conservatively, dorsal slitting of prepuce under local anesthesia by incising the constricting ring may be enough in an emergency
- Circumcision done later, after inflammation is subsided.

Index

Page numbers followed by *f* refer to figure.

A

Abdomen
   contrast-enhanced CT 318
   CT scan of 322
   erect, X-ray 318
Abdominal cavity 209, 225
Abdominal drain 92, 93*f*
Abdominal injuries, sustaining 312
Abdominal wall
   different incisions over anterior 210*f*
   rigidity 321
Abrahamson's nylon darn repair 232, 233*f*
Abscess
   appendicular 217
   cavity 260
   drainage of 259, 260
   incision of 259
   pelvic 317
   treatment of appendicular 217
Absorbable ligature 220
Absorbable suture 141, 213, 248
   materials 147
Acid-base balance 315
Adhesive obstruction, postoperative 319
Adrenaline 184
   injection 185
      tartrate 187, 188*f*
Advanced trauma life support system 307
Air embolism, risk of 284
Airways 159
Allie's tissue forceps 24, 25*f*, 26
Allison lung retractor 45, 46*f*
Ambu
   bag 165, 169, 169*f*
   valve 169
Ambulatory manual breathing unit 169
Anal canal, carcinoma of 276
Anal speculum 59, 276
Analgesia, postoperative 180
Anawin sensorcaine 181, 182
Anesthesia 207
   drugs in 181

   equipment 157
      for regional 177
   general 195, 222
   level of 181
   local 203
   maintenance of general 201
   spinal 179, 181, 203, 246
Anesthetic agents, inhalational 200
Anesthetic drug, local 179
Angle connector 171, 172*f*
Anoscope 59, 276
Anoscopy 59, 276
Antibiotics, injections of 178
Antiseptic solutions 207
Appendicectomy 209, 210, 211*f*, 318
   incisions for 213
   interval 318
Appendicitis
   acute 209, 316
      management of 318
   chronic 209
Appendicular mass, treatment of 216
Appendix
   dissection of 214
   masses 318
   mucocele of 209
Argon beam coagulation 303
Artery 21, 33
   forceps 19
Aspiration 167
   pneumonitis 275
Atmospheric oxygen 176
Atracurium 199
   besylate 199
Atraumatic grasping forceps 291
Atropine sulfate injection 189, 189*f*
Auchincloss procedure 252
Austin Moore's prosthesis 125, 126, 127*f*
Axillary abscess
   drainage of 261
   incision of 261
Axillary lymph nodes 42
   levels of 252

B

Babcock's tissue forceps 26, 26f, 212
Backhaus towel clip 19
Balanitis xerotica obliterans 222
Balfour's self-retaining retractor 49f
Bandage 136
    cotton 136
    crepe 136, 137f
Bard Parker's handle 11
    uses of 13
Basilic vein 265, 266f
Bassini's repair 230
    modified 230, 230f
Benzodiazepine 194
Benzyl alcohol 189, 194
Biflanged blade, uses of 42
Bipolar cautery forceps 304f
Bipolar diathermy 223
Bipolar instrument 294f, 303
    tip of 294f
Bipolar prosthesis 128, 129f
Black eye 308
Bladder 248
    stone 37
Blades 8
Blast injury 307
Bleeding vessels 21
Blood
    pressure, increase 188
    transfusion set 100, 101f
    vessels 311
Blumberg sign 316
Blunt trauma 307
Body temperature 217
Bohler's pin 134
Bohler's stirrup 135
Bone
    awl 115, 115f
    cutter 70
    cutting forceps 117, 118f
    gouge 114, 115f
    holding forceps 117
        types of 117f
    levers, types of 112f
    neurovascular bundle of 113
    nibbler 70, 118, 118f
    nibbling forceps 118
    shears 117
Bowel obstruction
    large 319, 320
    small 319
Boyle's machine 175

Bradawl 115
Bradycardia, treatment of 189
Brain injury 308
    primary 308, 309
    secondary 309
Breast tissue
    dissected 250
    whole 248, 251
Breathing unit, artificial manual 165
Brodie's abscess 119
Brodie's olive pointed fistula director 60, 61f
Bronchial asthma 195
Bronchospasm, treatment of 195
Building collapse 307
Bulldog vascular clamp 5, 56, 57f
Bupivacaine
    hydrochloride 181, 181f, 182
    injection 182f
Burn 314
    management of 315
Burr 70
Butterfly cannula 98

C

Calcified gallbladder 218
Calcium
    chloride 103
    sulfate 138
        hemihydrated salt of 137
Calmpose 194
Camera 283f
Camper's fascia 226
Cannula 63, 64, 64f, 83, 84f
    three-way 101, 101f
Capillaries 21
Carbon dioxide 171, 221, 285
    cylinder 285f
    insufflating 239
Carcinoma
    breast, removed in 252
    colon 319
Cardiac tamponade 312
    management of 312
Cardiopulmonary resuscitation 188
Catgut 147
    chromic 147, 215, 243, 244
    plain 147
    types of 148f
Catheter 75, 77
    diameter of 80
    silicone self-retaining 81, 81f
    suction 167, 168f
    suprapubic 80, 248

Cautery machine 304f
Cecum 212, 214
Cephalic vein 265
Cerebral edema 309
Cerebrospinal fluid 178, 308
    flow of 177
Cervical sympathetic trunk injury 256
Cetrimide spirit 207
Charged-coupled device 282
Cheatle forceps 30, 30f
Chemical peritonitis, stage of 321
Chemical sterilization 3
Chest 322
    injury 310
    pain 311
    X-ray 313
Chisel 114, 114f
Cholecystectomy 217
    complications of 222
Chromic catgut, uses of 148
Circumcision 222
    incision for 223f
Clamps 53
Clavicle fracture 125
Clip applicator 294, 295f
    handle of 295f
    tip of 295f
Clips of clip applicator 295f
Clutton's metallic bougie 73
Cobbler's needle 115, 296f
Colicky abdominal pain 319
Colles' fracture, percutaneous fixation of 131
Collingwood–Stewart cord holding 28
Common bile duct 220
Complete blood count 322
Confirmatory test 164
Conservative regimen 217
Conservative treatment 324
Cooper's ligament 231
    repair 231
Cord holding forceps 28, 28f
Corrugated antistatic rubber tube 173, 173f
Corrugated drainage sheet 90f
Corrugated rubber drain 90, 243, 244
Cotton bandage, open-weave 136f
Cotton crepe bandage 136
Cotton thread 152
Counter incision 260
Cranial fossa, fracture of anterior 308
Craniotomy 70
Cremasteric fascia 242
Crush injury 307
Cryotherapy 304
Crystalloid bottles 102

Curved blade 162
    skin retractor 47f
Cyanoacrylates 40
Cyanosis 311
Cyst 46
    excision of 267
    recurrent 252
Cystic duct 220
Cystography 78
Cystostomy 327
Cytotoxics, injections of 178
Czerny retractor 42, 42f

D

Darn repair 232
Dartos muscle 242
Davis mouth gag 52
Deaver's retractor 5, 44, 44f, 45
Deep fascia 260
Deep inguinal ring 225, 239
Deep vein thrombosis, chances of 266
Deming sign 325
Dental operation 164
Deriphyllin 195
Dermoid cyst 267
Desflurane 200, 201
Desjardin's choledocholithotomy forceps 35, 35f
Dexamethasone 192
    sodium phosphate injection 192, 192f
Dexon 149
Dexona 192
Dextrose 105f, 181
    injection 102, 103f, 181, 182, 183f
    normal saline 104
Diaphragm, right dome of 322
Diazepam 194
    injection 194f
Dinner knife position 11
Disinfection 3
    high level 3, 296, 297
Distal foreskin 328
Doyen's cross action towel clip 18
Doyen's gastrointestinal occlusion clamp 5, 53, 54f, 55
Doyen's mouth gag 51, 52f
Doyen's retractor 45, 45f
Doyen's rib raspatory 68
Doyen's towel clip 19
Drains 75, 90
Draping operative area 208
Drill bit guide 121, 122f
Drip chamber 99

Dunphy sign 317
Dura separator 72*f*
Duval lung forceps 29, 30*f*
Dynamic compression plate 125
Dyspnea 311

E

Echocardiography 312
Elastocrepe 136
Emergency laparotomy 63
Emergency room 305, 325
   acute abdominal conditions in 316
   trauma in 307
Empyema 63
   drainage of 262
Endogenous catecholamine 187
Endotracheal intubation 164
   insertion 87
Endotracheal tube 108, 163, 200, 307, 315
   intubation 165, 186
Epidural anesthesia 203, 214
   anesthetic effect of 179
   effect of 179
Epidural catheter 179
   set 180*f*
Epigastric artery, inferior 229
Epigastrium, pain in 321
Epistaxis 308
Ethanol 186
Ethicon 155
Ethilon 153
Etofylline injection 195, 195f
Exhaled air 171
Extracorporal knotting 215
Extradural hematoma 72
Extraperitoneal fat 247
Extraperitoneal repair 238
Eyeballs 174

F

Face mask 169, 173, 174*f*
   and tubing 175*f*
Facial nerves 174
Family planning 245
Farabeuf's raspatory 111
Fascia
   superficial 227
   transversalis 224, 233
Femoral shaft, fixation of diaphyseal fractures of 133
Fever 319
Fiberoptic bronchoscopy 164
Fibula 118

Finger bows 7
Fish mouth valve 170
Fistulectomy 62
Fistulotomy 61
Flat blade, uses of 43
Flatus tube 86, 86*f*
Fluid
   filter 99
   retention 191
Foil pack, suture material in 144
Foley's balloon 80
Foley's catheter 77, 81, 82, 108, 248, 273
   perurethral 248
   self-retaining balloon 79, 80*f*
Forceps 17
   dissecting 31
   plain dissecting 31, 31*f*
   right angle 33
   tips of
      atraumatic 291*f*
      traumatic 290*f*
Foreign bodies 179
Formaldehyde 4
Formalin chamber containing 297*f*
Formalin tablets 297*f*
French osteotomy 113
Frenulum slit 60
Fresh frozen plasma 315
Fundus first cholecystectomy 219
Furosemide 193
   injection 193*f*

G

Gallbladder
   congenital anomalies of 218
   stones 217
Gallstones 218
   indications in asymptomatic 218
Gangrene 328
Gangrenous contents, sliding of 324
Gas sterilization 3, 4, 296
Gastrectomy, partial 55
Gastric acid, effect of 321
Gastric clamp 55
Gastric contents, aspiration of 275
Gastric outlet obstruction 86
Gastroesophageal junction 85
Gastrointestinal clamps 53
General surgery 59
   advanced techniques in 279
   instruments in 9
Genitourinary emergencies 325
   acute 325

Gentle traction 220
Giant prosthetic reinforcement 235
Gigli's wire saw 119, 119*f*
Glans penis 328
Glasgow coma scale, examine 308
Glycopyrrolate 189
    injection 189, 190*f*
Goiter
    large 253
    pressure symptoms to 252
    retrosternal prolongation of 252
Graspers 290
Grasping forceps, traumatic 290
Great saphenous vein 265
Guedel's airway 159, 159*f*
Guidewire 120, 120*f*
Gypsum 138

H

Halothane 200, 201*f*
Halsted mosquito forceps 22, 22*f*
Halsted radical mastectomy 248, 250, 251
    disadvantages of 251
Hand apparatus
    irrigation 295
    suction 295
Hand drill 120, 121*f*
Hand instrument
    different handles of 292
    typical 290*f*
Handles of hand instruments, types of 293*f*
Harmonic scalpel 294, 294*f*, 304
Hartley-Dunhill procedure 253
Hartmann's pouch 220
    of gallbladder 18
Hasan's cannula 239, 287, 288*f*
Head injury 308
    management of 310
    mild 309
    minor 309
    moderate 309
    severe 309
    sustaining 308
Heart rate 188
Heath suture cutting scissor 16, 16*f*
Hematocele 246
Hematocrit 315
Hematoma 269, 270
Hematuria, bladder reveals 273
Hemiarthroplasty 128
Hemopneumothorax 262, 311
    traumatic 262
Hemorrhage 87, 255, 270
    from nose 308
    subconjunctival 308

Hemorrhoids 60, 276
Hemostatic forceps 19, 21, 212
    spencer Well's type of 19, 20*f*, 22, 23
Hemothorax 63, 262, 311
    management of 312
    traumatic 262
Hepatorenal pouch 82
Hernia
    contents 324
    forceps 28
    incision for repair of 228*f*
    incisional 281
    obstructed 319, 323
    orifice 239
    reduces 324
    repair 28
    ring 28
    strangulated 323
    surgery, complications of 237
Hernial sac 233
Hernioplasty 226, 228*f*, 233, 236
Herniorrhaphy 226, 228*f*, 236
Herniotomy 224, 225, 227, 233
    incision for 225*f*
Hilton's method 260
Hip hemiarthroplasty 115
    operation, disadvantage of 127
    prosthesis for 125
Hippocratic facies 322
Hook and spatula 294
Hook retractor, single 47, 47*f*
Hook, tip of 294*f*
Horner's syndrome 256
Horsley's dura mater 70, 71*f*
Hudson's brace 70, 71*f*, 118
Hudson's burr 70
Hudson's perforator 70
Human tissue 233
Humby's skin grafting knife 72, 73*f*
Humerus fracture, distal 125
Hydrocele 64, 64*f*
    repair of 64, 240, 240*f*, 244
    surgeries for 240
    treatment of congenital 245
Hydrocortisone sodium 191
    succinate injection 191, 191*f*
Hydrodissection 228
Hyperglycemia 191
Hypertension 188, 191
Hypertonic saline 310
Hypertrophic scar 258
Hypodermic needle 108
Hypokalemia 319
Hypoparathyroidism 256
Hypovolemic shock 101

I

Iliac fossa, right 316
Ilioinguinal nerve 227
Imaging system 281
Implants, orthopedics 109, 124
Incision 210
    lower midline 211, 213
Informed consent 206
Infusion tubing 99
Inguinal canal 224
    posterior wall of 224
Inguinal hernia 42
    direct 224, 227
    operations for repair of 224, 226
    repair of 224
Inguinal herniorrhaphy 227
Inguinal orchidectomy 236
Inguinal ring, internal 225
Injection, sterile water for 105f
Injury, closed 311
Instrument 289
    atraumatic forceps 289
    bipolar forceps 289
    clip applicator 289
    cutting 11
    grasping forceps 289
    irrigation 289
    laparoscopic 281, 296
    loop applicator 289
    monopolar instruments 289
    needle holder 289
    orthopedics 111
    parts
        of hand 290
        of surgical 1
    pencil-like 303
    retractors 289
    scissors 289
    sterilization of 3, 296
    tip of 8
    trackers 289
    trolley 285f, 286, 286f
    types of 5, 289
Insufflation cannulas 287
Insufflator 285, 285f
Intercostal drain, insertion of 262
Intercostal drainage trocar 84f
Intercostal space 262
Intercostal trocar cannula 83
Interfragmentary compression, lag screw for 125
Interlocking sutures, absorbable 243
Intestinal crushing clamp 56, 56f
Intestinal obstruction 86, 319
    diagnosis of 319
    management of 320
Intestine
    large 211
    small 211
Intra-abdominal injuries, management of 314
Intracranial tension 310
Intramedullary nails 128, 130f
Intravenous cannula 95, 97, 98f
    insertion 277
Intravenous fluid 95
    bottle 102, 102f
    resuscitation 315
Intravenous infusion set 99, 100f
Introducer 164
Isoflurane 200, 201
Isopropyl alcohol 207

J

Jaboulay's eversion of sac 242, 243f
    disadvantage of 243
Jennings mouth gag 52, 52f
Joint 8
Joll's thyroid retractor 51, 51f

K

Kelly's anal speculum 59, 60f
Kelly's rectal speculum 59
Keloid formation 258
Ketamine hydrochloride 197f
    injection 196
Kidney
    hilum retractor 47, 48f
    tray 66, 66f
K-nail 132f
Knife 307
Knot pusher 215
Kocher's forceps 56
Kocher's gastric occlusion clamp 55
Kocher's hemostatic forceps 22, 23f
Kocher's skin crease neck incision 254f
Kuntscher's intramedullary nail 132
Kuntz operation 236
    indications for 236
K-wire 131, 131f
    bender 122f, 123
        uses of 123
    cutter 122f, 123
    extraction of 123
    insertion 120

L

Labor analgesia 180
Lahey's forceps 5, 33, 34f
Lane's bone levers 112
Lane's tissue forceps 27, 27f
Langenbeck's right angled retractor 41, 41f, 42, 43, 46, 211, 247
Langer's line 268
Lanz's incision 211f, 214
Laparoscopes 281
Laparoscopic appendicectomy 214
    advantages of 216
    disadvantages of 216
    port sites for 215f
    postoperative complications of 216
Laparoscopic cholecystectomy 220
    advantages of 221
    contraindications for 222
    port sites for 221f
Laparoscopic hernia repair
    advantages of 239
    disadvantages of 239
    indications of 238
    port sites for 238f
Laparoscopic hernioplasty 237, 238
Laparoscopic surgery 281
    advantage of 281
Laparotomy 45, 207
Laryngeal mask airway 160, 161f
Laryngeal nerve palsy 256
Laryngoscope 162, 162f
Laryngoscopy 163
Latissimus dorsi, anterior border of 262
Lens, fogging of 281
Leukocyte count, differential 322
Leukocytosis 319
Lichtenstein tension free hernioplasty 233, 234f
Lidocaine 186
Light cable 284, 284f
Light source 283, 283f
    types of 283
Lignocaine 179, 184
    hydrochloride 182, 183, 183f, 185f
    gel 187, 187f
    injection 184f, 185, 186f
    sensitivity test 205
    spray 185
    topical aerosol 186f
    with adrenaline 184
Limb
    movements 309
    of T piece 176

Linen thread 152
Lipoma 46, 47, 268, 269
    excision of 268
Liquid crystal gel 284
Lister's metallic bougie 73
Lister's sinus forceps 23, 24f
Locking plate 125
Lord's plication 241, 241f, 242, 243
    advantage of 242
Lotheissen's repair 231
Low contact dynamic compression plate 125
LOX heavy 182
Lumbar puncture
    complications of 178
    contraindications for 178
Lymph node 46, 47
    biopsy 269
    capsule of 270
    mediastinal 251
    supraclavicular 251

M

Macintosh blade 162
Magill's blade 162
Magill's forceps 166, 167f
Malecot's catheter 82, 82f, 92
Malleable olive pointed probe 61, 62f
Malleable retractor 45, 45f
Mallet 116, 116f
Mammary fat 248, 251
Maryland forceps 291f
Mass, extent of 217
Mastectomy
    extended radical 251
    extended simple 251
    halsted 251
    simple 251
    super radical 251
    types of 251
Mastoid surgery 50
Mayo's pedicle clamp 57, 58f
Mayo's scissor 13, 14, 14f, 211
Mayo's towel clip 19
McBurney's grid iron incision 210, 211f
McBurney's incision 210
McBurney's point 210
McIndoe scissors 15, 15f
    uses of 14
McMurray's osteotomy 113
Meckel's diverticulum 212
Mersilk 151
    uses of 152

Mesh repair 233
Metacarpals 118
Metallic bougies, female 73
Metallic instruments, soakage of 297
Metallic urethral
   bougie 73, 74f
   catheter 77
      male 78f
Metatarsals 118
Methylparaben IP 192
Metzenbaum scissor 14, 15, 15f, 16
   uses of 14
Meyer's radical mastectomy 251
Mezolam 193
Microwave ablation 304
Micturating cystourethrogram 78
Midazolam 193
   injection 194f
Miller's bougie 73
Mini Vac suction drain 91, 92
Mixter forceps 33, 34f
Modular prosthesis 128
Mollison's self-retaining retractor 50, 50f
Monitor 284, 284f
Monofilament 142
   polyamide 153
   polypropylene 233
Monopolar cautery
   attachment for 294f
   cord 303f
Monopolar circuits 303
Monopolar diathermy 224
Morris retractor 5, 43, 43f, 45
Morrison's pouch 82, 92, 220
Mouth gags 51
Moynihan's gastric occlusion clamp 54, 54f
Multihole suction cannula 65, 66f
Multinodular goiter 253
Muscle 113, 118
   relaxants 198, 199f
   weakness 191
Myasthenia gravis, treatment of 200
Myocardial contractility 188

N

Nasal intubation, indications of 164
Nasogastric insertion 275
Nasogastric tube 85, 86f, 310
Nasopharyngeal airway 160, 160f
Neck abscess
   drainage of 261
   incision of 261

Neck humerus, fracture of surgical 131
Needle 107, 145
   classification 145
   description of 143
   types of 145f
   with needle protector 100
Needle holder 21, 38, 39f, 203f, 293
   handle of 293f
   tip of 293f
   typical 293f
Neoplasia 252
Neostigmine methylsulfate 199
   injection 200f
Neurosurgery, instruments in 70
Non-rebreathing valve 169f, 170, 171f
Non-toothed dissecting forceps 31
Nylon 153
   bundle 154f

O

Oblique elliptical incision 249f
Oblique end, telescope with 282f
Obstructive pulmonary disease, chronic 195
Obturator 59
   test 317
Omentum 214
Ondansetron 190
   injection 191f
Open appendicectomy 209, 216
Open cholecystectomy 218, 221
   different incisions for 219f
Open injury 311
Open pneumothorax 310
Operation bed, position of 245
Operation table 207
   position of 210, 245
Operative area
   antiseptic cleaning of 207
   preparation of 205
Operative hand instruments 286, 289
Operative intervention, urgent 324
Operative procedure 203
   major 209
   minor 259
   techniques 239
Oral cavity, retractors of 51
Oral operation 164
Oropharyngeal airway 159, 159f
   complications of 160
Oropharynx 167, 186
Osteomyelitic cavities 119
Osteomyelitis 115

Osteotome 113, 113*f*
Otorrhea 308
Oxygen 170
   mask and tubing 175
   reservoir 170
      bag 170*f*

P

Pain
   abdominal 217, 316
   excessive 187
   less postoperative 281
Pancuronium 199
Panda sign 308
Paramedian incision
   right 219*f*
      lower 211*f*, 213
Paraphimosis 327
   clinical features 328
   management 328
Parathyroid insufficiency 256
Patch and plug technique 234
Patey's mastectomy 248
Patey's modified radical mastectomy 250
   advantages of 250
Payr's gastric crushing clamp 5, 55, 55*f*
   uses of 55
Pectoralis major muscle 262
Pelvic appendix 317
Pelvic surgery 45
Pelvis, CT scan of 322
Penetrating trauma 307
Perforation peritonitis 321
Perforator 70
Periosteum
   advantages of separating 68
   elevator 111, 111*f*
Peritoneal cavity 53
   drainage of 213
Peritoneal lavage 313
Peritoneum 63, 211, 239, 321
Perurethral catheter 80, 273
   steps in 327
Pfannenstiel incision 247
Phalanges 118
Piles, diagnosis of 276
Plain catgut, uses of 148
Plaster of Paris bandage 136, 137, 138*f*
Plastic connectors 165*f*
Plastic disposable cannula 65
Plastic surgery, instruments in 72
Pleural effusion 262

Pneumoperitoneum 287
   gas for 284
Pneumothorax 262, 310
   closed 310
   management of 311
   traumatic 262
Pointing sign 316
Polyamide 154
Polyfilament 142
Polyglactin 910 141, 149, 150*f*
   910 sutures 149
Polyglycolic acid 141, 149
Polypropylene 155, 233
   sutures and mesh, types of 155*f*
Polytetrafluoroethylene 233
Polyvinyl chloride 85, 87, 90, 92, 167
Port closure instrument 295
Positive pressure ventilation, intermittent 163, 315
Postoperative drainage, thoracotomy for 262
Potassium
   chloride 103
   iodide solution 257
Povidine iodine 207
Predominantly tachycardia 189
Prehn sign 325
Preperitoneal repairs 234
Presterilized pack 177
Proctoscope 59, 276
Proctoscopy 59, 276
Prolene 155, 233
Prophylaxis 205, 257
Propofol injection 196, 197*f*
Prostate, benign hypertrophy of 326
Prostatic hyperplasia, benign 273
Psoas sign 317
Psychic disturbance 191
Pubic symphysis 246
Pulse rate 217
Punch 116, 116*f*
Pyelolithotomy forceps 36, 36*f*
Pyocele 246
Pyrolate injection 189

Q

Quadrant transverse incision, right upper 219*f*

R

Raccoon sign 308
Radial neck, fractures 131
Radical mastectomy, modified 248

Radiofrequency
    ablation 304
    electrosurgery 303
Rampley's swab holding forceps 17, 18f
Rectal polyps 276
Rectal ulcer 276
Repair of Shouldice's, layer by layer 231
Reservoir bag 171, 172f
Respiratory
    depression 196
    obstruction 256
Retractor 41
    right angled 5
    self-retaining 48, 49, 49f
Retrocecal appendix 317
Retrograde appendicectomy 214
Rhinorrhea 308
Rib raspatory 68f
Ringer lactate injection 102, 104f
Rive's preperitoneal prosthetic mesh repair 235
Road traffic accident 307
Rocuronium 199
Rovsing sign 317
Rubber catheter
    plain 78, 78f
    simple 78
Rule of Nine 314
Rush nail 129, 131f
Rutherford Morison incision 211f, 213
Ryle's tube 85
    insertion 275

S

Sac
    blind dissection of 243
    high ligation of 229
    jaboulay's eversion of 242
    over eversion 242
    subtotal excision of 244
Satinsky vascular clamp 56, 58f
Scalp vein set 98, 99f
Scarpa's fascia 226
Schoemaker rib shear 69, 69f
Scissors 13, 292, 292f
Screws 125, 126f
Scrotal hematoma 246
Sebaceous cyst 47, 267
Sensorcaine 178
Seroma 269, 270
Seton treatment 62
Sevoflurane 200, 201

Sexual contact 246
Shank 8
Sharma and Jhawer's technique 244
Sharp dissection, instruments for 292
Sheath, outer 293f
Shock 319
Shouldice's repair 231
Sigmoid volvulus 320
Silk 151
    uses of 151
Skin
    crease elliptical incision 267f
    cuts, risk of 205
    glues 40
        for wound closure 40
    incision 210, 211
    retractor 47
    stapler 40, 40f
    sutured 248
Sleeve, reducing 289, 289f
Sodium chloride 103, 105f
    injection 104f
    solution 103
Sodium lactate solution 103
Solitary nodular goiter 252
Solitary nodule 253
S-P nail 133, 133f
Specimen removal forceps 292f
Sperm granuloma 246
Spermatic fascia
    external 242
    internal 242
Spinal needle 177, 178f
Spinoumbilical line, right 210
Stab incision 260
Stainless steel wire 134, 134f, 156, 156f
Steam sterilization 3, 296
Steinmann pin 134, 135, 135f
    uses of 135
Sterile adhesive dressing 213
Sterile towels 270
Sterile tube 187
Sterile water vial 105
Sterilization 3, 296
Sterilized suture pack containing polyglactin 144f
Stitch granuloma 258
Stoma, infection of 88
Stone holding forceps 35
Stoppa's great 235
Stoppa's preperitoneal repair 237
Stylet 164, 166, 166f, 288f
Subcostal incision, right 219f

Subcutaneous tissue 177, 179, 260, 261, 268, 269
Succinylcholine 198
    injection 198*f*
Suction cannulas 65*f*, 211
Suction drain 91, 92*f*
Suction irrigation
    hand apparatus 295*f*
    machine 286
Suction tubings 88, 89*f*
Supine position 222
Suprapubic cystolithotomy 246
Suprapubic cystostomy 63, 83
Suprapubic puncture 327
Suprapubic route 83
Suprapubic trocar and cannula 63, 64*f*, 83
Surgery
    energy sources in 301, 303
    instruments in specialized 68
    position of 207
    types of 253
Surgical blades 11
    different sizes of 12f
    number of 12*f*
    uses of 13
Surgical instrument
    parts of typical 7, 7*f*
    right hand holding typical 5*f*
    sterilization of 1
    types of 1
Surgical practice, suture material in 139
Surgical procedures 203
    minor 203
    preoperative preparation of 205
Sutupak 151
Suture
    in pack, type of 143
    interrupted nonabsorbable 213, 248
    modern techniques of 40
    natural
        absorbable 141
        non-absorbable 142, 151
    non-absorbable 142, 151, 220, 233, 242, 270
    synthetic
        absorbable 141
        non-absorbable 142, 153
Suture material 141, 142
    characteristic of ideal 142
    classification of 141
    description of 141
    in pack, length of 143
    natural absorbable 147
    number of 143
    synthetic absorbable 149
    types of 141, 147
Syringes 107, 108*f*

T

T handle 121, 121*f*
T piece 175
T tube 176*f*
Tachycardia 188, 319
Tags
    black 307
    green 307
    red 307
    yellow 307
Tap 122, 122*f*
Technetium pertechnetate 326
Tension free mesh repair, anterior 233
Tension pneumothorax 311
Terminal ileum 214
Testes
    elevation of 325
    torsion of 325
Tetanus 205
    toxoid, injecting 205
Theophylline, injection of 195, 195*f*
Thiersch graft 72
Thiersch operation 156
Thiopentone sodium 195, 196*f*
Thiosol sodium 195
Thompson's prosthesis 125, 127, 128, 128*f*
Thoracotomy, instruments in 68
Thrombophlebitis 278
Thyroid
    capsule 254
    gland, surgeries for 252
    hormone 257
    insufficiency 256
    pole, inferior 255
    storm 257
    superior pole of 255
    swelling
        benign 253
        operations in 252
Thyroidectomy, bilateral subtotal 253
Thyrotoxic crisis 257
Thyroxine replacement 253
Tincture iodine and spirit 207
Tissue
    dissection, instruments for 31
    infected 147
    repairs
        commonly performed primary 229
        primary 227

Tongue holding forceps 29, 29f
Tooth dissecting forceps 32, 32f
Total thyroidectomy 253
Towel clips 18
    types of 19f
Towel holding forceps 18
Toxic adenoma 252
Trachea 276
Tracheal dilator 69, 70f
Tracheal intubation, equipment for 162
Tracheal stenosis 88
Tracheal tube 169
Tracheostomy 263
    complications of 87
    instruments in 69
    site 88
    tubes 87, 88f
Transabdominal preperitoneal approach 239
Transparent plastic tubing 85
Transverse suprapubic incision 247
Trauma, abdominal sonar for 313
Trendelenberg position 220
Trocar 63, 64, 64f, 83, 287, 288f
Tube 75, 85
    blockage of 88
    insulated outer 293
    misplacement 87
Tunica vaginalis 241-243
Turco's posteromedial release operation 132

U

Universal connector 171
Upper abdomen 322
    X-ray 313
Upper gastrointestinal
    endoscopy 186
    tract 275
Upper middle incision 219f
Urinary retention 326
    acute 327
    postoperative 200
Urinary tract injuries 273
Urine, acute retention of 326
Urology instruments 73
Urosac bag 93, 93f

V

Valve, unidirectional 170
Vas deferens, recanalization of 246
Vascular clamps 56
Vascular forceps 33, 33f
Vasectomy 245
Vecuronium 199
Vehicular accident 308
Vein 21, 33
Venesection 265
    cannula 266
    incision for 266f
Venotomy 265
Ventilation, equipment for 169
Ventricular ectopics 185
Ventricular tachycardia 185
Veress needle 287, 287f
Vesical calculus 37, 246
Vicryl 149
    ligatures 215
    rapide suture 150
Visceral
    blade 69
    sac 235
Volkmann's cat's paw retractor 46, 46f
Volkmann's scoop 67, 67f, 119, 119f

W

Whipple's procedure 44
Wound 250
    gape 269, 270
    infection 246, 258, 266, 269, 270
Written consent 206

X

Xylocaine 183, 184, 187, 205
Xylocard 185, 186

Y

Yankauer suction cannula 64, 65

Z

Z suture 212
Zachary cope 317

EU GSPR Authorised Reprsentative
Logos Europe, 9 rue Nicolas Poussin
1700, La Rochelle, France
Phone: +33 (0) 6 67 93 73 78
E-mail: contact@logoseurope.eu

www.ingramcontent.com/pod-product-compliance
Ingram Content Group UK Ltd.
Pitfield, Milton Keynes, MK11 3LW, UK
UKHW050454150426

5217IPUK00025B/1686